Practice Tests Answer Sheets[*]

Test A

1. ① ② ③ ④
2. ① ② ③ ④
3. ① ② ③ ④
4. ① ② ③ ④
5. ① ② ③ ④
6. ① ② ③ ④
7. ① ② ③ ④
8. ① ② ③ ④
9. ① ② ③ ④
10. ① ② ③ ④
11. ① ② ③ ④
12. ① ② ③ ④
13. ① ② ③ ④
14. ① ② ③ ④
15. ① ② ③ ④
16. ① ② ③ ④
17. ① ② ③ ④
18. ① ② ③ ④
19. ① ② ③ ④
20. ① ② ③ ④
21. ① ② ③ ④
22. ① ② ③ ④
23. ① ② ③ ④
24. ① ② ③ ④
25. ① ② ③ ④
26. ① ② ③ ④
27. ① ② ③ ④
28. ① ② ③ ④
29. ① ② ③ ④
30. ① ② ③ ④

Test B

1. ① ② ③ ④
2. ① ② ③ ④
3. ① ② ③ ④
4. ① ② ③ ④
5. ① ② ③ ④
6. ① ② ③ ④
7. ① ② ③ ④
8. ① ② ③ ④
9. ① ② ③ ④
10. ① ② ③ ④
11. ① ② ③ ④
12. ① ② ③ ④
13. ① ② ③ ④
14. ① ② ③ ④
15. ① ② ③ ④
16. ① ② ③ ④
17. ① ② ③ ④
18. ① ② ③ ④
19. ① ② ③ ④
20. ① ② ③ ④
21. ① ② ③ ④
22. ① ② ③ ④
23. ① ② ③ ④
24. ① ② ③ ④
25. ① ② ③ ④
26. ① ② ③ ④
27. ① ② ③ ④
28. ① ② ③ ④
29. ① ② ③ ④
30. ① ② ③ ④

Test C

1. ① ② ③ ④
2. ① ② ③ ④
3. ① ② ③ ④
4. ① ② ③ ④
5. ① ② ③ ④
6. ① ② ③ ④
7. ① ② ③ ④
8. ① ② ③ ④
9. ① ② ③ ④
10. ① ② ③ ④
11. ① ② ③ ④
12. ① ② ③ ④
13. ① ② ③ ④
14. ① ② ③ ④
15. ① ② ③ ④
16. ① ② ③ ④
17. ① ② ③ ④
18. ① ② ③ ④
19. ① ② ③ ④
20. ① ② ③ ④
21. ① ② ③ ④
22. ① ② ③ ④
23. ① ② ③ ④
24. ① ② ③ ④
25. ① ② ③ ④
26. ① ② ③ ④
27. ① ② ③ ④
28. ① ② ③ ④
29. ① ② ③ ④
30. ① ② ③ ④

*Practice tests are in Chapter 9, pages 129–158.

Practice Tests Answer Sheets[*]

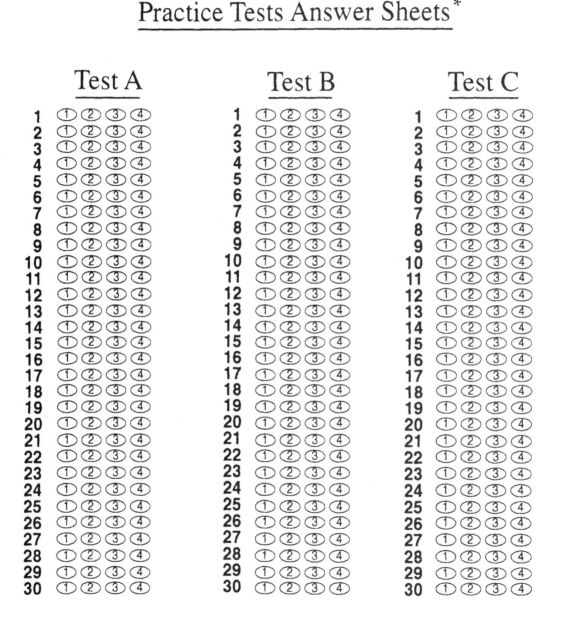

Test A

1	1	2	3	4
2	1	2	3	4
3	1	2	3	4
4	1	2	3	4
5	1	2	3	4
6	1	2	3	4
7	1	2	3	4
8	1	2	3	4
9	1	2	3	4
10	1	2	3	4
11	1	2	3	4
12	1	2	3	4
13	1	2	3	4
14	1	2	3	4
15	1	2	3	4
16	1	2	3	4
17	1	2	3	4
18	1	2	3	4
19	1	2	3	4
20	1	2	3	4
21	1	2	3	4
22	1	2	3	4
23	1	2	3	4
24	1	2	3	4
25	1	2	3	4
26	1	2	3	4
27	1	2	3	4
28	1	2	3	4
29	1	2	3	4
30	1	2	3	4

Test B

1	1	2	3	4
2	1	2	3	4
3	1	2	3	4
4	1	2	3	4
5	1	2	3	4
6	1	2	3	4
7	1	2	3	4
8	1	2	3	4
9	1	2	3	4
10	1	2	3	4
11	1	2	3	4
12	1	2	3	4
13	1	2	3	4
14	1	2	3	4
15	1	2	3	4
16	1	2	3	4
17	1	2	3	4
18	1	2	3	4
19	1	2	3	4
20	1	2	3	4
21	1	2	3	4
22	1	2	3	4
23	1	2	3	4
24	1	2	3	4
25	1	2	3	4
26	1	2	3	4
27	1	2	3	4
28	1	2	3	4
29	1	2	3	4
30	1	2	3	4

Test C

1	1	2	3	4
2	1	2	3	4
3	1	2	3	4
4	1	2	3	4
5	1	2	3	4
6	1	2	3	4
7	1	2	3	4
8	1	2	3	4
9	1	2	3	4
10	1	2	3	4
11	1	2	3	4
12	1	2	3	4
13	1	2	3	4
14	1	2	3	4
15	1	2	3	4
16	1	2	3	4
17	1	2	3	4
18	1	2	3	4
19	1	2	3	4
20	1	2	3	4
21	1	2	3	4
22	1	2	3	4
23	1	2	3	4
24	1	2	3	4
25	1	2	3	4
26	1	2	3	4
27	1	2	3	4
28	1	2	3	4
29	1	2	3	4
30	1	2	3	4

*Practice tests are in Chapter 9, pages 129–158.

Test Success

*Test-Taking Techniques for
Beginning Nursing Students*

Test Success

Test-Taking Techniques for Beginning Nursing Students

• • •

THIRD EDITION

Patricia M. Nugent, RN, MS, EdM, EdD
Department of Nursing
Nassau Community College
Garden City, New York

Barbara A. Vitale, RN, MA
Department of Nursing
Nassau Community College
Garden City, New York

F. A. Davis Company • Philadelphia

F. A. Davis Company
1915 Arch Street
Philadelphia, PA 19103

Printed in the United States of America

Last digit indicates print number: 10 9 8 7 6 5

Publisher, Nursing: Robert G. Martone
Production Editor: Jessica Howie Martin
Cover Designer: Louis J. Forgione

As new scientific information becomes available through basic and clinical research, recommended treatments and drug therapies undergo changes. The authors and publisher have done everything possible to make this book accurate, up to date, and in accord with accepted standards at the time of publication. The authors, editors, and publisher are not responsible for errors or omissions or for consequences from application of the book, and make no warranty, expressed or implied, in regard to the contents of the book. Any practice described in this book should be applied by the reader in accordance with professional standards of care used in regard to the unique circumstances that may apply in each situation. The reader is advised always to check product information (package inserts) for changes and new information regarding dose and contraindications before administering any drug. Caution is especially urged when using new or infrequently ordered drugs.

Library of Congress Cataloging-in-Publication Data

Nugent, Patricia Mary, 1944–
    Test success : test-taking techniques for beginning nursing students / Patricia M.
Nugent, Barbara A. Vitale.—3rd ed.
      p. ; cm.
    Includes bibliographical references and index.
    ISBN 0-8036-0524-2 (pbk.)
    1. Nursing—Examinations, questions, etc. 2. Practical nursing—Examinations,
questions, etc. 3. Test-taking skills. I. Title: Test-taking techniques for beginning nursing
students. II. Vitale, Barbara Ann, 1994– III. Title.
    [DNLM: 1. Nursing—Examination Questions. 2. Educational Measurement.
    WY 18.2 N967t 2000]
    RT55 .N77 2000
    610.73'076—dc21
                                                         99-052576

Dedicated to
KELLY MARIE DALL and HEATHER ANN McCORMACK
and
JOSEPH MICHAEL, JOHN ANDREW, and CHRISTOPHER NEIL VITALE
for all the joy they have
brought into our lives

Preface

· · ·

The increase in nursing knowledge and medical technology is accelerating at a breathtaking rate. This places greater stress on nursing students to learn what they need to know to provide safe patient-centered nursing care. Faculty and curricula are stretched to the limit to include all the information students must absorb to successfully complete the requirements to graduate as accountable practitioners. Attrition rates support the fact that academic demands are strenuous. This is compounded by the fact that nursing students arrive with more needs than ever before. An increasing percentage of nursing students are mature individuals who have been out of secondary education for years and need to relearn how to study and take tests, single parents who have the responsibility of supporting children and need to maximize their effectiveness when they study, or persons who speak English as their second language and demonstrate needs in reading and/or writing English. Beginning nursing students may be faced for the first time with multiple-choice questions that require not just regurgitation of information but comprehension, application, or analysis of information. Therefore the level of thinking on nursing examinations requires a high cognitive ability. Needless to say, testing situations induce anxiety for these test-takers. Nursing students need supportive textbooks to increase their chances of success.

This book is designed for beginning nursing students who are preparing to take tests at the end of a unit of instruction or at the completion of a fundamentals of nursing course. This book can also be used by students in licensed practical nurse programs to prepare for class examinations, NCLEX-PN, or advanced-standing examinations for entry into Registered Nurse programs. Students preparing for the NCLEX-RN may review this book to maximize their success on this national examination. Finally, nursing faculty members may find this book helpful when designing a test-taking workshop for student nurses.

The information presented in the book is designed to maximize success by helping students to develop a positive mental attitude; understand critical thinking; study and learn more effectively; become test-wise by identifying the step in the nursing process being tested to better establish what the question is asking and by exploring all testing formats, specifically multiple-choice questions; and appreciate computer applications in nursing education and evaluation. Because it takes nursing students at least 2 years of study to build a body of knowledge from which safe nursing judgments can be made, this book will present only content common to meeting patients' basic physical and psychosociocultural needs. In addition, such topics as ethics, rights, common theories, legal issues, the nursing process, pharmacology, community health nursing, and principles related to the management of nursing care are included on a fundamental level. Throughout the textbook the word "patient" is used to indicate the consumer of health care. It is recognized that consumers of health care may be referred to by such terms as "client" or "resident." Throughout the textbook the word "nurse" is used consistently to indicate a licensed nurse. It is recognized that this individual may be referred to by other titles such as Patient Care Coordinator, Nurse Manager, or Patient Care Associate. Throughout the textbook the words "Nurse Aide" or "Nursing Assistant" are used consistently to reflect unlicensed or credentialled supportive nursing staff. It is recognized that these individuals may be referred to by other titles such as Patient Care Assistant, Nurse Technician, or Comfort Care Associate.

In response to student and faculty input, the chapter on Critical Thinking (Chapter 2) has been expanded, particularly in relation to content concerning probability and risk as they relate to decision making. Chapter 10 has been enlarged to include four new sections: Meeting Patients' Physical Safety Needs, Meeting Patients' Microbiological Safety Needs, Meeting the Needs of the Patient in the Community Setting, and Pharmacology. In this edition, questions related to community health nursing, the management of nursing care, and pharmacology have been given greater emphasis because of the recent trends in the delivery of health care in the United States and the changing emphasis on credentialing/licensing examinations. In this edition, approximately 200 questions have been added for a total of 721 questions within the narrative content of Chapters 3 through 7, in three simulated tests in Chapter 9, and in content areas in Chapter 10.

All the multiple-choice questions in the book have been field tested, and the three simulated tests are designed to have an equal level of difficulty established at 76 percent. Rationales for the correct and incorrect answers are included for every question. These rationales should help the learner review some of the basic content in nursing theory and practice and contribute to mastery of answering questions. In addition, most questions in Chapter 10 include a Test-Taking Tip to emphasize one or more of the test-taking techniques that can be applied when answering a question.

There are some study guides on the shelves that provide students with practical skills to become more successful learners. However, few books exist that specifically aid beginning nursing students grappling with examination questions that test fundamental nursing theory and practice. This book was written to fill that void.

We want to thank Bob Martone, Publisher for Nursing, who guided and supported us through the publication process and Ruth DeGeorge for providing valuable editorial assistance. Thanks also go to the F. A. Davis staff, including Samuel A. Rondinelli, Assistant Director of Editing, Design, and Production; Jessica Howie Martin, Production Editor; Jamie Robinson, Copy Editor; and Louis Forgione, Cover Designer. Most importantly, we would like to thank our husbands and children—Neil, Kelly, and Heather and Joe, Joseph, John, and Christopher—for their love and support.

Contents

• • •

How to Use This Book to Maximize Success

• • •

It is amazing what **you** can achieve when **you** are tenacious, organized, and determined to attain a goal. By purchasing this book **you** have demonstrated a beginning commitment to do what **you** have to do to improve **your** success in nursing examinations. This book is designed to introduce **you** to various techniques that can contribute to a positive mental attitude, promote the development of critical thinking skills, and help **you** become test-wise. If you are beginning to get the feeling that "you" is an important word, "you" are right! Learning requires you to be an active participant in your own learning. Your ultimate success can be maximized if you progress through this book in a planned and organized fashion and are willing to practice the techniques suggested. Effort is directly correlated with the benefits you will derive from this book. Once you have determined that you are eager and motivated to learn, you are ready to begin.

Chapter content is organized in a specific order to provide you with techniques that will contribute to: developing a positive mental attitude; understanding critical thinking, studying and learning more effectively, exploring all testing formats with an emphasis on multiple-choice questions, identifying the nursing process as a form of problem solving, becoming test-wise, and appreciating computer applications in nursing education and evaluation. Over 700 questions will afford you the opportunity to practice test-taking techniques. The correct answers and the rationales for all the options are presented to reinforce the theories and principles of fundamentals of nursing practice that you have learned in your nursing program.

Three simulated tests of equal difficulty are included to provide you with a baseline score that reflects your general knowledge of nursing fundamentals and test-taking proficiency, afford you the opportunity to simulate a testing situation, demonstrate successful progress, and motivate you to continue practicing the learned techniques. These simulated tests were placed in Chapter 9 to avoid your inadvertently taking them before you understand their purpose. To use this book to its best advantage, take one of the simulated tests before reading Chapters 1 through 8. This is a pretest because the results will provide you with a baseline score for future comparison. After you have read Chapters 1 through 8, take another simulated test. Then practice the questions in Chapter 10. Be sure to read and study the rationales because this information will review and reinforce the material you are learning in your fundamentals of nursing course in your school of nursing. To maximize learning, it is suggested that you answer the questions in the specific categories in Chapter 10 after you have learned the content in class. When you finish Chapter 10, take the last of the simulated tests as a post-test. If you are employing the information presented in Chapters 1 through 8 and you practice the multiple-choice questions in Chapter 10, your test scores should improve from test to test.

You should be commended for your efforts to achieve success. It is hard work to take responsibility for your own learning. The magnitude of your learning will be in direct proportion to the amount of energy you are willing to expend in the effort to improve your skills. As you function from a position of strength, study more effectively, become test-wise, and are able to apply the nursing process to determine what the question is asking, you should become a more successful test-taker. Good luck on your nursing examinations!

Empowerment

Develop a Positive Mental Attitude

A positive mental attitude can help you control test anxiety by limiting anxious responses so that you can be a more successful test-taker. A positive mental attitude requires you to function from a position of strength. This does not imply that you have to be powerful, manipulative, or dominant. What it does require is that you develop techniques that put you in control of your own thoughts and behavior. To be in control of yourself, you need to operate from a position of positive self-worth with a feeling of empowerment. This begins with self-assessment.

You have both strengths and weaknesses. Both must be identified to maximize your potential. Strengths are easy to focus on because you feel safe and nonthreatened. Weaknesses are more difficult to focus on because you may feel inadequate and uncomfortable. When performing a self-assessment, be honest with yourself. You must separate your ego from your assessment. Only you will know the result. Remember, few people are perfect! Have the courage to be honest with yourself and recognize your imperfections. You can have weaknesses and imperfections and still have a positive self-concept.

To develop self-worth, you must be willing to look within yourself and recognize that you are valuable. Acting from a position of strength requires you to start saying and believing that you are worthwhile. Self-worth increases when you believe down to your very bones that you are important.

A feeling of empowerment arises when you are able to use all your available resources and learned strategies to achieve your goals. To achieve empowerment you need to develop techniques and skills that not only make you feel in control but actually position you in control. When you are in control, you function from a position of strength.

To achieve a sense of self-worth and a feeling of empowerment that will help you succeed in test taking, you must learn various techniques that must be practiced before taking the test. These techniques will help you to control stressful situations, reduce anxious responses, and enhance concentration, thereby improving your analytical and problem-solving ability and strengthening your test performance. By learning and practicing the following techniques, you will have a foundation on which to operate from a position of strength.

2

ESTABLISH A POSITIVE INTERNAL LOCUS OF CONTROL

Henry Ford once said, "Whether you think you can, or think you can't . . . you're right." In other words, what you think can be a self-fulfilling prophecy. It is important to recognize that the way you talk to yourself influences the way you think about yourself. The content of what you say indicates how you feel about the control of your behavior and your life. "I was lucky to pass that test." "I couldn't help failing because the teacher is hard." "I got test anxiety and I just became paralyzed during the test." Each of these internal dialogues indicates that you see yourself as powerless. When you say these things, you fail to take responsibility.

Identify your pattern of talking to yourself. Do you blame others, attribute failure to external causes, and use the words "I couldn't," "I should," "I need," or "I have to"? If you do, you are using language that places you in a position of impotence, dependence, defenselessness, and hopelessness. YOU MUST ESTABLISH A POSITIVE INTERNAL LOCUS OF CONTROL. You do this by replacing such language with language that reflects control and strength. You must say, "I want," "I can," and "I will." When you use these words, you imply that you are committed to a task until you succeed. Place index cards around your environment with "I WANT," "I CAN," and "I WILL" on them to cue you into a positive pattern of talking to yourself.

CHALLENGE NEGATIVE THOUGHTS

Your value as an individual should not be linked to how well you do on an examination. Your self-worth and your test score are distinctly isolated entities. If you believe that you are good when you do well on a test and are bad when you do poorly, you must alter your thinking. You need to work at recognizing that this is illogical thinking. Illogical thinking or negative thinking is self-destructive. Negative thoughts must be changed into positive thoughts to build confidence and self-worth. As confidence and self-worth rise, anxiety can be controlled and minimized.

Positive thinking focuses your attention on your desired outcomes. If you think you can do well on a test, you are more likely to fulfill this prophecy. It is critical that you control negative thoughts by developing a positive mental attitude. When you say to yourself, "This is going to be a hard test. I'll never pass," CHALLENGE THIS STATEMENT. Instead say to yourself, "This is a ridiculous statement: of course I can pass it. All I have to do is study hard to pass this test!" It is crucial that you challenge negative thoughts with optimistic thoughts. Optimistic thoughts are valuable because they can be converted into positive actions and feelings, which place you in a position of control.

For this technique to work, you must first be able to stop negative thoughts. To use the technique called ARREST NEGATIVE THOUGHTS, you must first identity the pattern of negative thinking that you use to defend yourself. Envision a police car with flashing lights that signifies ARREST NEGATIVE THOUGHTS. You could even place pictures of police cars around your environment to cue you to ARREST NEGATIVE THOUGHTS. Once you identify negative thoughts, handcuff them and lock them away so that they will no longer be a threat. Actually envision negative thoughts locked up in a cell with bars and throw away the key.

Once you stop a negative thought, replace it with a POSITIVE THOUGHT. If you have difficulty identifying a positive thought, praise yourself or give yourself a compliment. Tell yourself, "Wow! I am really working hard to pass this test." "Congratulations! I was able to arrest that negative thought and to be in control. "To increase your control, make an inventory of the things you can do, the things you want to achieve, and the feelings you want to feel that contribute to a positive mental attitude. Throughout the day take an "attitude inventory." Identify the status of your mental attitude. If it is not consistent with your list of the feelings you want to feel or the positive image you have of yourself, CHALLENGE YOUR ATTITUDE.

Compose statements that support the feelings that you want to feel and read them over and over, such as "I can pass this test!" or "I am in control of my attitudes, and my attitudes are positive!" Make sure that you end the day with a positive thought, and even identify something that you want to accomplish the next day. Forecasting positive events establishes a positive direction in which you can focus your attention.

USE CONTROLLED BREATHING (DIAPHRAGMATIC BREATHING)

An excellent way to reduce feelings of anxiety is to use the technique of controlled breathing. When you control your breathing, you can break the pattern of shallow short breaths associated with anxious feelings. Deep abdominal or diaphragmatic breathing enhances the relaxation response. When a person exhales, tense muscles tend to relax. You probably do this now unconsciously. Most people take a deep breath and exhale (sigh) several times an hour. When you "sigh," it is a form of diaphragmatic breathing. **Diaphragmatic breathing** causes the diaphragm to flatten and the abdomen to enlarge on inspiration. On exhalation the abdominal muscles contract. As you slowly let out this deep breath, the other muscles of the body will tend to "let go" and relax. This technique enables you to breath more deeply than if you just expand your chest on inspiration. Controlled breathing can be helpful to reduce anxious responses that occur at the beginning of a test, when you are stumped with a tough question, or when you are nearing the end of the test. During these critical times you can use controlled breathing to induce the relaxation response.

When practicing diaphragmatic breathing, place your hands lightly over the front of the lower ribs and upper abdomen so that you can monitor the movement you are trying to achieve. As you become accomplished in this technique, you will not need to position your hands on your body. Practice the following steps:

1. Gently position your hands over the front of your lower ribs and upper abdomen.
2. Exhale gently and fully. Feel your ribs and abdomen sink inward toward the middle of your body.
3. Slowly inhale, taking a deep breath through your nose and expanding your abdomen first and then your chest. Do this as you slowly count to four.
4. Hold your breath at the height of inhalation as you count to four.
5. Exhale fully by contracting your abdominal muscles and then your chest. Let out all the air slowly and smoothly through your mouth as you count to eight.

Monitor the pace of your breathing. Notice how your muscles relax each time you exhale. You may feel warm, tingly, and relaxed. Enjoy the feeling as you breathe deeply and evenly. You should practice this technique so that controlled breathing automatically induces the relaxation response after several breaths. Once you are able to induce the relaxation response with controlled breathing, you can effectively draw on this strategy when you need to be in control.

It is important not to do this exercise too forcefully or too rapidly because it can cause you to hyperventilate. Hyperventilation may cause dizziness and lightheadedness. If either of these occurs, cup your hands over your nose and mouth and slowly rebreathe your exhaled air. These symptoms should subside. Then you can continue the exercise less vigorously. Always monitor your responses throughout the exercise.

DESENSITIZE YOURSELF TO THE FEAR RESPONSE

Individuals generally connect a certain feeling with a specific situation. To learn to control your feelings, you must first recognize how you consider and visualize events. It is not uncommon to connect a feeling of fear with an event. In a testing situation, the examination is the event and the response of fear is the feeling. If this happens to you, you need to interrupt this fear response. You have the ability to control how you respond to fear. When you are able to sever the event from the feeling, you will establish control and become empowered. However, establishing control does not happen automatically. You need to desensitize yourself to the event to control the fear response.

Desensitization involves repeatedly exposing yourself to the identified emotionally distressing event in a limited and/or controlled setting until the event no longer precipitates the feeling of fear. Desensitization is dependent on associating relaxation with the fear response. To achieve this response you need to practice the following routine:

FIRST, you must practice a relaxation response. Controlled breathing is an excellent relaxation technique and has already been described. Once you are comfortable with the technique of controlled breathing, you can use it in the desensitization routine.

SECOND, you should make a list of five events associated with a testing situation that cause fear, and rank them starting with the one that causes the most anxiety and progressing to the one that causes the least anxiety. The following is an example:

1. Taking an important examination on difficult material

2. Taking an important examination on material you know well

3. Taking a small quiz on difficult material

4. Taking a small quiz on material you know well

5. Taking a practice test that does not count

Event number 5 should evoke the least amount of fear.

THIRD, you should practice the following routine:

1. Practice controlled breathing and become relaxed.

2. Now imagine event number 5. If you feel fearful, turn off the scene and go back to controlled breathing for about 30 seconds.

3. Once you are relaxed, again imagine scene number 5. Try to visualize the event for 30 seconds without becoming uncomfortable.

4. Once you have accomplished the previous step, move up the list of events until you are able to imagine event number 1 without feeling uncomfortable.

When you are successful in controlling the fear response in an imagined situation, you can attempt to accomplish the same success in simulated tests at home. Once you are successful in controlling the fear response in simulated tests at home, you can take some simulated tests in a classroom setting. Continue practicing desensitization until you have a feeling of control in an actual testing situation. This may take practice. It will not be accomplished in one practice session.

Another way you can use the concept of desensitization is to practice positive dialogue within yourself. For example, imagine the following internal dialogue within yourself.

"How are you feeling about the examination today?"	"A little uncomfortable and fearful."
"Do you want to feel this way?"	"Absolutely not!"
"How do you want to feel?"	"I want to feel calm, in control, and effective."
"What are you going to do to achieve that feeling?"	"I am going to practice relaxation and controlled breathing."

You might be saying to yourself, "I don't see myself doing this. This is silly." The resilient and tenacious individual who is flexible and willing to try new techniques is in a position of control. If your goal is to be empowered, you only have to be open and willing to learn.

PERFORM MUSCLE RELAXATION

This technique involves learning how to tense and relax each muscle group of your body until all of your muscle groups are relaxed. This technique requires practice. The basic technique involves assuming a comfortable position and then sequentially contracting and relaxing each muscle group in your body from your head to your toes. When a muscle group is tensed and then released, the muscle smooths out and relaxes. It is not a technique that can be quickly described in a short paragraph. However, the following brief exercise is included as an example:

EXAMPLE

Find a comfortable chair in a quiet place. Close your eyes and use diaphragmatic breathing, taking several deep breaths to relax. You are now ready to begin progressive muscle relaxation. Sequentially move from one muscle group in the body to another, contracting and relaxing each in an even manner. Contract and relax each muscle group for 10 seconds. After each muscle group is tensed and then relaxed, take a deep, slow breath using diaphragmatic breathing. As you are relaxing, observe how you feel. Experience the sensation. You may want to reinforce the feeling of relaxation by saying, "My muscles are relaxing. I can feel the tension flowing out of my muscles." Remember not to breathe too forcefully to avoid hyperventilation. The following is a sample of muscle groups that should be included in a progressive muscle relaxation routine:

1. Bend your head and try to rest your right ear as close as you can to your right shoulder. Count to 10. Assume normal alignment, relax, and take a deep breath.

2. Bend your head and try to rest your left ear as close as you can to your left shoulder. Count to 10. Assume normal alignment, relax, and take a deep breath.

3. Flex your head and try to touch your chin to your chest. Count to 10. Assume normal alignment, relax, and take a deep breath.

4. Make a fist and tense your right forearm. Count to 10. Relax and take a deep breath.

5. Make a fist and tense your left forearm. Count to 10. Relax and take a deep breath.

6. Tense your right biceps by tightly bending (flexing) the right arm at the elbow. Count to 10. Relax and take a deep breath.

Continue moving from the head to the arms, trunk, and legs by contracting and relaxing each of the muscle groups within these areas of your body. You can understand and master this technique by obtaining an audio or videotape that is designed to direct and instruct you through the entire routine of tensing and relaxing each muscle group. This technique should be practiced every day until the technique becomes natural. Once you have mastered this technique, you can use a shortened version of progressive relaxation along with controlled breathing at critical times during a test.

USE IMAGERY

Using imagery can help you to establish a state of relaxation. When we remember a fearful event, our heart and respiratory rates increase just as they did when the event occurred. Comparably, when we recall a happy, relaxing period, we can regenerate and re-create the atmosphere and feeling that we had during that pleasant event. This is not a difficult technique to master. Just let go and enjoy the experience.

Position yourself in a comfortable chair, close your eyes, and construct an image in your mind of a place that makes you feel calm, happy, and relaxed. It may be at the seashore or in a

6

field of wild flowers. Let your mind picture what is happening. Observe the colors of the landscape. Notice the soothing sounds of the environment. Notice the smells in the air, the shapes of objects, and movement about you. Recall the positive feelings that flow over you when you are in that scene and relax. You can now open your eyes relaxed, refreshed, and calm.

At critical times during a test, you can take a few minutes to use imagery to induce the relaxation response. To successfully reduce stress, you must position yourself in control. When you are in control, your test performance generally improves.

OVERPREPARE FOR A TEST

One of the best ways to reduce text anxiety is to be overprepared. The more prepared you are to take the test, the more confident you will be. The more confident you are, the more able you are to challenge the fear of being unprepared. Study the textbook, read your notes, take practice tests, and prepare with other students in a study group. Even when you think that you know the information, study the same information again to reinforce your learning. For this technique to be successful, you need to plan a significant amount of time for studying. Although it is time-consuming, it does build confidence and reduce anxiety. No one has said that learning would be easy. Any worthwhile goal deserves the effort necessary to achieve success. Being overprepared is the BEST way to place yourself in a position of strength.

Consider the following scenario: a student was not doing well in school and asked what she could do to improve her performance. The concept of being overprepared was discussed, and she worked out a study schedule of 2 hours a day for 2 weeks before the next test. After the test, the student said that she thought she did well because the test was easy. It had to be pointed out that she perceived the test as easy because she had attained the knowledge that enabled her to answer the questions correctly. Her eyes lit up as if someone had turned on a light bulb in her head! When you recognize that you have the opportunity to be in control and take responsibility for your own learning, you become all that you can be.

EXERCISE REGULARLY

Exercising regularly helps you to expend nervous energy. Walking, aerobics, swimming, bike riding, or running at least 3 times a week for 20 minutes is an effective way to maintain or improve your physical and mental status. The most important thing to remember about regular exercise is to slowly increase the degree and duration of the exercise. Your exercise program should not be so rigorous that it leaves you exhausted. It should serve to clear your mind and make you mentally alert and better able to cope with the challenge of a test. Exercise should not be performed just before going to bed because it can interface with sleep. Regular exercise should become a routine activity in your weekly schedule, not just a response to the tension of an upcoming test. Once you establish a regular exercise program, you should experience physical and psychological benefits.

Establish Control Before and During the Test

It is important to maximize your opportunities to feel in control in the testing situation. Additional techniques you can use to establish a tranquil and composed atmosphere require you to take control of your testing equipment, your activities before and during a test, and your immediate physical space. Techniques to help create this atmosphere are reinforced in Chapter 6, Test-Taking Techniques. However, they are also discussed here because they can be used to reduce anxiety and promote empowerment.

MANAGE YOUR DAILY ROUTINE BEFORE THE TEST

It is important to maintain your usual daily routine the day before the test. Eat normally, but avoid beverages with caffeine. Caffeine can lessen your attention span and reduce your concentration by overstimulating your metabolism. Avoid the urge to stay up late the night before a test. If you are tired when taking a test, your ability to concentrate and problem-solve may be limited. Go to bed at your regular time. Following your usual routines can be relaxing and can contribute to a feeling of control.

MANAGE YOUR STUDY HABITS BEFORE THE TEST

Do not stay up up late studying the night before the big test. Squeezing in last-minute studying may increase anxiety and contribute to feelings of powerlessness and helplessness. DO NOT CRAM. If you have implemented a study routine in preparation for the test, you should have confidence in what you have learned. Establish control by saying to yourself, "I have studied hard for this test and I am well prepared. I can relax tonight because I know the material for the test tomorrow and I will do well." Avoid giving in to the desire to cram. Instead, use the various techniques discussed earlier in this chapter to maintain a positive mental attitude.

MANAGE YOUR TRAVEL THE DAY OF THE TEST

Plan to arrive early the day of the test. It is important to plan for potential events that could delay you, such as traffic jams or a flat tire. The more important the test, the more time you should schedule for travel. If you live a substantial distance from the testing site, you might ask another student who lives closer to allow you to sleep over the night before the test. The midterm or final examination for a course may be held in a different location than the regularly scheduled classroom used for the lecture. If you are unfamiliar with the examination room, make a practice run to locate where it is and note how long it takes to get there. Nothing produces more anxiety than rushing to a test or arriving after the start of a test. A feeling of control reduces tension and the fear response. You can be in control if you manage your travel time with time to spare.

MANAGE THE SUPPLIES YOU NEED FOR THE TEST

The more variables you have control over, the more calm and relaxed you will feel. Compose a list of the items to bring with you to the test. They may include pencils, pens, scrap paper, erasers, a ruler, a watch, and even a lucky charm. It is suggested that you collect the items the day before the test. This eliminates a task so that you do not have to worry about it on the day of the test and contributes to your sense of control.

MANAGE YOUR PERSONAL COMFORT

Maslow's Hierarchy of Needs specifies that basic physiological needs must be met before you attempt to meet higher-level needs. Be aware of your own basic needs relating to factors such as nutrition, elimination, and physical comfort. Meet these basic needs before the test because unfulfilled needs will compete for your attention. For example, arrive early so that you can visit the restroom, wear layers of clothing so that you an adjust to various environmental temperatures, and eat a light, balanced meal to maintain your blood sugar. Once these basic needs are met, you can progress up the ladder of needs to self-actualization.

8

MANAGE THE TEST ENVIRONMENT

When you arrive early, you generally have the choice of where to sit in the room. This contributes to a feeling of control because you are able to sit where you are most comfortable. You might prefer to sit by a window, near a heat source, or in the back of the room. Generally it helps to sit near the administrator of the test. Directions may be heard more clearly, and the administrator's attention may be gained more easily if you need to ask a question. It is wise to avoid sitting by a door. The commotion made by people entering or exiting the room can be a distraction and interfere with your ability to concentrate. Take every opportunity to control your environment. Measures that help you feel in control contribute to a positive mental attitude.

MAINTAIN A POSITIVE MENTAL ATTITUDE

Remind yourself of how hard you worked and how well prepared you are to take this test. ESTABLISH CONTROL by arresting negative thoughts and focusing on the positive. Say to yourself, "I am ready for this test! I will do well on this test! I can get an A on this test!" These statements support a positive mental attitude and enhance a feeling of control.

MANAGE YOUR PHYSICAL AND EMOTIONAL RESPONSES

At critical times during the test, you may feel nervous, your breathing may become rapid and shallow, or you may draw a blank on a question. Stop and take a minibreak. Used controlled breathing to induce the relaxation response. You may also use a shortened version of progressive relaxation exercises to induce the relaxation response. Daily practice of breathing and relaxation exercises will enable you to quickly induce the relaxation response during times of stress. Once these techniques are implemented, you should again feel empowerment.

Summary

The techniques in this chapter are designed to increase your mastery over the stress of the testing situation. When you feel positive about yourself and have a strong self-image and a feeling of self-worth, you will develop a sense of control. When you are able to draw on various techniques that empower you to respond to the testing situation with a sense of calm, you will improve your effectiveness. Use these techniques along with the other skills suggested in this book, practice the questions, and take the simulated practice tests as instructed in the section "How to Use This Book to Maximize Success" at the beginning of the text. These activities will support your self-worth, provide you with a feeling of control, and increase your effectiveness in the testing situation.

Critical Thinking

Introduction

If your ultimate goal is to become a competent nurse, you have to first recognize what knowledge base and skills are needed to achieve this goal. Study skills, critical-thinking skills, and problem-solving skills are essential to achieve success as a learner. Your goal should be to develop skills that support your ability to use reasoning and not just react by rote (a fixed, routine, mechanical way of doing something). Several chapters in this book are designed to assist you in the journey toward this goal. General and specific study skills are addressed in Chapter 3, the nursing process as a problem-solving process is addressed in Chapter 5, and critical-thinking skills are addressed in this chapter. No one would argue with the statement that a nurse needs to be a safe, qualified, and technically proficient practitioner. Consumers of nursing care are most aware of the **actions** (psychomotor skills) that nurses engage in and generally rate the quality of nursing care in relation to the degree that their expectations are satisfied. However, the quality of nursing care is based on more than just what the nurse does. It is also based on how the nurse **thinks** (cognitive skills) in relation to how conclusions are drawn, decisions are made, and problems are resolved.

> *Thinking is the hardest work there is, which is the probable reason why so few engage in it.*
> HENRY FORD

The thinking skills that are rarely recognized by the consumer, such as reflecting, clarifying, analyzing, and reasoning, are crucial to the development of a competent nurse.

Historically, critical thinking in nursing has been associated with the nursing process (assessment, analysis/diagnosis, planning, implementation, and evaluation). This theoretical framework, which is used to identify and attain solutions to complex problems, has been the foundation for nursing education, practice, and research. It is a systematic, orderly, step-by-step progression with a beginning and an end (linear format). Problem solving in relation to the nursing process produces a nursing care plan or "product." Chapter 5 addresses the steps in the nursing process and provides many sample items that demonstrate application of information within the context of the nursing process.

Because nursing entails more than just the solving of problems, the concept of critical thinking as a "process" is receiving increasing attention. Various researchers believe that critical thinking in nursing is more than just a behavioral, task-oriented, linear approach demonstrated in problem solving and that critical thinking should be based on an emancipatory model. Emancipatory models embrace the concept of empowerment and autonomous action stemming from critical insights. Emancipatory models stress critical thinking as a process rather than just a problem-solving product or solution.

Definition of Critical Thinking

No one definition of critical thinking is agreed on by leaders in the field of nursing. However, the following excerpts may enhance your understanding of the concept. Chaffee (1990) defined critical thinking as "making sense of our world by carefully examining the thinking process in order to clarify and improve our understanding." Alfaro-LeFevre (1995) summarized that critical thinking:

- Entails purposeful, goal-directed thinking
- Aims to make judgments based on evidence (fact) rather than conjecture (guesswork)
- Is based on principles of science and scientific method
- Requires strategies that maximize *human potential* and compensate for problems caused by *human nature*

The Delphi Research Project characterized the ideal critical thinker as one who is habitually inquisitive, well informed, trustful of reason, open-minded in evaluation, honest in facing personal biases, prudent in making judgments, willing to reconsider, clear about issues, orderly in complex matters, diligent in seeking relevant information, reasonable in the selection of criteria, focused in inquiry, and persistent in seeking results which are as precise as the subject and the circumstances of inquiry permit (American Philosophical Association, 1990). Brookfield (1987) described four components of critical thinking: identifying and challenging assumptions; becoming aware of the importance of context in creating meaning; imagining and exploring alternatives; and cultivating a reflective skepticism. Pless (1993) identified the following critical-thinking cognitive skills and subskills as essential for critical thinking: INTERPRETATION—categorization, decoding significance, and clarifying meaning; ANALYSIS—examining ideas, identifying arguments, and analyzing arguments; EVALUATION—assessing claims and assessing arguments; INFERENCE—querying evidence, conjecturing alternatives, and drawing conclusions; EXPLANATION—stating results, justifying procedures, and presenting arguments; and SELF-REGULATION—self-examination and self-correction.

Critical Thinking in Nursing

Nursing requires not only the learning of facts and procedures but also the ability to evaluate each unique patient situation. In Chapter 3, Study Techniques, a section titled "Cognitive Levels of Nursing Questions" addresses the variety of thinking processes—knowledge, comprehension, application, and analysis—that the nurse uses when managing data and identifying and meeting a patient's nursing needs. Because these thinking processes are important to both the process and product inherent in nursing care, multiple-choice questions in this section are designed to test your knowledge base, comprehension of information, application of theory and principles, and analytical ability. In all but knowledge-type questions, intellectual skills are required that involve more than just the recall of information. In comprehension-type questions you are required to translate, interpret, and determine the implications, consequences, and corollaries of the effects of information. In application-type questions you are required to use information in a new situation. In analysis-type questions you are required to interpret a variety of data and recognize the commonalities, differences, and interrelationships among the ideas presented. Numerous sample items in this section challenge your analytical abilities, address the cognitive domains, and demonstrate the concepts being presented.

An understanding of the nursing process and the cognitive domains is important; however, critical thinking skills must be developed if you are going to be a successful thinker and ultimately an expert nurse. The first step is to build a foundation of knowledge and information that can eventually be applied in clinical situations.

> *Both minds and fountain pens will work when willed. But minds, like fountain pens, must first be filled.*
> ARTHUR GUITERMAN

Before you can apply knowledge, you need to know what needs to be known and how the knowledge can be applied. To do this you need to ask yourself serious questions such as: "What do I know?" "What do I need to know?" "How do I know it?" "What do I have to do to know it?" This is a new activity for some students. It can be threatening and even anxiety producing. It is not easy to acknowledge the degree of your own lack of knowledge or ignorance, and it can be a sobering experience.

> *The more I know I know, I know the less.*
> ROBERT OWEN

Therefore, to fill voids in your knowledge you need to study. Avoid the pitfall of being a superficial thinker. A superficial thinker devotes excessive time to memorization and rote learning. Become a deep thinker.

> *Many bring rakes but few shovels.*
> FRANK C. BROWN

A deep thinker develops a thorough understanding of the material studied. Chapter 3, Study Techniques, discusses strategies that will help you answer some of the above questions, and study more effectively and efficiently.

Once you know basic information, you are better able to recognize the significance of cue data. Multiple-choice questions are carefully designed to test your knowledge and comprehension of information regarding key concepts and your ability to analyze and apply this information in various situations. As you move from being a neophyte to a more experienced student, you are more able to recognize the significance of cues and respond readily in all situations, whether in a laboratory setting, computer simulation, clinical setting, or on a multiple-choice test. In multiple-choice questions you must recognize the key words and concepts being tested in the question. They require that you ask "What is happening?" and "What should I do?" Before you can answer these questions, it would be helpful to identify the information processing style that you use when confronted with a situation that requires a response.

LEFT-BRAIN AND RIGHT-BRAIN HEMISPHERE INFORMATION FUNCTIONING

Taggart and Torrance (1984) explored left-brain and right-brain hemisphere information processing. They found that individuals who used **left-brain hemisphere information processing** functions used rational problem-solving strategies and logical sequencing to problem-solve. Rational learners break down situations into components and look for universal rules and approaches that can be applied in all situations. Individuals who used **right-brain**

hemisphere information processing functions favored looking for main ideas to establish relationships that could be abstracted as the foundation for intuitive problem solving. The intuitive learner first learns from context and experience and then applies and analyzes principles. Additional research in this area demonstrates that, although both the novice and the expert used logical and rational problem-solving strategies, it is the expert who used a broad range of thinking skills that integrate both logical and intuitive thinking to address facts and feelings to achieve accurate decision making.

CLINICAL JUDGMENTS

The ability to build a foundation of data, inferences, and hypotheses for nursing decision making is dependent on your ability to use several types of clinical judgments. **Perceptual judgments** are judgments that you make regarding the data you need to collect and the validation of the importance of the data you collect within the context of the situation. **Inferential judgments** are judgments that you make when you determine which data are significant, eliminate data that are insignificant, and identify the relationship that exists among the data collected. **Diagnostic judgments** are judgments that you make when you link clusters of data with patterns affiliated with a specific nursing diagnosis.

INDUCTIVE AND DEDUCTIVE REASONING

The ability to make judgments relies on two types of reasoning, inductive and deductive. **Inductive reasoning** requires you to make generalizations from a set of facts or assessments. When a cluster of data is examined, it may suggest a specific interpretation. You move from considering the context of a situation to a theoretical basis for it. You move from considering particular facts or a specific scenario to making a general conclusion. In inductive reasoning you consider all of the possibilities. This method is more time consuming than deductive reasoning and is more often used by the novice critical thinker. **Deductive reasoning** requires you to move from examining a premise or an assumption to making a logical conclusion. You work at eliminating possible solutions at the same time that you continue to collect data. To use deductive reasoning successfully, you have to be able to separate relevant data from irrelevant data and separate plausible hypotheses from unlikely hypotheses. Inherent in this process is the ability to redefine hypotheses to arrive at the appropriate solution. Deductive reasoning is more often used by the expert nurse because the expert nurse has a larger knowledge and experiential background upon which to base judgments. Both inductive and deductive reasoning are necessary for you to think critically. Nurses use both types of reasoning and often shift from inductive to deductive reasoning depending on the situation.

LEVELS OF CRITICAL THINKING

As your knowledge of theory and experience increases, you will be constructing a scientific foundation to support critical thinking and clinical decision making. When developing critical thinking skills, you will advance through three levels of competence: basic, complex, and expert. As a student you are building a novice's database of information and experiential knowledge. When you are confronted with a situation, initially your response is based on recall and rote memory. As a **basic-level critical thinker,** you tend to guide your responses by rules and procedures and seek concrete actions. You reduce situations to their distinct and independent parts. For example, when performing a simple dry sterile dressing for an abdominal wound with approximated edges (healing by primary intention), you may use a procedure book and follow each step as outlined. As you acquire more knowledge and experience you will advance from basic-level thinker to complex-level thinker. As a **complex-level thinker** you will be guided by the need to explore options based on principles and patterns and an understanding of commonalities and differences. Your response will begin to be based on the ability to identify cue data, analyze clustered information, sort and choose the most appropriate action, and evaluate the client's response. For example, when performing a sterile dressing for an open wound where the edges are not readily approximated (healing by secondary intention), you may need to modify the procedure. Depending on the situation, you may need to reposition the patient, use additional sterile equipment, or irrigate the wound. The more knowledge and experience you gain, the more solid the connections will become between your knowledge base and the application of that knowledge. You are now becoming an expert critical thinker. As an **expert critical thinker,** you will develop reasoning based on models, patterns, and standards associated with the "uniqueness" and "wholeness" of each situation. For example, when performing a sterile dressing on a large gaping wound that has been purposely left open (healing by tertiary intention), your critical thinking will require a higher level of sophistication. You will need to consider concepts such as dehiscence, evisceration, fistula formation, sinus tracking, undermining, presence of infection, necrosis, factors that impair or facilitate wound healing, and dressing alternatives. The expert looks at the situation from an entire perspective that can only be accomplished with a broad and deep knowledge base and experience.

All critical thinkers should be asking, "What is wrong?" "Why?" "How?" "What else?" "What if?" and even "So what?" However, at each successive level of critical thinking, the degree of sophistication needed to explore these questions increases. These questions need to be asked when studying, when faced with a clinical situation (whether simulated or real), and when challenged by a multiple-choice question. As a beginning nursing student you are a novice, not an expert! Nursing school is several years long for a purpose. Be realistic with your self-expectations. It takes time to acquire and integrate the knowledge and experience necessary to be an expert critical thinker.

Practice Critical Thinking

Just as you first learned how to turn over, crawl, stand, walk, and then run by practicing balance and building strength and endurance, you must learn and practice critical-thinking and problem-solving skills until you are proficient in using these skills and can respond accurately and achieve your goal of being an expert critical thinker. To be able to tap your critical-thinking skills when taking an examination, your critical-thinking skills must be well entrenched in your approach to all professional endeavors. When challenged by any patient situation, you should employ these strategies.

- Identify assumptions.
- Use a method to collect and organize information.
- Validate the accuracy and reliability of collected information.
- Determine the significance of collected information.
- Determine inconsistencies in collected information.
- Identify commonalities and differences.
- Identify patterns of patient responses.
- Identify stressors and common adaptations to stressors.
- Identify discrepancies or gaps in information.
- Cluster information to determine relationships.

- Make inferences based on collected information.
- Identify actual problems and patients who may be at risk for problems based on common defining characteristics.
- Establish priorities. (Maslow's hierarchy is an excellent model to use to achieve this goal.)
- Formulate specific, patient-centered, realistic, measurable goals with a time frame.
- Identify appropriate nursing actions.
- Evaluate outcomes.
- Evaluate and modify critical-thinking activities.

This list of strategies reflects sophisticated, deep thinking. Critical thinking is a type of highly developed thinking and a learned skill. The learner has to be actively involved in the learning process. Critical thinking cannot be memorized; it must be practiced.

> *Knowledge is a treasure, but practice is the key to it.*
> THOMAS FULLER

To help you develop or refine thinking that can become more critical and automatic, it is suggested that you engage in the following activities while incorporating the strategies listed above.

THINKING ALOUD   The proficient thinker verbalizes thought processes and rationales. The actual expression of thoughts in words helps to clarify and solidify thinking. This strategy can be used while you are engaged in an activity or later when you review your performance. Clinical postconferences and individual mentoring experiences in which information is exchanged promote critical thinking.

REVIEW OF PATIENT SCENARIOS   Chart review, grand rounds, and case study approaches when performed in a group provide interdisciplinary exchanges, a variety of different thinking perspectives, and learning from role models. These approaches require a verbal exchange that includes reasoning, interpreting, identifying evidence, deducing, and concluding. In these situations you can examine your viewpoint in relation to the viewpoints of others. This exchange promotes learning and stimulates critical thinking.

WRITTEN ASSIGNMENTS   Written assignments are not just "busy work." Journal writing is an activity that requires you to log and respond to important and meaningful events and situations. Faculty review of your journal (with comments), and periodic study and review of it by you, will enable you to identify your progress and growth. Journal writing involves you in the process of learning. It encourages you to use abstract thinking and to conceptualize, elaborate, generalize, and interpret, all of which promote critical thinking. When you write a term paper, you are not only involved in the process of writing but in the development of a product. When this product is reviewed by the instructor, conclusions can be drawn regarding your command of the information and your ability to convey your knowledge to others. Written assignments require organizing, prioritizing, integrating, persuading, proving, and summarizing, which all require critical thinking.

COMPUTER-ASSISTED LEARNING   Computers provide an environment that enhances and challenges critical-thinking skills. Software offers a variety of critical-thinking programs from a simple lesson presenting content using an interactive linear approach to programs in which the learner is challenged to seek solutions to complex problems following a branching design. Computers allow for thinking and learning in a nonthreatening and safe environment. Refer to Chapter 8, Computer Applications in Education and Evaluation, for more details regarding the valuable use of computers to increase learning.

VIDEOTAPING   Videotaping can be used to record role-playing scenarios or the performance of a skill. Videotaping allows you to engage in an activity and then be able to review your performance. During this review, you as well as others can examine, analyze, rationalize, justify, and correct your performance, which can support critical thinking.

CLINICAL PROCESS RECORDS   A clinical process record is a focused writing assignment, similar to a case study, that centers on a simulated or specific patient experience. It requires you to use the problem-solving process, examine the scientific reasons for health care interventions, assess outcomes, and evaluate and modify the plan of care, which all contribute to critical thinking.

EXAMINATIONS   Examinations must be approached as learning opportunities. All examinations should be thoughtfully reviewed. Small groups of four or five students should review and discuss each question. Group members help each other to recognize the key concepts being tested and how to best answer the questions "What is happening?" and "What should I do?" When reviewing examination questions, be willing to listen to other people's interpretation of the question. If all of your energy is spent defending your response, your mind is not open to different perspectives, which limits your learning. Reviewing examinations requires you to integrate information, apply theory and principles, analyze content, compare and contrast information, and rationalize your response, which all contribute to critical thinking.

APPLY CRITICAL THINKING TO MULTIPLE-CHOICE QUESTIONS

To develop critical thinking skills when practicing multiple-choice questions, examine, reframe, critique, and evaluate the stem of each question. Then try to construct the correct answer before looking at the options. When assessing the options in a multiple-choice question, manipulate the information by cognitive activities such as organizing, correlating, differentiating, reasoning, and evaluating against standards of practice, criteria, and critical elements. When reviewing test questions, study the rationales offered as to why the correct answers are correct and the rationales as to why the wrong answers are wrong. See if you can identify other situations in which the same principle would apply and situations in which it would be different. A great way to explore additional situations using multiple-choice questions is to change one of the key facts in the stem of a question or eliminate or change one of the distractors to alter the focus of the question. When the context of the problem is altered even slightly, the contour or territory around it changes, which may significantly rearrange the internal structure of the entire question. When a question is altered, the meaning of the situation may require a distinctly different nursing assessment or action.

Another critical thinking study technique using multiple-choice questions is to explore not only the rationales for the options, but the consequences of each nursing action presented in the alternatives. You can ask many different questions: "Is the action safe or unsafe?" "Is the statement true or false?" "Is it fact or inference?" "Why is it wrong?" and "How can I make it into a correct answer?" This is particularly effective when conducted in a study group because different people bring different perspectives and thinking styles to the sharing that enrich the learning experience. More perspectives produce a variety of contextualizations of the problem and generate more approaches to selecting the most accurate response.

> *Where all think alike, no one thinks very much.*
> WALTER LIPPMANN

In addition, studying in groups contributes to building a body of knowledge that increases your perspective and context when you are faced with seeking a solution to a highly discriminating multiple-choice question.

Highly discriminating questions are questions that are answered correctly by the test-taker who scored in the top percent of the class versus the test-taker who answered the question incorrectly and scored in a lower percent of the class on the same examination. It is believed that the student who answers a highly discriminating question correctly is generally responding to subtle cues based on more highly developed critical-thinking skills. However, students who come to the testing situation with an in-depth perspective sometimes will "read into" the question because of the "context" they bring to the test item. It is often frustrating for students who are sophisticated, deep thinkers to accept lost points on an examination because they "read into" the question or "knew too much." Analyze questions you answer incorrectly and determine why by asking questions such as: "Did I add information to the stem?" "Did I have difficulty deciding among the options presented because I would have done something completely different?" "Did I delete an option because my experience was different from the patient situation presented?" "Did I view the question in light of a more sophisticated level of curricular content than that being tested?" "Did I view the patient scenario in more depth and breadth than was necessary?" Multiple-choice questions provide all the data necessary to permit you to answer the question. Your job is to use critical thinking to answer the question, not rewrite the question.

Case (1994) explored the concept of critical thinking as a journey, not a destination. Case stated, "We cannot stand in the same river twice, because water rushes away as new water takes its place and the rushing water changes the river bed. The decisions we make today may not fit circumstances that change tomorrow." This concept applies not only to clinical situations but to answering multiple-choice questions. Each question scenario is different and requires that the test-taker use critical-thinking skills to identify the key concept being tested and to answer the questions "What is happening?" and "What should I do?" Examine the following question using critical-thinking skills.

SAMPLE ITEM 2–1

A patient has just returned from the operating room with a retention (Foley) catheter, an IV, and an oral airway, and is still unresponsive. Which assessment should be made first?

(1) Check the surgical dressing to ensure that it is intact.

(2) Confirm the placement of the oral airway.

(3) Examine the IV site for infiltration.

(4) Observe the Foley for drainage.

First you need to identify the key concept being tested in the question. The key concept in this question is that the **postoperative care of the unresponsive patient takes priority.** The key words in the question that asks "What is happening?" are **postoperative patient, oral airway, and unresponsive.** The key words in the question that asks "What should I do?" are **assessment** and **should be made first.** The question being asked is: **What assessment takes priority when caring for an unresponsive postoperative patient with an oral airway?** Although the IV, the retention catheter, and surgical dressing are important and must be assessed, it is ensuring the correct placement of the oral airway that takes priority. To answer this question you need to know:

- The normal anatomy and physiology associated with the respiratory system and the body's essential need for a continuous exchange of oxygen and carbon dioxide
- That a patent airway is essential to the exchange of oxygen and carbon dioxide
- The ABCs of life support, which refer to Airway, Breathing, and Circulation, and make the connection that maintaining an airway takes priority
- That a common response to anesthesia is lack of a gag reflex
- That a correctly placed oral airway will contribute to maintaining an open airway

Rationales for Sample Item 2–1

An asterisk (*) is in front of the rationale that explains the correct answer.

2–1   ① Although this is important, it is not life threatening.

    *② Confirming the placement of the oral airway ensures a patent air passage. An oral airway displaces the tongue and prevents obstruction of the trachea, permitting free passage of air to and from the lungs. Oxygen is essential for life, and this action takes priority

    ③ Although this is important, an infiltration can be tolerated for a few minutes while higher-priority assessments are made.

    ④ Although this is important, urinary output at this time is less critical than assessing airway, breathing, and circulation.

To answer this question you need to use critical-thinking skills to identify the cue data that establish the uniqueness of the situation being presented in the question, the key concept being tested in the question, and what nursing action takes priority. Maintaining a patent airway always takes priority.

18 ## Conclusions

With our informational society, there is no way you can know or experience everything. With the explosion of knowledge and technology and changes in the role of the nurse within a fluid health care delivery environment, what is learned today may be obsolete tomorrow. Consequently, an integral part of your continuing education is the development and refinement of critical-thinking skills. To be a critical thinker you must be intellectually humble, able to listen, dissatisfied with the status quo, creative, flexible, self-confident but aware of your limitations, and willing to change. Take time to cultivate your critical-thinking skills because they will be the ultimate tool you bring to patient care situations—the therapeutic use of self. When you can think critically, you are empowered to maximize your abilities to meet patient needs.

Bibliography

Adams, AK: The Home Book of Humorous Quotations. New York, Dodd, Mead & Company, 1969.

Alfaro-LeFevre, R: Critical Thinking in Nursing: A Practical Approach. Philadelphia, W. B. Saunders Company, 1995.

American Philosophical Association: Critical Thinking: A Statement of Expert Consensus for Purposes of Educational Assessment and Instruction. The Delphi Report: Research Findings and Recommendations Prepared for the Committee on Pre-College Philosophy. (ERIC Document Reproduction Service No. ED 315-423), 1990.

Bowers, B, and McCarthy, D: Developing analytic thinking skills in early undergraduate education. J Nurs Educ 32:107–113, 1993.

Brookfield, DD: Developing Critical Thinkers. San Francisco, Jossey-Bass, 1987.

Case, B: Walking around the elephant: A critical-thinking strategy for decision making. The Journal of Continuing Education in Nursing 25:101–109, 1994.

Chaffee, J: Thinking Critically, ed. 3. Boston, Houghton Mifflin, 1990.

Kataoka-Yahiro, M, and Saylor, C: A critical thinking model for nursing judgment. J Nurs Educ 33:351–356, 1994.

Loving, GL: Competence validation and cognitive flexibility: A theoretical model grounded in nursing education. J Nurs Educ 32:415–421, 1993.

Paul, RW, and Heaslip, PH: Critical thinking and intuitive nursing practice. J Adv Nurs 22:40–47, 1995.

Pless, BS: Clarifying the concept of critical thinking in nursing. J Nurs Educ 32:425–428, 1993.

Pond, EE, and Bradshaw, MJ: Teaching strategies for critical thinking. Nurse Educator 15:18–22, 1991.

Safire, W, and Safir, L: Good Advice. New York, Times Books, 1982.

Snyder, M: Critical thinking: A foundation for consumer-focused care. The Journal of Continuing Education in Nursing 24:206–210, 1993.

Stevenson, B: The Home Book of Questions Classical and Modern, ed 10. New York, Dodd, Mead, & Company, 1967.

Taggart, W, and Torrance, PE: Administrator's Manual for the Human Information Processing and Survey. Bensenville, IL, Scholastic Testing Service, 1984.

Study Techniques

3

Learning is the activity by which knowledge, attitudes, and/or skills are acquired. Learning is a complex activity that is influenced by various factors such as genetic endowment, level of maturation, experiental background, effectiveness of formal instruction, self-image, readiness to learn, level of motivation, and extent of self-study. Although some of these factors are unchangeable, others you can control.

Learning is an active process that takes place within the learner. Therefore, the role of the learner is to participate in or initiate activities that promote learning. Like test taking, learning is a learned skill. This chapter presents both general and specific study techniques that should increase your ability to learn. The general study techniques presented include skills that facilitate learning regardless of the topic being studied. The specific study techniques are presented in relation to levels of thinking processes that are required to answer multiple-choice questions in nursing: knowledge, comprehension, application, and analysis. Use of these techniques when studying will help you to comprehend more of what you have studied and retain the information for a longer period of time. This information should increase your success in answering multiple-choice questions.

General Study Techniques

ESTABLISH A ROUTINE

Set aside a regular time to study. Learning requires consistency, repetition, and practice. Deciding to sit down to study is the most difficult part of studying. We tend to procrastinate and think of a variety of things we must do instead of studying. By committing yourself to a regular routine, you eliminate the repetitive need to make the decision to study. If you decide that every night from 7:00 PM to 8:30 PM you are going to study, you are using your internal locus of control and establishing an internal readiness to learn. You must be motivated in order to learn.

Your study schedule must be reasonable and realistic. Shorter, more frequent study periods are more effective than long study periods. For most people, 1- to 3-hour study periods with a 10-minute break each hour are most effective. Periods of learning must be balanced with adequate rest periods because energy and endurance decrease over time and limit learning efficiency. Physical and emotional rest make you more alert and receptive to new information.

When planning a schedule, involve significant family members in the decision making. Because a family is an open system, the action of one family member will influence the other family members. If they are involved in the decision making, they will have a vested interest and probably be more supportive of your need to study.

SET SHORT- AND LONG-TERM GOALS

A goal is an outcome that a person attempts to attain, and it may be long term or short term. A long-term goal is the eventual desired outcome. A short-term goal is a desired outcome that can be achieved along the path leading to the long-term goal. In other words, a long-term goal is your destination, whereas each short-term goal is an objective that must be attained to help you eventually reach your destination. Each long-term goal may have one or more short-term goals. Goals should be formulated to promote learning that is purposeful, to serve as guides for planning action, and to establish standards so that learning can be evaluated. Goals must be specific, measurable, and realistic, and must have a time frame. A specific goal states exactly what is to be accomplished. A measurable goal sets a minimum acceptable level of performance. A realistic goal must be potentially achievable. A goal with a time frame states the time parameters in which the goal will be achieved.

A typical long-term goal would be to correctly answer 90 percent of the study questions at the end of Chapter 1 in a fundamentals of nursing textbook within 7 hours. Typical short-term goals might be to read and highlight important information in Chapter 1 within 2 hours, to list the principles presented in Chapter 1 within 1 hour, and to compare and contrast information in your class notes with information in the textbook within 2 hours. Each of these short-term goals can be achieved as a step toward attaining the long-term goal. It is wise to break a big task into small manageable tasks because it is easier to learn small bits of information than large blocks of information. The most effective learning is goal-directed learning because it is planned learning with a purpose. In addition, when goals are attained, they increase self-esteem and motivation.

SIMULATE A SCHOOL ENVIRONMENT

The familiar is generally less stressful than the unfamiliar. Therefore, your posture, surroundings, and equipment should be similar to those in the school or testing environment. Study at a desk or table and chair. Avoid the temptation to study in a reclining chair, on the couch, or in bed. If you are too comfortable, you may become too relaxed or even fall asleep. Gather all the necessary equipment for studying, such as your textbook, class notes, paper, pens, a highlighter, a dictionary, and so on. Use the same tools you plan to use when you take your examinations. Control other factors that reflect the testing environment such as ensuring adequate light and avoiding eating while you are studying. The study environment should be comfortable enough to promote learning while strict enough to keep you alert and focused.

CONTROL INTERNAL AND EXTERNAL DISTRACTORS

Stimuli, both internal and external, must be controlled to eliminate distractions. External stimuli are environmental happenings that interrupt your thinking and should be limited. Select a place to study where you will not be interrupted by family members, phone calls, the doorbell, or family pets. Do not study while watching television or listening to the radio. These stimuli compete for your attention when you need to be focusing on your work. Internal stimuli are your inner thoughts, feelings, or concerns that interfere with your ability to study. Internal stimuli are often more difficult to control than external stimuli because they involve attitudes. Review the techniques in Chapter 1 that promote a positive mental attitude. By limiting or eliminating internal and external distractors, you should improve your ability to concentrate.

PREPARE FOR CLASS

To prepare adequately for class, you need to know the content that will be addressed. Look at the course outline or ask your instructor. "If you don't know where you're going, you can't get there!" Once you know the topic, identify the appropriate content in your textbook. To pre-**pare** for class you must **pare** down the written information in your textbook. To **pare** means to cut, clip, shave, or whittle away. When reviewing textbook material before class, it is not always necessary to read every word. First, read the chapter headings. This will give you an overview of the topic presented. Second, look at tables and figures and read their captions. These provide visual cues. Third, skim the chapter content but read information that is CAPITALIZED, **boldfaced,** or *italicized*. These formats indicate important information; use a highlighting marker to accentuate these and other meaningful content. Fourth, list the questions you may want to ask in class. You are now minimally prepared for class. Finally, to be well prepared, read the chapter thoroughly to gain an in-depth understanding of the content.

TAKE CLASS NOTES

Taking notes in class is critical. Class notes are valuable because they provide you with a blueprint for study when preparing for an examination. The following are note-taking tips.

- **Stay focused on the topic being presented.** Generally, instructors present material that they believe is important. Compare this information to the material you highlighted in your textbook.

- **Use your notebook creatively.** Open your notebook so that you have facing sheets. Use the page on the left side for class notes. Save the page on the right side for adding information from the textbook or other sources that clarify the class notes.

- **Use an outline format and abbreviations.** There is no way that you can write down every word that comes out of your instructor's mouth. Focus on concepts because you can expand on the content later. For example, if an instructor is talking about abnormal respiratory rates such as apnea, bradypnea, and tachypnea, write these words down and listen to the instructor's presentation. The definitions can be added at a later time to the page on the right side of your notebook.

- **Ask questions to clarify information.** Your goal is not to be a stenographer. Your goal is to understand the information. Ask questions that you have prepared before class or that you may have as a result of the discussion in class. If you have a question, there are probably other students who have the same question. Have the courage to ask questions. Some of the roles of the instructor are to make the information more understandable and clarify misconceptions. Your tuition pays the instructor's salary, so get your money's worth!

- **Review your notes after class.** You should review your notes within 48 hours after class. Reviewing, reorganizing, and rewriting class note are techniques of reinforcement. Repetition helps commit information to memory. Some instructors allow you to use a tape recorder in class. Reviewing class tapes is particularly helpful to students who are auditory learners, those who have difficulty grasping complex material the first time, and those for whom English is a second language.

IDENTIFY LEARNING DOMAINS

How we learn is never identical for two different people, nor is it identical for one person in different situations. Over the years you have developed a learning style with which you feel comfortable and that has proved successful. It is in your best interest, however, to be open to a variety of learning approaches.

Learning is the process by which you attain new information (cognitive domain), acquire new physical skills (psychomotor domain), or form new attitudes (affective domain).

Cognitive Domain

New information is usually learned through symbols such as words or pictures. We read them, see them, or hear them. Use all your senses to acquire new information. The more routes information takes to travel to your brain, the greater are the chances that you will learn the information. For example, when reading information about positioning patients, learning is reinforced by viewing pictures of patients in the various positions.

Psychomotor Domain

New skills involve the physical application of information. It is possible for a person to understand all the goals and steps of a procedure and yet not be able to perform the procedure. For information to get from the head to the hands, the learner must do more than read a book, look at pictures, view a video, or watch other people. The learner must become actively involved. Physical skills are not learned by osmosis or diffusion; they are learned by doing. For example, when learning how to change a sterile dressing, the learner can read a book and look at a video, but it is essential that the learner actually practice changing a sterile dressing.

Affective Domain

Learning new attitudes represents an increasing internalization of or commitment to a feeling, belief, or value. This is the most difficult type of learning because attitudes result from lifelong experiences and tend to be well entrenched. For example, a student may know and understand the theory concerning why a person should be nonjudgmental and yet in clinical situations be judgmental toward the patient. The development of new attitudes is best learned in an atmosphere of acceptance by exploring feelings, becoming involved in group discussions, and observing appropriate role models. For example, before providing physical hygiene for a patient for the first time, it is beneficial to explore feelings about invading a patient's personal space.

CAPTURE MOMENTS OF TIME

Using your spare moments for reviewing information is a method of maximizing your time for constructive study. We all have periods during the day that are less productive than others, such as waiting at a red light or standing in line at a store. Also, there are times when you engage in repetitive tasks such as vacuuming a rug or raking the leaves. Capture these moments of time and use them to study. Carry flash cards, a vocabulary list, or categories of information that you can review when you have unexpected time. These captured moments should be in addition to, rather than a replacement for, your regularly scheduled study periods. There is an old saying that "**Time is on your side.**" Capture spare moments of time and use them to your advantage.

USE APPROPRIATE RESOURCES

The theories and principles of nursing practice are complex. They draw from a variety of disciplines (psychology, sociology, anatomy and physiology, microbiology, and so on), use new terminology, and require unique applications to clinical practice. When you study, you will find that your learning will not proceed in a straight line, moving progressively forward. You may experience plateaus, remissions, and/or periods of confusion when dealing with complex material. When your forward progress is slowed, identify your needs and immediately seek help. Your instructor, another student, a study group, or a tutor may be beneficial. When studying with another student, make sure that the person is a source of correct information. When studying in groups, three to five students are ideal because a group of more than five people becomes a "party." The group should be heterogeneous; that is, there should be a variety of academic abilities, attitudes, skills, and perspectives among the members. This variety should enrich the learning experience and provide checks and balances for the sharing of correct information. Remember, you learn not only from the instructor but also from yourself and your classmates.

Generally, people do not like to admit that they have learning difficulties because they think it makes them look inadequate in the eyes of others. For this reason, people may be embarrassed to ask for help. This can be self-destructive because it denies people the opportunity to use resources that support growth. Be careful that you do not fall into this trap! To obtain access to the appropriate resources, you must be willing to be open to yourself and others. Resources (e.g., extra help sessions; computer labs; reading, writing, and math centers; psychological counseling; and availability of faculty during office hours) are there to be used. Have the courage to acknowledge to yourself and others that you need help. Seeking help is a sign of maturity rather than a sign of weakness. When you ask for help, you are in control because you are solving problems in order to meet your own needs.

BALANCE SACRIFICES AND REWARDS

When you decided to enter nursing school, no one promised you a rose garden. Your commitment to become a nurse requires sacrifice. Your time and energy are being diverted from your usual activities related to a job, family members, friends, and pleasurable pastimes. Rigorous activity, whether physical or mental, requires concentration and endurance. However, too much work hinders productivity. You must establish a balance between energy expenditure and rewards for your efforts. Rewards can be internal or external. Internal rewards are stimulated from within the learner and relate to feelings associated with meaningful achievement. Learning something new, achieving a goal, or increasing self-respect are examples of internal rewards. External rewards arise from outside the learner. A grade of 100 percent, respect and appreciation from others, or a present for achieving a goal are examples of external rewards.

Unfortunately, the rewards for studying are usually not immediate but in the extended future. Graduating from nursing school, passing the NCLEX-RN, earning a paycheck, and enjoying the prestige of being a nurse are future-oriented rewards. Therefore, you should be the one to provide immediate rewards for yourself for studying. During study breaks or at the completion of studying, reward yourself by thinking about how much you have learned, reflecting on the good feelings you have about your accomplishments, relaxing with a significant other, having a cup of coffee, watching a favorite television show, calling a friend on the telephone, or taking a weekend off. Short-term rewards promote a positive mental attitude, reinforce motivation, and provide a respite from studying.

SET REALISTIC DEMANDS ON TIME AND ENERGY

Your course of study to become a nurse is demanding and will take much of your time and energy. Generally, you should study 1 to 2 hours a week for every hour you are in class. For example, if you are in school 12 hours a week, you should be studying 12 to 24 hours a week. To be successful, school should be viewed as a full-time job! If you work several days a week, manage a home with several children, or are involved in community activities, the demands on your time and energy may be excessive. This may not be the time to go to school. Only you can decide what you are capable of doing. To manage your time and responsibilities efficiently and fairly, you may have to make difficult decisions. Reducing work hours, sharing household chores, hiring a babysitter, or limiting your social life may be necessary strategies to help you manage study time. Sacrifices in and of themselves should not be viewed negatively. Often these sacrifices promote growth in the student and family. Involve your family in your decisions.

Specific Study Techniques

COGNITIVE LEVELS OF NURSING QUESTIONS

The nurse uses a variety of thinking processes when caring for patients. Therefore, nursing examinations must reflect these thinking processes to effectively evaluate the safe practice of nursing. There are four types of thinking processes that are incorporated into multiple-choice questions concerning the delivery of nursing care: **knowledge, comprehension, application, and analysis.** These thinking processes are within the cognitive domain and are ordered according to complexity. That is, a knowledge question requires the lowest level of thinking (recalling information), whereas an analysis question requires the highest level of thinking (comparing and contrasting information).

In this section of the book each cognitive level (knowledge, comprehension, application, or analysis) is discussed and sample items are presented to illustrate the thinking processes involved in answering the item. In addition, specific study techniques are presented to help you to strengthen your thinking abilities.

The correct answers for the sample items in this chapter and the rationales for all the options are at the end of this chapter.

KNOWLEDGE QUESTIONS

Knowledge questions require you to **recall** or **remember** information. To answer a knowledge question, you need to commit facts to memory. Knowledge questions expect you to know terminology, specific facts, trends, sequences, classifications, categories, criteria, structures, principles, generalizations, or theories. This basic information is necessary before you can think critically.

SAMPLE ITEM 3–1

When you are administering medications, *qid* means:

(1) Once a day

(2) Twice a day

(3) Three times a day

(4) Four times a day

To correctly answer this question, you have to know the meaning of the abbreviation *qid*.

SAMPLE ITEM 3–2

The first step of the procedure for making an unoccupied bed is:

(1) Pulling the curtain

(2) Washing your hands

(3) Collecting the clean linen

(4) Placing the bottom sheet

To correctly answer this question, you need to know the sequence of steps in the procedure of making an unoccupied bed or the basic principle that your hands must be washed before all procedures.

SAMPLE ITEM 3–3

What is the normal range of a radial pulse in an adult?

(1) 50 to 65

(2) 70 to 85

(3) 90 to 105

(4) 110 to 125

To answer this question correctly, you have to know the normal range of a radial pulse for an adult.

Memorization/Repetition

Knowledge questions require you to remember information that forms the foundation of nursing practice. Initially, information can be learned by memorization. Memorization is committing information to the brain through repetition for recall at a later time. Repeatedly studying information by reciting it out loud, reviewing it in your mind, or writing it down increases your chances of remembering the information because a variety of senses are used. Memorization can be facilitated by using lists of related facts, flash cards, or learning wheels. For example:

- On an index card you can list the steps of a procedure. This can be carried with you to study when you capture moments of time.

- On the front of an index card you can write a word and on the back define the word. An entire deck of cards can be developed for the terminology within a unit of study. Again, use the flash cards when you have unexpected time to study.

- To make a learning wheel, cut a piece of cardboard into a circle and draw pie-shaped wedges on the front and back. On a front wedge write a unit of measure, such as 30 ml, and on the corresponding back wedge write its conversion to another unit of measure, such as 1 ounce. Then, on individual spring clothespins, write each of the units of measure that appear on the back of the wheel. When you want to study approximate equivalents, mix up the clothespins and attempt to match each one of its corresponding unit of measure. You can turn the wheel over and evaluate your success by determining if the clothespin you attached to the wheel matches the unit of measure on the back of the wheel.

These memorization techniques reinforce learning by the use of repetition, but the information is learned by rote memorization without any in-depth understanding of the information learned. Information learned by repetition uses short-term memory and is generally quickly forgotten unless reinforced through additional study techniques or application in your nursing practice.

Alphabet Cues

The memorization of information can be facilitated if the information is associated with letters of the alphabet. Each letter serves as a cue that stimulates the recall of information. The most effective alphabet cues are those you make up yourself. They meet a self-identified need, and you must review the information before you can design the alphabet cue. You can use any combination of letters as long as they have meaning for you and your learning. Examples of alphabet cues include:

- The **ABCs** of cardiopulmonary resuscitation are: **Airway**—clear the airway; **Breathing**—initiate artificial breathing: **Circulation**—initiate cardiac compression.
- Identify patients at high risk for injury through the letters **A, B, C, D, E, F, G: Age**—the young and very old; **Blindness**—lack of visual perception; **Consciousness**—decreased level of consciousness; **Deafness**—lack of auditory perception; **Emotional state**—reduced perceptual awareness; **Frequency of accidents**—previous history of accidents; and **Gait**—impaired mobility.
- The **Three P's** for the cardinal signs of diabetes mellitus are: **Polyuria, Polydipsia,** and **Polyphagia.**

Acronyms

An acronym is a word formed from the first letters of a series of statements or facts. Each part of the acronym relates to the information it represents. It is useful to learning because each letter of the word jolts the memory to recall information. An acronym is a technique used to retrieve previously learned information. Examples of acronyms include the following:

- The American Cancer Society teaches the early warning signs of cancer through the acronym of **CAUTION.**

  Change in bowel and bladder habits

  A sore that does not heal

  Unusual bleeding or discharge

  Thickening or a lump

  Indigestion or difficulty in swallowing

  Obvious change in a wart or mole

  Nagging cough or hoarseness

- When assessing a patient for adaptations indicating the presence of infection, remember the acronym **INFECT.**

  Increased pulse and respirations

  Nodes are enlarged

  Function is impaired

  Erythema, edema, exudate

  Complaints of discomfort or pain

  Temperature—local and/or systemic

Acrostics

An acrostic is a phrase, motto, or verse in which a letter of each word (usually the first letter) prompts the memory to retrieve information. A variation of an acrostic is a sentence with content that jogs the memory. Memorizing information can be difficult and boring. This technique is a creative way to make learning more effective and fun. Examples of acrostics include:

- When studying the fat-soluble vitamins, recall this motto, "**All** **D**ieters **E**at **K**ilocalories." This should help you remember that **A, D, E,** and **K** are the fat-soluble vitamins.
- When studying apothecary and metric equivalents, remember this verse. "There are **15 grains** of sugar in **1 graham (gram)** cracker." This sentence should help you remember that **15 grains** are equivalent to **1 gram.**

COMPREHENSION QUESTIONS

Comprehension questions require you to **understand** information. To answer a comprehension question, you must commit facts to memory as well as translate, interpret, and determine the implications of that information. You demonstrate understanding when you translate or paraphrase information, interpret or summarize information, or determine the implications, consequences, corollaries, or effects of information. Comprehension questions expect you not only to know but also to understand the information being tested. Once you understand basic information, you can recognize the significance of data, an initial step in critical thinking.

SAMPLE ITEM 3–4

To evaluate the therapeutic effect of a cathartic, the nurse should assess the patient for:

    (1) Increased urinary output

    (2) A decrease in anxiety

    (3) A bowel movement

    (4) Pain relief

To answer this question, you have to know not only that a cathartic is a potent laxative that stimulates the bowel but also that the increase in peristalsis will result in a bowel movement.

SAMPLE ITEM 3–5

When clarifying is used as a therapeutic communication tool, the nurse is:

    (1) Summarizing the patient's communication

    (2) Verifying what is implied by the patient

    (3) Restating what the patient has said

    (4) Paraphrasing the patient's message

To answer this question, you not only have to know that clarifying is a therapeutic tool that promotes communication between the patient and nurse, but you must also explain why or how this technique facilitates communication.

SAMPLE ITEM 3–6

After administering an intramuscular injection, the nurse should massage the needle insertion site to:

    (1) Limit infection

    (2) Prevent bleeding

(3) Reduce discomfort

(4) Promote absorption

To answer this question, you not only have to know that massage is one step of the procedure for an intramuscular injection, but you must also understand the consequence of massaging the needle insertion site once the needle is withdrawn.

Explore "Whys" and "Hows"

The difference between knowledge questions and comprehension questions is: to answer knowledge questions, you must know facts; to answer comprehension questions, you must understand the significance of facts. Facts can be understood and retained longer if they are relevant and meaningful to the learner. When studying information, ask yourself why or how the information is important. For example, when learning that immobility causes pressure ulcers, explore *why* they occur. Pressure compresses the capillary beds, which interferes with the transport of oxygen and nutrients to tissues, resulting in ischemia and necrosis. When studying a skill such as bathing, explore how soap cleans the skin. Soap reduces the surface tension of water and helps remove accumulated oils, perspiration, dead cells, and microorganisms. If you interpret information and identify **why** or **how** the information gained is relevant and useful, then the information has value. When information increases in value, it also increases in significance and is less readily forgotten.

Study in Small Groups

Once you have studied by yourself, it is usually valuable to study the same information with another person or in a small group. The sharing process promotes your comprehension of information because you listen to the impressions and opinions of others, learn new information from a peer tutor, and reinforce your own learning by teaching others. In addition, the members of the group reinforce your interpretation of information and correct your misunderstanding of information. The value of group work is in the exchange process. Group members must listen, share, evaluate, help, support, reinforce, discuss, and debate to promote learning. There is truth in the saying **"One hand washes the other."** Not only do you help the other person when you study together, but you also help yourself.

APPLICATION QUESTIONS

The application of information demonstrates a higher level of understanding than just knowing or comprehending information because it requires the learner to **show, solve, modify, change, use,** or **manipulate** information in a real situation or presented scenario. To answer an application question, you must apply concepts you learned previously to concrete situations. The concepts may be theories, technical principles, rules of procedures, generalizations, or ideas that have to be applied in a presented scenario. Application questions test your ability to use information in a new situation. The making of rational and reflective judgments, which are part of the critical-thinking process, results in a course of action.

SAMPLE ITEM 3-7

An elderly patient's skin looks dry, thin, and fragile. When providing back care, the nurse should:

(1) Apply a moisturizing body lotion

(2) Wash the back with soap and water

(3) Massage using short, kneading strokes

(4) Leave excess lubricant on the patient's skin

To answer this question, you must know that dry, thin, fragile skin is common in elderly people and that moisturizing lotion helps the skin to retain water and become more supple. When presented with this patient scenario, you have to apply your knowledge concerning developmental changes in elderly persons and the consequences of the use of moisturizing lotion.

SAMPLE ITEM 3–8

When caring for several patients on bladder-retraining programs, the nurse should recognize that an intervention that is always implemented during a bladder-retraining program is toileting:

(1) Every 2 hours when awake

(2) At 8 AM, 2 PM, 8 PM, and 2 AM

(3) Every 4 hours and through the night

(4) When the patient goes to bed at night

To answer this question, you have to understand the principle that nursing care should be individualized. You also must understand the commonalities within the procedure of bladder retraining. When presented with this concrete situation, you have to apply your knowledge about patient-centered care and the theoretical components of bladder-retraining programs.

SAMPLE ITEM 3–9

To prevent self-injury when lifting a heavy patient higher in bed, the nurse should:

(1) Keep the knees and ankles straight

(2) Straighten the knees and bend at the waist

(3) Place the feet together with the knees bent

(4) Position the feet apart with one placed forward

To answer this question, you have to understand the principles of body mechanics. You also need to apply these principles in a particular patient care situation, moving a heavy patient higher in bed.

Relate New Information to Prior Learning

Learning is easier when the information to be learned is associated with what you already know. Therefore, relate new information to your foundation of knowledge, experience, attitudes, and feelings. For example, when studying the principles of body mechanics, review which principles are used when you carry a heavy package, move from a reclining to a standing position, or assist an elderly person to walk up a flight of stairs. When studying the principles of surgical asepsis, recall and review the various situations when you performed sterile technique and identify the principles that were the foundation of your actions. Applying concepts, such as principles and theories, in concrete situations reinforces your ability to use them in future circumstances.

30 Recognize Commonalities

To facilitate learning to apply information, identify commonalities when studying principles and theories that can be used in a variety of situations. A commonality exists when two different situations require the application of the same or similar principle. For example, when studying the principle of gravity, you must understand that it is the force that draws all mass in the earth's sphere toward the center of the earth. Now try to identify situations that employ this principle. As a nurse, you apply this principle when you place a urine collection bag below the level of the bladder, hang an intravenous bag higher than the needle insertion site, raise the head of the bed for a patient with dyspnea, and raise the foot of the bed for a patient with edema of the feet. This study technique is particularly effective when working in small groups because it involves brainstorming. Others in the group may identify situations that you would not consider. Recognizing commonalities reinforces information and maximizes the application of information in patient care situations.

ANALYSIS QUESTIONS

Analysis questions require you to **interpret a variety of data** and **recognize the commonalities, differences,** and **interrelationships among presented ideas.** Analysis questions make the assumption that you know, understand, and can apply information. Now you must identify, examine, dissect, evaluate, or investigate the organization, systematic arrangement, or structure of the information presented in the question. This type of question tests your analytical ability and requires higher-level critical-thinking processes.

SAMPLE ITEM 3–10

A patient has dependent edema of the ankles and feet and is obese. Which diet should the nurse expect the physician to order?

(1) Low in salt and high in fat
(2) Low in salt and low in calories
(3) High in salt and high in protein
(4) High in salt and low in carbohydrates

To answer this question, you have to understand the relationships between salt in the diet and fluid retention, and between obesity and caloric intake. You must also understand the impact of carbohydrates, proteins, and fats in a diet for a patient with edema and obesity. When you answer this question, you must understand and examine the information presented, identify the interrelationships among the elements, and arrive at a conclusion.

SAMPLE ITEM 3–11

A patient who is undergoing cancer chemotherapy says to the nurse, "This is no way to live." Which response uses reflective technique?

(1) "Tell me more about what you are thinking."
(2) "You sound discouraged today."
(3) "Life is not worth living?"
(4) "What are you saying?"

To answer this question, you must understand the communication techniques of reflection, clarification, and paraphrasing. You also must analyze statements and identify the use of these techniques in presented conversations. This question requires you to understand, interpret, and differentiate information.

The physician orders 500 mg of an antibiotic to be administered via an intramuscular injection. A 1-gram vial of the medication, which needs to be reconstituted, carries the statement: Add 2.7 mL of solution to yield 3 mL. How much solution should the nurse administer?

(1) 0.5 mL

(2) 1 mL

(3) 1.5 mL

(4) 2 mL

To answer this question, you must understand the relationship of milligrams to grams (1000 mg = 1 gram; therefore, 500 mg = 0.5 gram) and use a formula for ratio and proportion. This question requires you to identify the various components of the problem, select the appropriate formula required to solve the problem, place the correct elements within the formula, and then do the mathematical calculation to arrive at the answer.

Recognize Differences

Analysis questions require an ability to examine information, which is a higher thought process than knowing, understanding, or applying information. For example, when studying blood pressure, you first memorize the parameters of a normal blood pressure (knowledge). Then you develop an understanding of what factors influence and produce a normal blood pressure (comprehension). Then you identify a particular patient situation that would necessitate obtaining a blood pressure (application). Finally, you must differentiate among a variety of situations and determine which has the highest priority for assessing the blood pressure (analysis). Analysis questions are difficult because they demand scrutiny of a variety of complex data presented in the stem and options.

To study for complex questions, you cannot just memorize and understand facts or recognize the commonalities among facts; you must learn to discriminate. Analysis questions often require you to use differentiation to determine the significance of information. When studying the causes of an elevated blood pressure, identify the different causes and why they would result in an increased blood pressure. For example, a blood pressure can rise for a variety of reasons: infection causes an increased metabolic rate; fluid retention causes hypervolemia; anxiety causes an autonomic nervous system response that constricts blood vessels. In each situation the blood pressure increases but for a different reason. Recognizing differences is an effective study technique to broaden the interrelationship and significance of learned information.

Practice Test Taking

Taking practice tests is an excellent way to improve the effectiveness of your learning. Reviewing rationales for the right and wrong answers serves as an effective study technique. It reinforces learning, and it can help you identify areas that require additional study.

As you practice test taking, not only do you increase your knowledge but you also become more emotionally and physically comfortable in the testing situation and better at selecting the correct option when answering a multiple-choice question. It is most effective if you gradually increase the time you spend taking practice tests to 2 to 3 hours. This will help build stamina, enabling you to concentrate more effectively during a shorter test. Marathon runners have long recognized the value of building stamina and the need for practice to achieve a "groove" that enhances performance. Marathon runners also manage their practice so that they "peak" on the day of the big event. The same principles can be applied to the nursing student preparing for an important test. You are at your peak and can achieve a groove when you feel physically, emotionally, and intellectually ready for the important test.

Practicing test taking should assist you to learn by:

- Acquiring new knowledge
- Comprehending information
- Understanding concepts
- Identifying rationales for nursing interventions
- Applying theories and principles
- Identifying commonalities and differences in situations
- Analyzing information
- Reinforcing previous learning
- Applying critical thinking

In addition, practicing test taking should assist you to:

- Use test-taking techniques
- Effectively manage time during a test
- Control your environment
- Control physical and emotional responses
- Feel empowered and in control
- Develop a positive mental attitude

Answers and Rationales for Sample Items in Chapter 3

An asterisk (*) is in front of the rationale that explains the correct answer.

3–1 ① The abbreviation for once a day is qd. (L. *quaque die*).
② The abbreviation for twice a day is bid. (L. *bis in die*).
③ The abbreviation for three times a day is tid. (L. *ter in die*).
* ④ The abbreviation for four times a day is qid. (L. *quater in die*).

3–2 ① Pulling the curtain is unnecessary when making an unoccupied bed; this is required to provide for privacy when making an occupied bed.
* ② Washing your hands removes microorganisms that can contaminate clean linen.
③ Collecting the clean linen is done after your hands are washed to prevent contamination of the linen.
④ Placing the bottom sheet is done after your hands are washed and you have collected the sheets.

3–3 ① 50 to 65 beats is below the normal range for the pulse in an adult.
* ② 70 to 85 is within the normal range of 60 to 100 beats for the pulse of an adult.
③ Although 90 beats is within the high end of the normal range for the pulse of an adult, 105 beats is above the normal range.
④ 110 to 125 beats is above the normal range for the pulse of an adult.

3–4 ① Diuretics produce an increase in urinary output.
② Antianxiety agents (anxiolytics) reduce anxiety.
* ③ Cathartics stimulate bowel evacuation; therefore, the patient should be assessed for a bowel movement.
④ Analgesics alter the perception and interpretation of pain.

3–5 ① Summarizing involves reviewing the main points in a discussion; this is useful at the end of an interview or teaching session.
* ② Clarifying (verifying) is a method of making the patient's message more understandable; it is an attempt to obtain more information without interpreting the original statement.
③ Restating, also called "paraphrasing," is a technique that repeats the patient's basic message in similar words.
④ Same as #3.

3–6 ① Using sterile equipment and sterile technique limits infection.
② Removing the needle along the line of insertion and pressure at the site prevent bleeding.
③ Removing the needle along the line of insertion and depressing the skin with a swab while the needle is withdrawn reduce discomfort.
* ④ Massage disperses the medication in the tissues and facilitates its absorption.

3–7 * ① Moisturizing lotion limits dryness and reduces the friction of the hands against the skin, which prevents skin trauma.
② Soap should be avoided because it can further dry the skin.
③ Massaging with short, kneading strokes can cause injury to delicate, thin skin; light, long strokes should be used.
④ Excess lubricant on the skin can promote skin maceration, and it also provides a warm, moist environment for the growth of microorganisms, which should be avoided.

3–8 ① This may not be appropriate for all patients; a bladder-retraining program must be based on individual needs.
② Same as #1.
③ Same as #1.
* ④ All patients, regardless of the specifics of each individual bladder-retraining program, will be toileted before going to bed at night and after awakening in the morning.

3–9 ① This places strain on the muscles of the back and should be avoided.
② Same as #1.
③ Keeping the feet together produces a narrow base of support that can result in a fall.
* ④ Both actions provide a wide base of support that promotes stability; placing one foot in front of the other facilitates bending at the knees, which permits the muscles of the legs, rather than the back, to bear the patient's weight.

3–10 ① Although a low-salt diet would be appropriate to limit edema, a diet high in fat should be avoided by an obese individual because fats are high in calories.
* ② Salt promotes fluid retention and increased calories add to body weight; therefore, both should be avoided by an obese patient with edema.
③ Salt promotes fluid retention and should be avoided by a patient with edema; protein may or may not be related to this patient's problem.
④ Although carbohydrates may be restricted in an obese individual to facilitate weight loss, a high-salt diet would promote fluid retention and should be avoided.

3–11 ① This response is using the technique of clarification and asks the patient to expand on the message so that it becomes more understandable.
* ② This response is using reflective technique because it attempts to identify feelings in the patient's message.
③ This response is using the technique of paraphrasing; this response restates the patient's basic message in similar words.
④ Same as #1.

3–12 ① This is less than the ordered dosage of medication.
② Same as #1.
* ③ Use ratio and proportion to solve for x by cross-multiplying:

$$\frac{0.5 \text{ g (desired dosage)}}{1.0 \text{ g (supplied dosage)}} = \frac{x \text{ ml}}{3 \text{ mL}}$$

$$1.0\, x = 3 \times 0.5$$
$$x = 1.5 \text{ mL}$$

④ This is more than the ordered dosage of medication.

The Multiple-Choice Question

In our society, success is generally measured in relation to levels of achievement. Before you entered a formal institution of learning, your achievement was subjectively appraised by your family and friends. Success was rewarded by smiles, positive statements, and perhaps favors or gifts. Lack of achievement or failure was acknowledged by omission of recognition, verbal corrections, and possibly punishment or scorn. When you entered school, your performance was directly measured against acceptable standards. In an effort to eliminate subjectivity, you were exposed to objective testing. These tests included true/false questions, matching columns, and multiple-choice questions. Achievement was reflected by numerical grades or letter grades. These grades indicated your level of achievement and by themselves provided rewards and punishments.

In nursing education, achievement can be assessed in a variety of ways: a patient's physiological response (did the patient's condition improve?), a patient's verbal response (did the patient state improvement?), student nurses' clinical performance (did the students do what they were supposed to do?), and student nurses' levels of cognitive competency (did the students know what they were supposed to know?). You must pass the National Council Licensing Examinations, also known as NCLEX-PN and NCLEX-RN, to legally work as a nurse. These examinations consist entirely of multiple-choice questions. Consequently, multiple-choice questions are frequently used in schools of nursing to evaluate student progress throughout the nursing curriculum. They are also used because they are objective, time efficient, and can comprehensively assess the understanding of curriculum content that has depth and breadth. Therefore, it is important for you to understand the components and dynamics of multiple-choice questions early in your nursing education.

A multiple-choice question is an objective test item. It is objective because the perceptions or opinions of another person do not influence the grade. In a multiple-choice question, a question is asked, three or more potential answers are presented, and only one of the potential answers is correct. The student answers the question either correctly or incorrectly.

Components of a Multiple-Choice Question

The entire multiple-choice question is called an **item.** Each item consists of two parts. The first part is known as the **stem.** The stem is the statement that asks the question. The second part contains the possible responses offered by the item, which are called **options.** One of the options answers the question posed in the stem and is the **correct answer.** The remaining options are the incorrect answers and are called **distractors.** They are referred to as "distractors" because they are designed to distract you from the correct answer.

The correct answers and the rationales for all the options of the sample items in this chapter are at the end of the chapter. Test yourself and see if you can correctly answer the sample items.

SAMPLE ITEM 4–1

What should the nurse do immediately before performing any procedure?		STEM
(1) Shut the door	DISTRACTOR	
(2) Wash the hands	CORRECT ANSWER	OPTIONS
(3) Close the curtain	DISTRACTOR	
(4) Drape the patient	DISTRACTOR	

(STEM and OPTIONS together form the ITEM)

SAMPLE ITEM 4–2

When providing care to a patient with a nasogastric tube, the nurse recognizes that the tube goes into the:		STEM
(1) Stomach	CORRECT ANSWER	
(2) Bronchi	DISTRACTOR	OPTIONS
(3) Trachea	DISTRACTOR	
(4) Duodenum	DISTRACTOR	

(STEM and OPTIONS together form the ITEM)

SAMPLE ITEM 4–3

A man describes his son as being difficult to get along with and concerned about what his friends think about him. How old is the son?		STEM
(1) 3 years old	DISTRACTOR	
(2) 7 years old	DISTRACTOR	OPTIONS
(3) 14 years old	CORRECT ANSWER	
(4) 22 years old	DISTRACTOR	

(STEM and OPTIONS together form the ITEM)

The Stem

The stem is the initial part of a multiple-choice item. The purpose of the stem is to present a problem in a clear and concise manner. The stem should contain all the details necessary to answer the question. The stem of an item can be a **complete sentence** that asks a question. It can also be presented as an **incomplete sentence** that becomes a complete sentence when it is combined with one of the options of the item. In addition to sentence structure, a characteristic of a stem that must be considered is its polarity. The polarity of the stem can be formulated in either a positive or negative context. A stem with a **positive polarity** asks the question in relation to what is true, whereas a stem with a **negative polarity** asks the question in relation to what is false.

THE STEM THAT IS A COMPLETE SENTENCE

A complete sentence is a group of words that is capable of standing independently. When a stem is a complete sentence, it will pose a question and end with a question mark (?). It should clearly and concisely formulate a problem that could be answered before reading the options.

SAMPLE ITEM 4–4

What should be the first action of the nurse when a fire alarm rings in a health care facility?

    (1) Close all doors on the unit.

    (2) Take an extinguisher to the fire scene.

    (3) Move patients laterally toward the stairs.

    (4) Determine if it is a fire drill or a real fire.

SAMPLE ITEM 4–5

What is the most common reason why elderly patients become incontinent of urine?

    (1) The muscles that control urination become weak.

    (2) The aged tend to drink less fluid than younger patients.

    (3) Their increase in weight places pressure on the bladder.

    (4) They use incontinence to manipulate and control others.

SAMPLE ITEM 4–6

What part of the body requires special hygiene when a patient has a nasogastric feeding tube?

    (1) Rectum

    (2) Abdomen

    (3) Oral cavity

    (4) Perineal area

THE STEM THAT IS AN INCOMPLETE SENTENCE

When a stem is an incomplete sentence, it is a group of words that forms the beginning portion of a sentence. The sentence becomes complete when it is combined with one of the options in the item. Some tests will have a period at the completion of each option and others will not. Whether there is a period or not, each option should complete the sentence with grammatical accuracy. However, the answer is the only option that correctly completes the sentence in relation to the informational content. When reading a stem that is an incomplete sentence, it is usually necessary to read the options before the question can be answered.

SAMPLE ITEM 4–7

To best understand what a patient is saying, the nurse should:
- (1) Demonstrate interest
- (2) Listen carefully
- (3) Remain silent
- (4) Employ touch

SAMPLE ITEM 4–8

People should be encouraged not to smoke in bed because it could:
- (1) Result in a fire
- (2) Upset a family member
- (3) Trigger a smoke alarm
- (4) Precipitate lung cancer

SAMPLE ITEM 4–9

When assisting a female patient with dementia to groom her hair, the nurse should:
- (1) Offer constant support and encouragement
- (2) Set time aside for a long teaching session
- (3) Alternate using a brush and a comb
- (4) Teach her how to braid her hair

THE STEM WITH A POSITIVE POLARITY

The stem with a positive polarity is concerned with truth. It asks the question with a positive statement. The correct answer is accurately related to the statement. It is in accord with a fact or principle, or it is an action that should be implemented. A positively worded stem attempts to determine if you are able to understand, apply, or differentiate correct information.

SAMPLE ITEM 4–10

An elderly patient who is dying starts to cry and says, "I was always concerned about myself first, and I hurt many people during my life." What is the underlying feeling being expressed by the patient?
- (1) Ambivalence
- (2) Sadness
- (3) Anger
- (4) Guilt

SAMPLE ITEM 4–11

Which intervention most accurately supports the concept of informed consent?

(1) Obtaining the patient's signature

(2) Explaining what is being done and why

(3) Involving the family in the teaching plan

(4) Teaching preoperative deep breathing and coughing

SAMPLE ITEM 4–12

What should the nurse do when a patient appears to be asleep but does not react when called by name?

(1) Loudly say, "Are you awake?"

(2) Tell the patient, "Squeeze my hand."

(3) Inform the nurse in charge immediately.

(4) Gently touch an arm and say the patient's name.

THE STEM WITH A NEGATIVE POLARITY

The stem with a negative polarity is concerned with what is false. It asks the question with a negative statement. The stem usually incorporates words such as "except," "not," or "never." These words are obvious. However, sometimes the words that are used are more obscure, for example, "contraindicated," "further," "unacceptable," "least," and "avoid." When a negative term is used, it may be emphasized by an underline (<u>except</u>), italics (*least*), dark type (**not**), or capitals (NEVER). A negatively worded stem requires you to recognize exceptions, detect errors, or identify interventions that are unacceptable or contraindicated. NCLEX-RN does not emphasize the negative word when used in a stem, and many nursing examinations do not have questions with a negative polarity. However, this information has been included in the event that you may be challenged by questions with a negative polarity.

SAMPLE ITEM 4–13

On what part of the body should the nurse <u>avoid</u> using soap when bathing a patient?

(1) Eyes

(2) Back

(3) Under the breasts

(4) Glans of the penis

SAMPLE ITEM 4–14

Range-of-motion (ROM) exercises should NOT be done:

(1) For comatose patients

(2) On limbs that are paralyzed

(3) Beyond the point of resistance

(4) For patients with chronic joint disease

SAMPLE ITEM 4–15

Which suggestion would be the **least** therapeutic when teaching the patient about promoting personal energy?

(1) Eat breakfast every day.

(2) Exercise three times a week.

(3) Get adequate sleep each night.

(4) Drink a cup of coffee each morning.

SAMPLE ITEM 4–16

What position would be *contraindicated* for the patient who has dyspnea?

(1) Supine

(2) Contour

(3) Fowler's

(4) Orthopneic

SAMPLE ITEM 4–17

Which action by the nurse would be unacceptable during a bed bath?

(1) Uncover the area being washed

(2) Use long, firm strokes toward the heart

(3) Wash from the rectum toward the pubis

(4) Remove the top sheets and use a bath blanket

The Options

All of the possible answers offered within an item are called "options." One of the options is the best response and is therefore the correct answer. The other options are incorrect and distract you from selecting the correct answer. These options are called "distractors." An item must have a minimum of three options to be considered a multiple-choice item, but the actual number varies among tests. The typical number of options is four or five responses, which reduces the probability of guessing the correct answer while limiting the amount of reading to a sensible level. Options are usually listed by number (1, 2, 3, and 4), lowercase letters (a, b, c, and d), or uppercase letters (A, B, C, and D). The grammatical presentation of options can appear in four different formats. An option can be a **sentence, complete the sentence begun in the stem,** an **incomplete sentence**, or a **single word.**

THE OPTION THAT IS A SENTENCE

A sentence is a unit of language that contains a stated or implied subject and verb. It is a statement that contains an entire thought and stands alone. Options can appear as complete sentences. Some tests have a period at the end of these options and others do not. Whether there is a period or not, each option should be grammatically correct. When the option is a verbal response, it should be grammatically correct and incorporate the appropriate punctuation, such as quotation marks (" "), comma (,) exclamation point (!), question mark (?), or period (.).

SAMPLE ITEM 4–18

Before performing a procedure, what should the nurse do first?

    (1) Raise the patient's bed to its highest position.

    (2) Collect the equipment for the procedure.

    (3) Position the patient for the procedure.

    (4) Explain the procedure to the patient.

SAMPLE ITEM 4–19

A Catholic patient tells the nurse, "Before being hospitalized I went to Mass and received Communion every morning." What should the nurse do to meet this patient's spiritual needs?

    (1) Encourage the patient to say the rosary every day.

    (2) Make arrangements for the patient to receive Communion.

    (3) Transfer the patient to a room with another Catholic patient.

    (4) Have a priest administer the Sacrament of the Sick to the patient.

SAMPLE ITEM 4–20

A male patient is crying, and the only word the nurse understands is "wife." What should the nurse say?

    (1) "I'm sure that your wife is fine."

    (2) "You are concerned about your wife?"

    (3) "What did your wife do to upset you?"

    (4) "Your wife will be visiting later today."

THE OPTION THAT COMPLETES THE SENTENCE BEGUN IN THE STEM

When the option completes the sentence begun in the stem, the stem and the option together should form a sentence. Some tests have correct punctuation at the end of these options and others do not. Whether or not there is a period, each option should complete the stem in a manner that is grammatically accurate.

SAMPLE ITEM 4–21

The primary etiology of obesity is a:

    (1) Lack of balance in the variety of nutrients

    (2) Glandular disorder that prevents weight loss

    (3) Caloric intake that exceeds metabolic needs

    (4) Psychological problem that causes overeating

SAMPLE ITEM 4–22

The nurse can best prevent the patient from getting a chill during a bed bath by:

(1) Rubbing briskly to cause vasodilation

(2) Exposing only the area being washed

(3) Giving a hot drink before the bath

(4) Pulling the curtain around the bed

SAMPLE ITEM 4–23

The nurse is to assist a patient with a bed bath; however, the patient has just returned from x-ray, is in pain, and refuses the bath. The nurse should:

(1) Cancel the bath today

(2) Delay the bath until later

(3) Give a partial bath quickly

(4) Encourage a shower instead

THE OPTION THAT IS AN INCOMPLETE SENTENCE

When an option is an incomplete sentence, it does not contain all the parts of speech (e.g., subject and verb) necessary to construct a complete, autonomous statement. The option that is an incomplete sentence is usually a phrase or group of related words. Although not a complete sentence, it conveys a unit of thought, an idea, or a concept.

SAMPLE ITEM 4–24

Which intervention is the most effective way to prevent the spread of microorganisms?

(1) Donning a mask

(2) Wearing a gown

(3) Washing the hands

(4) Keeping visitors out

SAMPLE ITEM 4–25

When should mouth care be administered to an unconscious patient?

(1) Whenever necessary

(2) Every 4 hours

(3) Once a shift

(4) Twice a day

SAMPLE ITEM 4–26

Which action by the nurse would help meet a patient's basic need for security and safety?

(1) Addressing the patient by name

(2) Explaining what is going to be done

(3) Accepting a patient's angry behavior

(4) Ensuring the patient gets adequate nutrition

THE OPTION THAT IS A WORD

A word is a series of letters that form a term. It is the most basic unit of language and is capable of communicating a message. The option that is a single word can be almost any part of speech (e.g., noun, pronoun, verb, or adverb) as long as it conveys information.

SAMPLE ITEM 4–27

Which of the following is a primary source for obtaining information related to the independent functions of a nurse?

(1) Chart

(2) Patient

(3) Physician

(4) Supervisor

SAMPLE ITEM 4–28

What approach should be used by the nurse caring for a patient who is grieving?

(1) Confronting

(2) Supporting

(3) Avoiding

(4) Limiting

SAMPLE ITEM 4–29

What is the nurse doing when formulating a nursing diagnosis?

(1) Planning

(2) Assessing

(3) Analyzing

(4) Implementing

SAMPLE ITEM 4–30

Which word best describes feelings associated with a child in Erikson's stage of autonomy versus shame and doubt?

(1) Hers

(2) Mine

(3) Theirs

(4) Nobody's

44 Answers and Rationales for Sample Items in
Chapter 4

An asterisk (*) is in front of the rationale that explains the correct answer.

4-1 ① This is unsafe; this should be done before washing the hands.
*   ② Before touching the patient, the nurse should wash his or her hands to remove microorganisms.
③ Same as #1.
④ This is done after handwashing.

4-2 * ① The tube enters the nose, passes through the posterior nasopharynx and esophagus, and enters the stomach through the cardiac sphincter.
② The bronchi are passages between the trachea and bronchioles and are part of the respiratory system.
③ The trachea is a passage between the posterior nasopharynx and bronchi and is part of the respiratory system.
④ The duodenum is distal to the stomach and is the first portion of the small intestine; a nasogastric tube is designed to be advanced into the stomach, not the duodenum.

4-3 ① Toddlers are concerned about themselves and their autonomy, not others.
② School-age children are easy to get along with and are concerned about performing and achieving.
* ③ Adolescents are concerned about their identity, independence, and peer relationships; this causes tension between them and their parents.
④ Young adults are developing intimate relationships and becoming socially responsible.

4-4 * ① This should be the initial action. A closed door provides patient safety.
② The location of the fire must be identified before an extinguisher can be taken to the scene.
③ This is unnecessary; patients need to be moved only if they are in danger.
④ Whenever the fire alarm rings, it should always be considered an indication of a real fire.

4-5 * ① Muscles, particularly the perineal muscles, tend to lose strength as people age.
② Incontinence is unrelated to fluid intake.
③ The elderly do not necessarily gain weight; many lose weight because of the loss of subcutaneous fat associated with aging. Body weight does not influence incontinence.
④ This is untrue; most elderly people want to be independent and in control of their bodily functions.

4-6 ① Special care of this area of the body is unnecessary; care provided during a routine bed bath is adequate.
② Same as #1.
* ③ A nasogastric tube feeding generally negates the need to chew; with lack of chewing, salivation decreases, which causes the mucous membranes to become dry.
④ Same as #1.

4-7 ① While this may indicate acceptance and encourage ventilation of feelings, it does nothing to promote understanding.

    * ② Attentive listening is important so that the nurse can pick up key words and iden-
tify emotional themes within the message.

    ③ Same as #1.

    ④ Touch is used to communicate a message, not to receive, understand, or interpret
a message from another person.

4-8   * ① Confused, weak, or lethargic individuals may drop lighted cigarettes or ashes,
which can ignite bed linens.

    ② Although smoking can physically and emotionally disturb a family member,
safety is the priority.

    ③ Smoke from a cigarette will not trigger a smoke alarm.

    ④ Although smoking may precipitate lung cancer, safety is the priority.

4-9   * ① People with dementia become easily confused and need support and encouragement to stay focused and motivated.

    ② People with dementia cannot concentrate long enough for a prolonged teaching
session; learning occurs best with short, frequent teaching sessions.

    ③ Alternating a brush and a comb could promote confusion; patients with demen-
tia need consistency.

    ④ Braiding the hair involves cognitive and psychomotor skills that the patient with
dementia probably does not possess.

4-10   ① Ambivalence would demonstrate two simultaneous conflicting feelings.

    ② Although the patient may be unhappy about past behaviors, it is the underlying
thoughts about hurting others that precipitated the patient's statement.

    ③ Anger is a feeling of displeasure caused by opposition or mistreatment and is
demonstrated by the words or gestures used by the patient in an effort to fight
back at the cause of the feeling.

    * ④ Guilt is a painful feeling of self-reproach resulting from the belief that one has
done something wrong.

4-11   ① Although obtaining the patient's signature is part of consent, the signature by itself does not imply that the patient understands.

    * ② The patient's knowledge and understanding of what is going to be done, why it is
being done, and what the outcomes will be is what constitutes being informed before giving consent.

    ③ Although the family may be involved, it is the patient who must sign the informed
consent.

    ④ Preoperative teaching is necessary only if the patient consents to surgery.

4-12   ① Speaking loudly could frighten the patient; one of the patient's other senses
should be stimulated because the patient previously has not responded to a verbal intervention.

    ② The nurse must get the patient's attention before giving a direction.

    ③ The nurse needs to assess the patient further before informing the nurse in charge.

    * ④ This action is the first step to further assess this patient. Touch and sound stimu-
late two senses, and using the patient's name is individualizing care.

4-13   * ① Soaps usually contain sodium or potassium salts of fatty acids, which are irritating and can injure the sensitive tissues of the eyes.

    ② The back needs soap and water to remove perspiration that collects on the skin.

    ③ Body surface areas that touch are dark, warm, and moist areas and must be
washed with soap and water to limit the growth of microorganisms.

④ The glans of the penis needs soap and water to remove perspiration, urine, and smegma.

4-14　① ROM should be performed for unconscious patients because they are usually immobile and are at risk for developing contractures.

② Paralyzed limbs must be moved through full ROM by the nurse to prevent loss of range secondary to inactivity.

* ③ Resistance indicates that there is strain on the muscles or joints; continuing ROM beyond the point of resistance could cause injury.

④ People with chronic joint disease usually need gentle ROM to keep the joints mobile.

4-15　① Food contains nutrients and calories, which provide energy.

② Exercise promotes muscle tone and energy.

③ Sleep is restful and restorative.

* ④ Caffeine, although a stimulant, can be harmful to the body.

4-16　* ① In the supine position the abdominal contents press against the diaphragm, impeding expansion of the lungs.

② This position is desirable because the abdominal contents drop by gravity, permitting efficient contraction of the diaphragm and expansion of the thoracic cavity.

③ Same as #2.

④ Same as #2.

4-17　① Only the area being washed should be exposed, to permit adequate bathing and inspection.

② Using long, firm strokes toward the heart is desirable because it promotes venous return.

* ③ This is unsafe; it would contaminate the urinary meatus with microorganisms from the perianal area.

④ Using a bath blanket is desirable; it absorbs moisture, provides warmth, and promotes privacy.

4-18　① This could be frightening if the patient does not know why the action is being done; this also would be unsafe.

② Collecting equipment would be done after the patient agrees to the procedure.

③ Same as #1.

* ④ Explaining the procedure meets the patient's right to know why and how care will be provided.

4-19　① This focuses on a different ritual and denies the patient's concerns about missing Mass and not receiving Communion.

* ② This helps to meet the patient's spiritual needs and is easily accomplished in a hospital setting.

③ The nurse, not other patients, must assist the patient to meet spiritual needs.

④ Same as #1.

4-20　① This statement offers false reassurance and draws a conclusion based on insufficient information.

* ② This response encourages further communication, which is necessary to obtain more information about what is upsetting the patient.

③ This is a judgmental statement that is not based on fact.

④ This is not an open-ended question that allows the patient to express concerns; this is a statement that may or may not be true.

4-21 ① A lack of balance in nutrients would result in malnutrition, not necessarily obesity; it could also result in weight loss.

② Although glandular disorders such as hypothyroidism may result in obesity, they are not the primary causes of obesity.

* ③ If more calories are ingested than the body requires for energy, they will be converted to adipose tissue, which causes weight gain.

④ A psychological problem is only one of many factors that influence overeating; it is not the primary etiology of obesity.

4-22 ① Vasodilation promotes heat loss.

* ② Exposing only the area being washed limits the evaporation of fluids on the skin and radiation of heat from the body, which prevents the patient from getting a chill.

③ A hot drink will not prevent a chill.

④ Although this may prevent drafts, it will not prevent the patient's getting a chill from the environmental temperature, excessive exposure, or evaporation of water from the skin.

4-23 ① The bath may eventually be canceled, but it should be delayed first.

* ② Delaying the bath accepts the patient's present refusal to bathe; rest and pain reduction may make the patient more amenable to hygiene later in the day.

③ This ignores the patient's right to refuse care and the fact that the patient is in pain.

④ Same as #3.

4-24 ① This personal protective equipment is not necessary for all standard and transmission-based precautions.

② Same as #1.

* ③ Washing the hands before and after patient care and whenever contaminated is the most important action for preventing the spread of microorganisms.

④ After they have been taught how to use standard and transmission-based precautions, people are permitted to visit patients with infections.

4-25 * ① Unconscious patients usually have dry mucous membranes of the oral cavity because they frequently breathe through the mouth, are not drinking fluids, and may be receiving oxygen; oral hygiene is required whenever necessary, which is usually at least every 2 hours.

② This is too long; drying, sordes, and lesions of the mucous membranes can occur.

③ Same as #2.

④ Same as #2.

4-26 ① This action meets the patient's need for self-esteem.

* ② Knowing what will happen and why provides for the patient's security needs; it is also a patient's right. The unknown can be frightening.

③ Same as #1.

④ This action meets the patient's basic physiological need for adequate nutrients for body processes.

4-27 ① The chart is a secondary source; it also contains physicians' orders, which are dependent functions of the nurse.

* ② The primary and most important source for obtaining information referring to the patient is the patient. The independent functions of the nurse include interven-

tions that relate to human responses, which are identified by direct contact with the patient.

③ The physician is a secondary source of information; when the nurse follows a physician's order, it is a dependent function of the nurse.

④ The supervisor is a secondary source; independent functions of the nurse can be performed independently of others.

4-28 ① A confrontation could take away the patient's current coping mechanisms and leave the patient defenseless.

* ② A patient who is grieving is using defenses to deal with the crisis; these defenses should be supported.

③ Avoiding the patient is a form of abandonment; the nurse should be present to provide support.

④ Setting limits would take away the patient's coping mechanisms and leave the patient defenseless.

4-29 ① A nursing diagnosis should be made during the analysis phase before planning nursing care because the interventions should be appropriate for the focus of concern.

② Assessing involves collecting the data, which must be gathered before it can be analyzed and nursing diagnoses formulated.

* ③ Data must be clustered and interpreted to identify human responses that indicate potential or actual health problems that can be treated by the nurse; statements that indicate actual or potential health problems treatable by the nurse are nursing diagnoses. These actions require analysis.

④ Implementation is putting the plan of care into action, which occurs after analysis and planning.

4-30 ① This word is associated with others rather than the self or self-interests.

* ② Toddlers are developing a sense of autonomy and are discovering the difference between independence and dependence; they are concerned about themselves and their mastery over their environment.

③ Same as #1.

④ Same as #1.

The Nursing Process

Problem solving is a process that provides a framework for identifying solutions to complex problems. It is a step-by-step process that uses a systematic approach. One might say that problem solving is a "blueprint" that can be followed to identify and solve problems. The concept of problem solving is not used exclusively by nurses. It is used by other professionals to find solutions within the context of their own job responsibilities. Nurses use the problem-solving process to identify human responses and to plan, implement, and evaluate nursing care. When scientific problem solving is used within the context of nursing, it is known as the nursing process. The **nursing process** contains five steps: **assessment, analysis, planning, implementation,** and **evaluation.**

Because the nursing process incorporates critical thinking used by nurses to meet patients' needs, items on nursing examinations are designed to test the use of this process. Test items are not written haphazardly. They are carefully designed to test your knowledge of a specific concept, skill, theory, or fact, from the perspective of one of the five steps of the nursing process. When reading an item, being able to identify its place within the nursing process should contribute to your ability to recognize what the test item is asking. To do this, you must focus on the critical words within the item.

This chapter explores the five steps of the nursing process: assessment, analysis, planning, implementation, and evaluation. Sample items are presented to demonstrate item construction as it relates to each step. Critical words associated with each step of the nursing process are illustrated within the sample items. Attempt to identify variations of critical words within the sample items indicating activities associated with each step of the nursing process. Practice answering the questions. The correct answers and the rationales for all the options of the sample items in this chapter are at the end of the chapter. The better you understand the focus of the item you are reading, the better you will be at identifying what is being asked and the greater your chances of identifying the correct answer.

Assessment

During assessment, data must be accurately collected, verified, and communicated. Assessment items are designed to test your knowledge of information, theories, principles, and skills related to the assessment of the patient. This establishes the foundation on which nurses base the subsequent steps in the nursing process. Assessment questions ask you to:

- Obtain vital statistics
- Perform a physical assessment
- Collect specimens
- Identify patient adaptations that are objective or subjective
- Identify patient adaptations that are verbal or nonverbal
- Identify adaptations that are normal or abnormal
- Use various data collection methods
- Identify sources of data
- Verify critical findings
- Identify commonalities and differences in response to illness
- Communicate information about assessments to appropriate members of the health team

The critical words within a test item that indicate that the item is focused on assessment include these: inspect, identify, verify, observe, notify, check, inform, question, communicate, verbal and nonverbal, signs and symptoms, stressors, adaptations, sources, perceptions, and assess. See whether you can identify variations of these critical words in the sample items in this chapter. Most testing errors occur on assessment items because options are selected that:

- Collect insufficient data
- Have data that are inaccurately collected
- Use unscientific methods of data collection
- Rely on a secondary source rather than the primary source, the patient
- Contain irrelevant data
- Fail to verify data
- Reflect bias or prejudice
- Fail to accurately communicate data

COLLECT DATA

Collecting data is the first part of assessment. The nurse collects data through specific **methods of data collection,** such as performing a physical examination, interviewing, and reviewing records. A **physical examination** includes the assessment techniques of inspection, palpation, auscultation, and percussion. It also includes obtaining the vital signs and recognizing normal and abnormal parameters of obtained values. **Interviewing** is done to collect data using a formal approach (e.g., obtaining a health history) or an informal approach (e.g., exploring feelings while providing other nursing care). **Review of records** includes consideration of reports such as the results of laboratory tests, diagnostic procedures, as well as assessments or consultations by other members of the health team.

SAMPLE ITEM 5–1

While making rounds, the nurse finds a patient on the floor in the hall. What should be the nurse's initial response?

(1) Inspect the patient for injury.

(2) Transfer the patient back to bed.

(3) Move the patient to the closest chair.

(4) Report the incident to the nursing supervisor.

This item tests your ability to recognize that, in an emergency situation, the nurse must first assess the condition of the patient. This principle is basic to any emergency response by a nurse. Moving a patient before an assessment could worsen any injury. This item demonstrates how a basic concept related to assessment can be tested.

SAMPLE ITEM 5–2

What should the nurse do to avoid patient accidents?

(1) Assess the strength of a patient before walking.

(2) Keep an overbed table in front of a sitting patient.

(3) Provide a cane for ambulation if the patient is weak.

(4) Apply a vest restraint when a patient uses a wheelchair.

This item tests your ability to recognize the concept that the nurse must assess a patient before implementing care. The three distractors are all concerned with implementing care. This question also tests your ability to recognize physical examination as a method of collecting data about the status of a patient.

SAMPLE ITEM 5–3

Which assessment would most likely indicate that a patient is having difficulty breathing?

(1) 18 breaths per minute and inhaled through the mouth

(2) 20 breaths per minute and shallow in character

(3) 16 breaths per minute and deep in character

(4) 28 breaths per minute and noisy

This item tests your ability to identify the option that reflects a respiratory rate and characteristic that is outside normal parameters. To successfully answer this question, you need to know the rate and characteristics of normal and abnormal respirations.

SAMPLE ITEM 5–4

What should the nurse always do when taking a rectal temperature?

(1) Allow the patient to insert the thermometer.

(2) Position the patient on the left side.

(3) Use an electronic thermometer.

(4) Lubricate the thermometer.

Option 4 identifies what must be done (a critical element) to safely take a rectal temperature. The three distractors may or may not be done when obtaining a rectal temperature. Although this appears to be an implementation question because it involves an action, it is actually an assessment question because it is concerned with collecting data.

SAMPLE ITEM 5–5

When determining if a person's body weight is appropriate, it is important to also assess the person's:

(1) Body height

(2) Daily intake

(3) Clothing size

(4) Food preferences

This item tests your ability to recognize that, to calculate the patient's ideal body weight, the nurse must also know the patient's height. The ideal body weight is the measurement that reflects the range of weight that would be considered appropriate in relation to the patient's height. The ideal body weight is the measurement against which the patient's present weight is compared to determine if the patient is underweight or obese. Although the question does not address these concepts, the nurse must also know the patient's age and extent of bone structure.

The **types of data** collected when assessing a patient can be objective or subjective. **Objective data** are measurable assessments collected when the nurse uses sight, touch, smell, or hearing to acquire information. Examples of objective data include an excoriated perineal area, diaphoresis, ammonia odor to urine, crackles, and vital signs. **Subjective data** can be collected only when the patient shares feelings, perceptions, thoughts, and sensations about a health problem or concern. Examples of subjective data include patient statements about pain, shortness of breath, or feeling depressed.

SAMPLE ITEM 5–6

A patient with painful terminal cancer is depressed and withdrawn. During a conversation with the nurse, the patient states, "Life is not worth living. I'm going to kill myself." The nurse recognizes that the patient's statement is:

(1) Primary data

(2) Objective data

(3) Subjective data

(4) Secondary data

This item tests your ability to differentiate the types of information collected during the assessment phase of the nursing process. The nurse should know the type of data collected for the purposes of future clustering and determining its significance. Any information that a patient shares regarding feelings, thoughts, and concerns is subjective.

Data can be gathered not only by different methods but also from different sources. **Sources of data** available to the nurse include those that are primary, secondary, and tertiary. There is only one **primary source,** the patient. The patient is the most valuable source of information because the data collected are the most current and specific to the patient.

A **secondary source** produces information from someplace other than the patient. A family member is a secondary source who can contribute information about the patient's likes and dislikes, ethnic and cultural background, similarities and differences in behavior, and functioning before and during the health problem. The patient's medical record (chart) is another example of a secondary source. It is a legal document containing information that concerns the patient's physical, psychosocial, religious, and economic history and documents the patient's physical and emotional adaptations. Controversy surrounds the labeling of diagnostic test results in a chart as being from either primary or secondary sources. Although the chart itself is a secondary source, diagnostic test results are direct objective measurements of the patient's status and therefore are considered by some health care providers to be a primary source. The nurse must remember that the information in a chart is history and does not reflect the current status of the patient because the patient is dynamic and constantly changing. Secondary sources are valuable for gathering supplementary information about a patient.

A **tertiary source** provides information from outside the specific patient's frame of reference. Examples of tertiary sources include textbooks, the nurse's experience, and accepted commonalities among patients with similar adaptations. The nurse's or other health team members' responses to the patient are tertiary sources of patient data.

SAMPLE ITEM 5-7

The nurse asks a patient's wife specific questions about the patient's health complaints before admission. When collecting this information, the nurse is seeking information from a:

(1) Primary source

(2) Tertiary source

(3) Subjective source

(4) Secondary source

This item tests your ability to recognize that a family member is a secondary source of information. Secondary sources provide information that is supplemental to the information collected from the patient.

Data transmitted via communication can be verbal or nonverbal. **Verbal data** are collected via the spoken or written word. For example, statements to the nurse by the patient are verbal data. **Nonverbal data** are collected via transmission of a message without words. Crying, a fearful facial expression, the appearance of the patient, and gestures are all examples of nonverbal data.

SAMPLE ITEM 5-8

What is an example of nonverbal communication?

(1) A letter

(2) Holding hands

(3) Noise in the room

(4) A telephone message

This item tests your ability to recognize that holding hands is a form of nonverbal communication. Nonverbal communication does not use words. Touch, gestures, posture, and facial expressions are examples of nonverbal communication.

Reasoning is essential when assessing and collecting data. Nurses should use both deductive and inductive reasoning. **Deductive reasoning** moves from the general to the specific. For example, the nurse can use deductive reasoning when collecting data about a patient who has a body cast. If it is accepted that patients in a body cast are generally at risk for altered skin integrity, the nurse should recognize the need to assess this specific patient's skin for early signs of impaired skin integrity. **Inductive reasoning** moves from the specific to the general. For example, the nurse uses inductive reasoning when collecting data related to a specific postoperative patient's weak, thready pulse. The nurse is aware that a weak, thready pulse can indicate postoperative hemorrhage. From this specific assessment the nurse recognizes the need to further assess for additional general signs of hemorrhage such as a drop in blood pressure, increased respirations, and cold clammy skin. Effective inductive and deductive reasoning are based on a strong theoretical foundation of knowledge that is drawn on when collecting data.

SAMPLE ITEM 5–9

A patient is drinking 3000 mL of fluid a day. When assessing the patient's urine, the nurse can expect the urine to be:

(1) Light yellow

(2) Dark yellow

(3) Light amber

(4) Dark amber

This item tests your ability to use deductive reasoning (moving from the general to the specific) to identify an expected common response to fluid intake of 3000 mL of fluid a day. It is a known fact that the more fluid a person drinks, the lighter the color of the urine. Light yellow is the only option that is within normal parameters.

VERIFY DATA

Once data are collected, they must be verified. To **verify data** is to confirm information by collecting additional data, questioning orders, obtaining judgments and/or conclusions from other team members when appropriate, and by collecting data oneself rather than relying on technology. Verifying data ensures authenticity and accuracy. For example, when a vital statistic is outside the normal range or is a measurement that is unexpected, the nurse must substantiate the results by collecting the data again and/or collecting additional data to supplement the original information.

SAMPLE ITEM 5–10

The nurse takes the patient's blood pressure and records a diastolic pressure of 120. What should the nurse do first?

(1) Retake the blood pressure.

(2) Take the other vital signs.

(3) Notify the nurse in charge.

(4) Notify the physician.

This item tests your ability to recognize that you need to verify data when they are unexpected or outside the normal range. Your first action should be to wait a minute and then retake the blood pressure. An error may have been made when taking the blood pressure.

COMMUNICATE INFORMATION ABOUT ASSESSMENTS

The last component of assessment includes the nurse's ability to communicate information obtained from assessment activities. Sharing vital information about a patient is essential if members of the health team are to be alerted to the most current status of the patient. Communication methods vary (e.g., progress notes, verbal notification, flow sheets); however, they all share the need to be accurate, concise, thorough, current, organized, and confidential.

What should the nurse do immediately after a patient drinks 8 oz of apple juice?

(1) Record 240 cc on the I&O sheet.

(2) Assess the patient's skin turgor.

(3) Offer the patient a bedpan.

(4) Provide oral hygiene.

This item tests your ability to assess that the patient ingested 240 cc of fluid and document this information on a flow sheet so that it can be communicated to other health team members.

Analysis

Analysis, the second step of the nursing process, is the most difficult component. Analysis requires that data be validated and clustered and that its significance be determined. To analyze data, you need a strong foundation in scientific principles related to nursing theory, social sciences, and physical sciences, and you need to know the commonalties and differences in patients' responses to various stresses. You need to use deductive and inductive reasoning to apply your knowledge and experience when answering analysis items. After the initial analysis of data, sometimes additional data need to be collected and analyzed. Only after all the data have been analyzed should a nursing diagnosis be made. Analysis questions ask you to:

- Validate data
- Cluster data
- Identify clustered data as meaningful
- Identify when additional data are needed to validate clustered data
- Interpret validated and clustered data
- Identify nursing diagnoses
- Communicate nursing diagnoses to others
- Ensure that the patient's health care needs will be appropriately met

The critical words within a test item that indicate that the item is focused on analysis include these: valid, organize, categorize, cluster, reexamine, pattern, formulate, nursing diagnosis, reflect, relate, problem, interpret, contribute, relevant, decision, significant, deduction, statement, and analysis. See whether you can identify variations of these critical words in the sample items in this chapter. Testing errors occur on analysis items when options are selected that:

- Omit data
- Cluster data prematurely
- Make a nursing diagnosis before all significant data have been clustered
- Force the nursing diagnosis to fit the signs and symptoms collected

INTERPRET DATA

Interpretation of data is a critical step in the process of analysis. It is related to the nurse's ability to validate, cluster data, determine the significance of clustered data, and come to a conclusion. Conclusions are the opinions, decisions, or inferences made after careful analysis of data. In analysis the nurse validates data to determine their accuracy and significance. Information is more meaningful when its relationship to other data is established. Clustering enables the nurse to organize data; eliminate that which is insignificant, irrelevant, or redundant; and reduce the remaining data into manageable categories. To cluster data, the nurse needs to group related information. Data must first be organized into general categories such as physical, sociocultural, and psychological. Once grouped into general categories, data can be further grouped into specific categories such as nutrition, mobility, and elimination. Data can be obvious and easy to cluster or obscure and difficult to cluster. Some data are easily clustered because the information collected is clearly related to only one system of the body. For example, hard stool, a feeling of rectal fullness, and straining on defecation all relate to intestinal elimination. These adaptations are easy to group and indicate constipation. Other data are more difficult to cluster because the patient's adaptations may involve a variety of systems of the body. Hypotension; a weak, thready pulse; weight loss; and dry mucous membranes are characteristics of dehydration. These adaptations cross several body systems and their relationship to each other is not clear; therefore, they are more difficult to cluster. At first the information collected may not appear to be related. However, with a thorough analysis the nurse should recognize the data that are interrelated. After data are clustered, the significance of the clustered data must be determined. "Significance" in this context refers to some consequence, importance, implication, or gravity connected to the cluster as it relates to the patient's health problem. Finally, the interpretation of the clustered data should lead to a conclusion.

SAMPLE ITEM 5–12

The patient had a stroke that resulted in paralysis of the right side. When clustering data, the nurse grouped the following data together: drooling of saliva and slurred speech. Which information would be most significant to include with this clustered data?

(1) Expressive aphasia

(2) Difficulty swallowing

(3) Inability to perform ADLs

(4) Incontinence of urine and stool

This item tests your ability to recognize a cluster of data that indicates that a patient is at risk for aspiration. Oxygenation is a basic physiological need. A patient who is drooling saliva and has slurred speech, right-sided paralysis, and difficulty swallowing would be at serious risk for aspiration of material into the respiratory tract. Although the other options are all problems that must be addressed by the nurse, they are not data related to oxygenation and have no significance to this specific cluster.

SAMPLE ITEM 5–13

Pressure ulcers are most often associated with patients who:

(1) Are immobilized

(2) Have psychiatric diagnoses

(3) Experience respiratory distress

(4) Need close supervision for safety

This item tests your ability to recognize the relationship between immobility and the formation of pressure ulcers. It is designed to test your knowledge of the fact that prolonged pressure on a site interferes with cellular oxygenation, which causes cell death resulting in a pressure ulcer.

SAMPLE ITEM 5–14

A patient has a loss of appetite (anorexia), has difficulty falling asleep (insomnia), and has lost interest in activities of daily living. Which feeling reflects these adaptations?

    (1) Anger

    (2) Denial

    (3) Depression

    (4) Acceptance

This item tests your ability to come to a conclusion based on a cluster of data. The word "reflect" in the stem cues you to the fact that this is an analysis question. You need to draw from your knowledge of commonalities of human behavior and theories of grieving to arrive at the conclusion that the patient is probably depressed.

SAMPLE ITEM 5–15

A patient who is debilitated and unsteady when standing insists on walking to the bathroom without calling for assistance. This behavior reflects a need to be:

    (1) Alone

    (2) Accepted

    (3) Independent

    (4) Manipulative

This item also tests your ability to come to a conclusion based on a cluster of data. To answer this question, you must analyze and interpret the information in the stem and come to a conclusion. Your knowledge of human behavior should enable you to select the correct answer.

COLLECT ADDITIONAL DATA

After arriving at an initial conclusion, additional data collection might be indicated to provide more information to support the suspected conclusion. This is done to establish and ensure the relationship among the original data. The nurse continually reassesses the condition of the patient and the presence of needs, recognizing that the patient is dynamic and ever changing throughout all phases of the nursing process.

SAMPLE ITEM 5–16

The nurse assesses that a postoperative patient has a decreased blood pressure and weak, thready pulse. The nurse should reassess the patient for additional signs of:

    (1) Hemorrhage

    (2) Infection

    (3) Anxiety

    (4) Pain

This item is designed to test your ability to recognize that the nurse needs to reassess a patient for additional data to reinforce the proposed conclusion. Hypotension and a weak, thready pulse are related to a decreased blood volume that is associated with postoperative hemorrhage.

IDENTIFY AND COMMUNICATE NURSING DIAGNOSES

Converting a conclusion into a diagnostic statement changes it from a general statement of a problem into a specific statement, or a nursing diagnosis. A **nursing diagnosis** is a statement of a specific health problem that a nurse is legally permitted to treat. The diagnostic statement should include the problem and the factors that contributed to the development of the problem.

It is important to include the contributing factors because, although two patients may have the same problem, it may have been caused by different stresses. This concept is important because the nature of the contributing factors generally drives the choice of interventions being planned. For example, two patients have impaired skin integrity. However, one patient's skin problem is related to incontinence and edema, and the other patient's skin problem is related to immobility and pressure. The interventions may be very different because the factors contributing to the problem are different. This is discussed in more detail in the section in this chapter titled "Planning." Nurses use the taxonomy of nursing diagnoses developed by the North American Nursing Diagnosis Association (NANDA) as a blueprint. This taxonomy provides for classifying nursing problems, standardizing language, facilitating communication, and focusing on an individualized approach to identifying and meeting a patient's nursing needs. The following are examples of nursing diagnoses:

- Risk for impaired skin integrity related to incontinence
- Feeding self-care deficit related to bilateral arm casts
- Ineffective airway clearance related to excessive secretions

Nurses need to communicate nursing diagnoses to other nurses via a written plan of care. The plan should include the nursing diagnosis, expected outcomes, and planned interventions. The section of this chapter titled "Planning" discusses outcomes and planned nursing interventions in more detail.

SAMPLE ITEM 5–17

The patient has suffered a cerebrovascular accident (CVA, stroke), has left-sided hemiparesis, and is incontinent. Which is an appropriately worded nursing diagnosis for this patient?

(1) The patient has a need to maintain skin integrity.

(2) The patient will be clean and dry and will receive range-of-motion exercises every 4 hours.

(3) The patient has a stroke evidenced by hemiparesis and incontinence secondary to a cerebrovascular accident.

(4) The patient is at risk for impaired skin integrity related to left-sided hemiparesis and incontinence secondary to a CVA.

This item tests your ability to recognize language used by the NANDA taxonomy. To answer this item correctly, you must be able to recognize the differences between a patient need, an expected outcome, a nursing intervention, and a properly stated nursing diagnosis associated with a cluster of data.

Planning

Planning is the third step of the nursing process. It involves setting goals, establishing priorities, identifying expected outcomes, identifying interventions designed to achieve goals and outcomes, modifying the plan as necessary, and collaborating with other health team members to ensure that care is coordinated. Goals, outcomes, and identified interventions are formulated in response to the nursing diagnoses that were identified in the previous step (analysis) of the nursing process. A plan of care consists of nursing diagnoses, goals, outcomes, and identified interventions. The plan outlines the nursing care for each patient. To plan care, you will need to have a strong foundation of scientific theory, know the commonalities and differences in response to nursing interventions, and know theories related to establishing priority of needs. You will need to use your knowledge and clinical experience when answering planning questions. Planning questions will ask you to:

- Involve the patient in the planning process
- Set goals
- Establish expected outcomes against which results of care can be compared for the purpose of evaluation
- Establish priorities
- Plan appropriate interventions
- Anticipate patient needs
- Recognize the need to collaborate with others
- Recognize the need to coordinate planned care with other disciplines
- Recognize that plans must be flexible and modified based on changing patient needs

The critical words within a test item that indicate that the item is focused on planning include these: achieve, desired, plan, effective, desired result, goal, priority, develop, formulate, establish, design, prevent, strategy, select, determine, anticipate, modify, collaborate, arrange, coordinate, expect, and outcome. See whether you can identify variations of these critical words in the sample items in this chapter. Testing errors occur during the planning phase when options are selected that:

- Do not include the patient in setting goals and priorities
- Are inappropriate goals
- Misidentify priorities
- Reflect goals that are unrealistic
- Reflect goals that are unmeasurable
- Reflect planned interventions that are inappropriate or incomplete
- Fail to include family members and significant others when appropriate
- Fail to coordinate and collaborate with other health team members

The planning component of the nursing process generates a statement of goals and expected outcomes, as well as interventions that are planned to meet these goals and outcomes. This plan becomes the blueprint for nursing interventions that are dictated by the patient's individual needs and preferences.

IDENTIFY GOALS

Goals are general statements that direct nursing interventions, provide broad parameters for measuring results, and stimulate motivation. Goals can be long term or short term. A **long-term goal** is one that will take time to achieve (weeks to months). A **short-term goal** is one that can be achieved relatively quickly (usually within a week or two). Goals should be:

- Patient centered
- Specific (measurable)

- Realistic
- Achievable within a time frame

A long-term goal for a patient who has a respiratory tract infection might be, "Mr. Brown will be free of infection within 3 weeks." "Mr. Brown" is the subject of the statement and therefore the goal is patient centered. Being "free of infection" is specific and realistic. The phrase "within 3 weeks" indicates the time frame in which the goal should be achieved. Eventually a goal can be further developed to become an expected outcome. An outcome provides a standard of measure that can be used to determine whether the goal has been reached. An expected outcome for the long-term goal listed above might be, "Mr. Brown's vital signs will be within normal limits and breath sounds will be clear." Outcomes are discussed in more detail later in this chapter.

SAMPLE ITEM 5–18

The nurse is caring for a patient with a new temporary colostomy. Which would be a realistic short-term goal for this patient?

(1) The patient's bowel will function within 2 days.

(2) The patient will have regular bowel elimination.

(3) The patient will be at risk for impaired skin integrity.

(4) The patient's skin will remain intact around the stoma.

This item tests your ability to recognize a short-term goal. To answer this question, you need to know commonalities related to caring for a patient with a new temporary colostomy and be able to recognize the differences between short- and long-term goals, a nursing diagnosis, and an outcome statement.

SET PRIORITIES

Setting priorities is an important step in the planning process. Once nursing diagnoses and goals are identified, they must be ranked in order of importance. Maslow's hierarchy of needs is helpful in establishing priorities. Basic physiological needs are ranked first, with the need for safety and security, belonging and love, self-esteem, and self-actualization following in rank order. It is important, however, to recognize that at one point in time any one of Maslow's needs may take priority depending on the needs of the individual patient. Obviously, if someone is choking on food, clearing the airway would take priority. However, there are times when the emergency or immediate need of the patient is in the psychological dimension. The nurse must be aware of the patient's perceptions and perspective when setting priorities because patients are the center of the health team. When possible, the patient should always be involved in setting priorities.

SAMPLE ITEM 5–19

A patient has just returned from surgery with an IV and does not have a gag reflex. Which planned intervention takes priority?

(1) Ensure adequacy of air exchange.

(2) Observe the dressing for drainage.

(3) Check for IV infiltration.

(4) Monitor vital signs.

This item tests your ability to prioritize care. All of these planned interventions are important. However, oxygenation is essential to sustain life, and therefore maintaining a patent airway is the priority.

IDENTIFY INTERVENTIONS

After priorities are established, a plan for nursing action must be formulated. To plan appropriately, the nurse must rely on scientific knowledge, clinical judgment, and knowledge about the patient. Relying on this background, the nurse determines what nursing measures would be most effective in assisting the patient to achieve a goal or outcome. For example, when caring for a patient with a pressure ulcer, the nurse reasons, "If I turn and reposition the patient and massage around the area with lotion every 2 hours, then circulation will increase and healing will be promoted." When planning care, the nurse must know the scientific rationales for nursing interventions so that the interventions selected are the most appropriate for the patient care situation. It is not enough to just know **how,** you must also know **why.**

When making decisions, the nurse must consider the concepts of "cause and effect," "risk and probability," and "value of the consequence to the patient." The action you plan is the "cause." The patient's response is the "effect." The likelihood of the occurrence of either a positive or negative effect is the "probability." The probability of the patient suffering harm from the action is the "risk." The value of the effect, in relation to its probability of occurring, influences the degree of risk one is willing to take to achieve the effect. To facilitate this process of problem solving, an **information-processing model of decision making** should be used. It requires you to first identify all the possible nursing actions (cause) that may help the patient. Second, you need to identify all possible positive and negative consequences (effect) associated with each action. Third, you need to determine the odds (probability) that each consequence will occur. This includes determining the probability of a negative effect occurring (risk). Fourth, you need to arrive at a judgment based on the value of each effect to the patient. Once all these steps are completed, you must choose the action that is "best" for the patient. The "best" action is one that has the lowest risk and the highest probability of helping the patient achieve the expected outcome (effect).

The concept of probability versus risk can be applied to buying a lottery ticket. If you buy one lottery ticket, your chances of winning are small (low probability). If you do not win, your risk will be small because you will lose only one dollar (low risk). On the other hand, if you spend your entire paycheck on lottery tickets you will not dramatically increase your chances of winning (low probability). However, if you do not win, you will lose your whole paycheck and have no money to pay your bills (high risk). When making clinical decisions, you want to choose an action that has the highest probability of being successful with the lowest risk to the patient.

Also, the appropriateness of clinical decisions depends on the quality of the data collected and the inferences made in the earlier steps of the nursing process. Each step of the nursing process relies on the quality and accuracy of the preceding step.

SAMPLE ITEM 5–20

What is the most effective way to prevent the spread of microorganisms in a hospital?

(1) Washing the hands

(2) Implementing contact precautions

(3) Administering antibiotics to sick patients

(4) Using linen hampers with foot-operated covers

This item tests your ability to recognize that handwashing is the single most effective measure to prevent the spread of microorganisms. This is a question that focuses on a specific action that can contribute to the protection of all patients from the risk of infection.

SAMPLE ITEM 5–21

A patient on bed rest needs a complete change of linen. What should the nurse plan to do?

(1) Make an occupied bed.

(2) Change the draw sheet and top sheet.

(3) Raise the patient with a mechanical lift.

(4) Transfer the patient to a chair during the linen change.

This item tests your ability to recognize the needs of a patient on bed rest and, therefore, to plan to make an occupied bed. The word "plan" used in the stem is an obvious clue that this is a planning question.

SAMPLE ITEM 5–22

An occupied bed must be made for a patient who is:

(1) Obese

(2) In a cast

(3) Immobile

(4) On bed rest

This item is similar to sample item 5–21; however, the content of the stem and the correct option are reversed. This item is more difficult to identify as a planning item because the word "plan" is not in the stem.

PROJECT EXPECTED OUTCOMES

Expected outcomes are the changes in the patient's condition that are expected in response to care given. Expected outcomes are derived from goal statements, but they are more specific because they describe the behavior to be demonstrated or data to be collected once the goal is achieved. Expected outcomes are the benchmarks against which the actual outcomes are compared to determine the effectiveness of the interventions provided. To be meaningful, they must be patient centered, realistic, measurable, and within a certain time frame. The process of comparing actual outcomes with expected outcomes occurs in the evaluation phase, which is the next step in the nursing process. Examples of outcomes are, "The patient states a reduction in anxiety in 1 week," and "The patient's diastolic blood pressure is below 90 mm Hg by discharge." Sometimes the nurse may state goals and outcomes together. For example, "The patient will continuously maintain an effective airway clearance as evidenced by expectoration of sputum, clear lung fields, and noiseless breathing." The first part of the statement is the goal and what follow "as evidenced by" are the expected outcomes. The first part of the statement is general and the second part is specific.

A nurse is caring for a patient experiencing loss of appetite (anorexia) and nausea. Which statement includes an expected outcome?

(1) The patient will eat 50 percent of every meal during the next week.

(2) The patient has altered nutrition less than body requirements.

(3) The patient's privacy will be maintained when providing care.

(4) The patient's mouth will be cleaned every 4 hours.

This item tests your ability to recognize a statement that reflects an expected outcome. To answer this question, you need to know commonalities of caring for a patient with anorexia and nausea. You also need to recognize the differences among a goal, an expected outcome, a nursing diagnosis, and a nursing intervention.

ENSURE THAT PATIENTS' HEALTH CARE NEEDS WILL BE APPROPRIATELY MET

During the analysis phase of the nursing process the nurse must identify whether or not the patient's health care needs can be met. If adequate care cannot be provided because the provider's expertise is unrelated to the patient's needs, the provider is inexperienced for caring for a patient with a particular problem, or there is inadequate staffing, a patient may be placed at risk. The nurse is obligated to take an action that will ensure that appropriate care will be provided. This might necessitate rearranging the assignment, or it might require intervention by the nurse supervisor. Once the nurse embarks on a "duty of care," the nurse is obligated to provide a standard of care defined by the Nurse Practice Act in the state in which the nurse works.

SAMPLE ITEM 5–24

The nurse manager arrives on duty and discovers that several staff members have just called in sick. What would be the nurse's most appropriate response?

(1) Inform the supervisor and ask for additional staff

(2) Identify which patients need care and assign staff accordingly

(3) Explain to patients that when the unit is short staffed, only essential care can be provided

(4) Provide the best care possible, but refuse to accept responsibility for the standard of care delivered

This item tests your ability to recognize your responsibility to ensure that patients' needs are appropriately met. Once the nurse perceives a risk to patient safety, the nurse is obligated to take action that will ensure that appropriate care will be provided.

MODIFY THE PLAN OF CARE AS NEEDED

Planning generally takes place before care is given. However, patient needs sometimes change while the nurse is in the process of implementing care, and a plan must be immediately modified. Modification of the plan of care also may take place after evaluation. The original plan may have been inadequate or inappropriate, or the patient's condition may have improved. It is important to recognize that plans of care are not set in stone but are modified in response to the changing needs of the patient. Because a patient's needs are dynamic, the nursing plan is also dynamic. It must be continually changed to be kept current, substituting new nursing diagnoses, goals, expected outcomes, and planned interventions as indicated by the patient's changing needs.

SAMPLE ITEM 5–25

A patient is receiving oxygen by nasal cannula. After morning care, the patient experiences dyspnea and complains of feeling tired. When planning for this patient's bath the next day, the nurse should plan to:

    (1) Give a complete bath quickly

    (2) Bathe only the body parts that need bathing

    (3) Arrange for several rest periods during morning care

    (4) Continue with the same plan because dyspnea is unavoidable

This item tests your ability to recognize the need to modify a plan of care based on new data. The words "planning" in the stem and "arrange" in the correct answer are obvious clues that this is a planning question.

COLLABORATE WITH OTHER HEALTH TEAM MEMBERS

Another component of planning is consultation and collaboration with other health team members to brainstorm, seek additional input, and delegate and coordinate the delivery of health services. The nurse is responsible for coordinating the members of the nursing team as well as the entire health team. The nurse manages the members of the nursing team by appropriately delegating and supervising nursing interventions. The plan also identifies and coordinates the services of other health care professionals. The nurse is responsible for ensuring that services such as laboratory tests, radiological studies, and physical therapy are performed within the context of the patient's physical and emotional abilities. For example, the nurse may arrange for a patient to go to physical therapy in the morning before the patient tires, or the nurse may consult with the dietitian for help with designing a menu that incorporates a patient's preferences. Effective planning contributes to the delivery of patient care that has continuity and is patient centered, coordinated, and individualized.

SAMPLE ITEM 5–26

The nurse is caring for a patient with a large pressure ulcer that has not responded to common nursing interventions. To best deal with this problem, the nurse should consult with the:

    (1) Plastic surgeon

    (2) Physical therapist

    (3) Attending physician

    (4) Clinical nurse specialist

This item is designed to test your ability to recognize that planning nursing care may require the nurse to seek the expertise of a specialist. A clinical nurse specialist is educated and prepared to provide expert advice and lend problem-solving and educational skills to seek solutions to difficult clinical nursing problems. Although the nurse consults with health team members of other disciplines for various reasons, the nurse should consult with a clinical nurse specialist or other resources in nursing for assistance with solving nursing problems.

Implementation

Effective implementation of nursing care is based on:

- Reassessing the patient
- Reviewing and modifying the plan of care when indicated
- Identifying when additional help in either staff or resources is needed to safely implement the plan
- Implementing types of interventions
- Using methods of intervention
- Documenting and reporting patient care and responses

The first three actions listed above have been discussed in detail in previous steps from the perspective of assessment, analysis, and planning. When they are considered from the perspective of intervention, the nurse must remember that the principles described in the preceding sections apply here as well. The concept for the nurse to internalize is that these actions are ongoing throughout the nursing process. The last three actions for the nurse listed above are discussed in more detail in the next section.

Implementation is the step of the nursing process whereby planned actions are initiated and completed. It includes tasks such as organizing and managing planned care; providing total or partial assistance with activities of daily living (ADLs); counseling and teaching the patient and significant others; providing planned care; supervising, coordinating, and evaluating the process of the delivery of care by the nursing staff (this does not include the actual delegation of care that occurs in planning or the evaluation of the patient's response to care that occurs in evaluation); and recording and sharing data related to the care implemented.

To implement safe nursing care designed to achieve goals and expected outcomes, the nurse must understand and follow the implementation process. In addition, the nurse must have knowledge of scientific rationales for nursing procedures; psychomotor skills to implement procedures safely; and the ability to use different strategies to effectively implement nursing care. Implementation questions will ask you to:

- Recognize steps in the implementation process
- Identify independent, dependent, and interdependent actions of the nurse
- Implement a procedure or treatment
- Identify and respond to common or uncommon outcomes in response to interventions
- Identify or respond to life-threatening or adverse events
- Prepare a patient for a procedure, treatment, or surgery
- Choose an approach that is most appropriate when implementing care
- Identify safe or unsafe practice
- Rationalize a step in a procedure
- Identify or use concepts associated with teaching
- Identify or use concepts associated with counseling
- Identify or use principles associated with motivation
- Identify or use techniques for therapeutic communication
- Recognize the relationship between a procedure and an expected outcome
- Identify when an intervention must be modified in response to a change in the patient's condition

- Identify when additional assistance is required to provide safe care
- Recognize the nurse's responsibility associated with supervising and evaluating care delivered by those to whom interventions have been delegated
- Recognize how and when to document or report care given along with the patient's response.

The critical words within a test item that indicate that the item is focused on implementation include these: dependent, independent, interdependent, change, assist, counsel, teach, give, supervise, perform, method, procedure, treatment, instruct, strategy, reassess, facilitate, provide, inform, refer, technique, motivate, delegate, and implement. See whether you can identify variations of these words indicating implementation activities in the sample items. Testing errors occur on implementation items when options are selected that:

- Implement actions outside the definition of nursing practice
- Fail to identify or appropriately respond to an adverse or life-threatening situation
- Fail to reassess the patient
- Fail to modify interventions in response to the changing needs of the patient
- Fail to identify when additional assistance is required for the delivery of safe care
- Reflect a lack of knowledge to safely implement interventions
- Do not accurately document the patient's response to the care given
- Fail to supervise and evaluate the delivery of delegated interventions

IMPLEMENT NURSING CARE

Implementation occurs when the nurse uses an intervention to help a patient meet expected outcomes. Nursing interventions can be dependent, independent, or interdependent in nature. **Dependent interventions** (physician prescribed) are interventions that require a physician's order. Administering a medication, providing IV fluids, and inserting a nasogastric tube are examples of dependent interventions because they all require a physician's order. When implementing a dependent intervention, the nurse does not blindly follow the order, but determines whether the order is correct or appropriate. A nurse who does not question and carries out an incorrect or inappropriate order is contributing to the initial error and will be held accountable.

Independent interventions (nurse prescribed) are those actions that a nurse is legally permitted to implement with no direction or supervision from others. Independent interventions do not require a physician's order. Tasks related to collecting data, providing assistance with ADLs, teaching regarding health, and counseling are in the realm of independent legal nursing practice. Encouraging coughing and deep breathing, encouraging verbalization of fears, teaching principles related to nutrition, and providing a bed bath also are examples of specific independent nursing interventions.

Interdependent interventions (collaborative) are actions implemented in partnership with other appropriate professionals. An example of an interdependent intervention is implementing actions identified in standing orders or a protocol. These situations delineate the parameters within which the nurse is permitted to administer to the patient. Protocols and standing orders are commonly found in emergency and critical care areas. Another example of an interdependent intervention would be when a physician orders, "Out of bed as tolerated." When ambulating this patient, the nurse must assess the patient's response to the activity. Based on the patient's response, the nurse can decide to terminate the activity or to increase the time and/or distance to be ambulated.

The primary nurse assigns a staff nurse to insert an indwelling urinary (Foley) catheter. What is the first thing the staff nurse should do?

    (1) Explain the procedure to the patient.

    (2) Gather all equipment at the bedside.

    (3) Check the physician's order.

    (4) Wash hands thoroughly.

This question is designed to test your ability to recognize that the insertion of a urinary catheter is a dependent nursing intervention that requires a physician's order.

Nursing care is delivered by using **implementation methods.** These methods include:

- **Assisting with Activities of Daily Living (ADLs):** Assisting with ADLs refers to activities associated with eating, dressing, hygiene, grooming, toileting, transfer, and locomotion. Situations associated with needs addressing ADLs can be acute, chronic, temporary, permanent, or related to maintaining or restoring function. ADLs are an integral part of daily life, and therefore their implementation is often tested.

- **Teaching:** To effectively teach in the cognitive (learning new information), psychomotor (learning new skills), and affective (developing new attitudes, values, and beliefs) domains, the nurse must apply teaching-learning principles to motivate patients to learn and grow. Health teaching activities are incorporated throughout the health-illness continuum, in a variety of health care delivery settings, and across the age span. For these reasons, teaching principles are often incorporated into patient situations in test questions.

- **Responding to Life-Threatening Situations:** Responding to adverse or life-threatening situations requires the use of clinical judgment and decision making. Activities such as stopping the administration of an antibiotic in response to a patient's allergic reaction, initiating cardiopulmonary resuscitation, implementing the abdominal thrust procedure (Heimlich maneuver), and administering emergency medication are examples of measures that can be implemented in life-threatening situations. Most of these interventions address the basic physiological needs required for survival and are therefore frequently tested.

- **Implementing Preventive Actions:** These actions are activities that help the patient to avoid a health problem. Administering immunizations, applying an allergy bracelet, and leading a group on weight reduction are examples of preventive measures. Because today's society emphasizes health, wellness, and illness prevention, these topics are often tested.

- **Performing Technical Skills:** The nurse must know how and when to implement a procedure and the expected outcomes of the procedure. Inserting a urinary catheter, providing a tube feeding, administering an enema, and preparing a patient for a diagnostic test are examples of procedures implemented by the nurse. Steps, principles, rationales, and expected outcomes associated with procedures are concepts that are often tested in multiple-choice questions.

- **Implementing Interpersonal Interventions:** These activities help the nurse to assist a patient to adapt to changes that are caused by loss, illness, disability, or stress. Emotional care can be provided by activities such as promoting a supportive environment, motivating a patient, providing for privacy, addressing spiritual needs, and accepting feelings. Counseling is also a component of interpersonal interventions. To effectively counsel, the nurse must apply therapeutic communication principles to explore patients' feelings and meet their emotional needs. Another aspect of interpersonal interventions is coordinating health care activities. When the nurse collaborates with others and coordinates health care activities, the nurse functions as the patient's advocate. People are complex human beings, and nursing care must address the mental, physical, emotional, and spiritual realms. Because these realms are so important, associated nursing interventions are often tested in multiple-choice questions.

- **Supervising and Evaluating the Effectiveness of Delegated Interventions:** Occasionally, the nurse who formulates the plan of care delegates all or part of the implementation of the plan to other members of the nursing team. Uncomplicated and basic interventions, particularly those associated with ADLs, are often delegated to a nursing assistant or licensed practical nurse. The nurse who delegates is responsible for the plan of care and is accountable for ensuring that the care is delivered according to standards of the profession. With the changing rules in healthcare delivery, the importance of the nurse as manager is increasing and is therefore tested.

- **Reporting and Recording:** Once care is given, it is recorded along with an assessment of the patient's response to care. Written communication establishes a permanent document of the care patients receive and their responses. In addition to documenting, the nurse may verbally report to other health team members the care that was provided along with the patients' responses. Also, verbal reports are given at the change of shifts and when responding to an emergency. Because communication is essential to the provision of quality care, it is a method of implementation that is often tested.

The following sample items are examples of multiple-choice questions that test concepts associated with methods of implementation.

SAMPLE ITEM 5–28

A patient has an order for a 2-gram sodium diet. What should the nurse teach this patient to avoid?

    (1) Salt

    (2) Sugar

    (3) Liquids

    (4) Margarine

This item tests your ability to identify a principle that needs to be taught to a patient. Teaching is an implementation method used by the nurse to assist a patient to meet a health need. Mainly, this question tests your ability to recognize that salt is sodium, and therefore, a patient on a 2-gram sodium diet should be taught to avoid it.

SAMPLE ITEM 5–29

What should the nurse do when a patient vomits while in the supine position?

    (1) Position the patient's head between the knees.

    (2) Raise the patient to a high-Fowler's position.

    (3) Transfer the patient to the bathroom.

    (4) Turn the patient on the side.

This item is designed to test your ability to appropriately respond to an event. To answer this question, you need to recognize that it is important to quickly assist the patient to expectorate the vomitus to avoid aspiration. In addition, you need to know that turning the patient on his or her side is putting the patient in the best position to facilitate drainage of matter from the mouth. Responding to an event by implementing an action is an implementation question.

SAMPLE ITEM 5–30

What should the nurse do to provide support for the patient who complains of nausea?

(1) Give mouth care every hour.

(2) Delay meals until the nausea passes.

(3) Position the emesis basin in easy reach.

(4) Explain that the nausea will lessen with time.

Implementing actions that anticipate an event is a step of implementation. The word "provide" in the stem gives you a clue that this is an implementation question. To answer this question correctly, you need to know that a complaint of nausea is a precursor to vomiting and that providing an emesis basin will support the nauseated patient.

SAMPLE ITEM 5–31

What is the underlying rationale for turning a patient every 2 hours?

(1) To relieve pressure

(2) To assess skin condition

(3) To ensure that skin is clean and dry

(4) To provide massage to bony prominences

This item tests your ability to recognize the correct rationale for a nursing procedure. Relieving pressure is the rationale for regularly turning a patient. To implement safe and effective care, nurses need to have a strong understanding of the scientific rationales for nursing actions.

SAMPLE ITEM 5–32

When administering medications, the safest way to identify a patient is to:

(1) Ask the patient his or her name.

(2) Check the identification bracelet.

(3) Call the patient's name and observe the response.

(4) Double-check the medication administration record.

This test item is designed to see if you can correctly identify a step in a procedure. Although more than one of the options might be an action implemented by the nurse, the question is asking you to choose the best answer from all the options offered. In this set of options, checking the identification bracelet is the most reliable and safest method to verify a patient's identity.

SAMPLE ITEM 5–33

To provide aseptically safe perineal care to all female patients, what should the nurse do?

(1) Use different parts of the washcloth with each stroke.

(2) Apply deodorant spray to the perineal area.

(3) Sprinkle talcum powder on the perineum.

(4) Cleanse the labia in a circular motion.

This item tests your ability to identify a step in a procedure based on a specific scientific principle (asepsis). To answer this question correctly, you need to know that medical asepsis is promoted when the spread of microorganisms is limited. Using one area of the washcloth for each stroke when washing the perineum contributes to aseptically safe perineal care. Identifying a step in a procedure is an implementation question.

SAMPLE ITEM 5–34

The registered nurse (RN) delegates the implementation of a nasogastric tube feeding to a licensed practical nurse (LPN). Which statement is accurate in terms of the responsibility of the RN?

(1) The RN should implement the planned care and not delegate.

(2) The LPN should respectfully refuse to implement this care.

(3) The LPN is accountable for his or her own actions.

(4) The RN is responsible for delegated care.

This item tests your ability to recognize that a nurse who delegates care to another nursing staff member is responsible for supervising and evaluating the delivery of that care. This is an important component of implementation and is a concept that may be tested.

SAMPLE ITEM 5–35

When the nurse signs a turning and positioning schedule form, it indicates that the patient:

(1) Received a backrub with lotion

(2) Was turned at the time initialed

(3) Received range-of-motion (ROM) exercises

(4) Was encouraged to turn to a different position

This question tests your ability to recognize the purpose of a turning and positioning flow sheet. Documenting the care given is a component of the step of implementation.

Evaluation

Evaluation is the fifth and final step of the nursing process. Evaluation is a process that consists of four steps that must be implemented after care is delivered if the effectiveness of the nursing care is to be determined. The evaluation process includes identifying patient responses to care, comparing a patient's actual responses to the expected outcomes, analyzing the factors that affected the outcomes for the purpose of drawing conclusions about the success or failure of specific nursing activities, and modifying the nursing care plan when necessary. Evaluation questions will ask you to:

- Identify the steps in the evaluation process
- Identify actual outcomes as being desirable or undesirable
- Identify whether an outcome in a situation is met or not met
- Identify progress or lack of progress toward an expected outcome
- Recognize the need to modify the plan of care in response to a change in the status of the patient or a plan that is ineffective
- Recognize that the process of evaluation is continuous
- Recognize that the nursing process is dynamic and cyclical

The critical words within a test item that indicate that the item is focused on evaluation include these: expected, met, desired, compared, succeeded, failed, achieved, modified, reassess, ineffective, effective, response, compliance, noncompliance, and evaluate. See whether you can identify variations of these words indicating evaluation activities in the sample items. Most testing errors occur on evaluation items when options are selected that:

- Do not thoroughly and accurately reassess the patient after care is implemented
- Fail to appropriately cluster new data
- Fail to determine the significance of new data
- Come to inappropriate or inaccurate conclusions
- Fail to modify the plan of care in response to the changing needs of the patient or in response to an ineffective plan.

IDENTIFY PATIENT RESPONSES

The process of evaluation begins with a reassessment that collects new information. Once nursing care is implemented, the patient is reassessed and new clusters of data are identified and their significance determined. In the nursing literature, the term "evaluation" has often been used interchangeably with the term "assessment," which causes confusion. It is important to remember that assessment is only one component in the process of evaluation. The nurse needs to first reassess to identify the patient's responses (outcomes). Patient outcomes are the actual patient responses to nursing care. These data are then clustered and their significance determined before the actual patient outcomes can be compared with expected outcomes.

SAMPLE ITEM 5-36

A patient on a bland diet complains about a poor appetite. What would be the MOST effective way to determine whether the patient's nutritional needs have been met?

    (1) Institute a 3-day food intake study.

    (2) Weigh the patient at the end of the week.

    (3) Request an order for a dietary assessment.

    (4) Compare a current weight with the weight history.

This item is designed to test your ability to identify a common way to evaluate a patient's nutritional status. In this situation, the results of nutritional care are determined by comparing a current weight assessment with a previous weight assessment in an effort to identify any gain or loss in the patient's weight. Once a change in status is identified, a conclusion about the effectiveness of care can be determined from the data.

72 COMPARE ACTUAL OUTCOMES WITH EXPECTED OUTCOMES

Patient outcomes are the criteria that are established for the evaluation of nursing care. A comparison is made between the actual outcomes and the expected outcomes to determine the effectiveness of nursing interventions. By comparing the new data with expected outcomes it is possible to determine which outcomes have been achieved and which have not been achieved. The closer the patient's actual outcomes are to expected outcomes, the more positive the evaluation. Negative evaluations reflect situations in which the expected outcomes were not achieved. Negative evaluations indicate that an error occurred in the implementation of the nursing process or that nursing care was ineffective. An example of a positive evaluation would be: A nurse crushes and mixes medication with applesauce, expecting that the patient will have less difficulty swallowing the medication, and following administration, the nurse determines that this intervention was effective because the patient had no difficulty swallowing the medication.

SAMPLE ITEM 5–37

The nurse would know that the patient understood the teaching about a 2-gram sodium diet when from a menu that patient selects:

    (1) Milk

    (2) Fruit

    (3) Celery

    (4) Vegetables

This item is designed to test your ability to recognize that of all the options presented, fruit has the least amount of sodium. In addition, the stem is worded in such a way that it requires the nurse to evaluate the correctness of the patient's response. The action described in the stem is an attempt to evaluate the patient's understanding of the teaching provided.

ANALYZE FACTORS THAT AFFECT ACTUAL OUTCOMES OF CARE

Once a determination of whether care is effective or not is made, the nurse must come to some conclusions about the potential factors that contributed to the success or failure of the plan of care. If a plan of care is ineffective, the nurse must examine what contributed to its failure. This requires the nurse to start at step one of the nursing process with assessment and work through the entire process again in an attempt to identify why the plan was ineffective. Questions the nurse must ask include these: "Was the original assessment accurate?" "Was the nursing diagnosis accurate, and did it include all the *related-to* factors?" "Was the goal realistic?" "Were the outcomes measurable?" "Were the interventions consistently implemented?" When plans of care fail because *related-to* factors used in the NANDA terminology were incorrectly identified or omitted, then nursing strategies generally were inappropriate or were never implemented.

SAMPLE ITEM 5–38

A patient returns to the clinic after taking a 7-day course of antibiotic therapy and is still exhibiting signs of a urinary tract infection. What should be the nurse's initial action?

    (1) Arrange for the physician to order a different antibiotic.

    (2) Obtain another urine specimen for a culture and sensitivity.

(3) Determine if the patient took the medication as prescribed.

(4) Make an appointment for the patient to be seen by the physician.

This item is designed to test your ability to recognize that the nurse must analyze the factors that influence outcomes of care. Options 1, 2, and 4 can be eliminated because these actions immediately move to an intervention before collecting more information. They may be unnecessary, depending on the information gleaned from option 3. Option 3 is the correct answer because compliance with a medication administration schedule will influence the effectiveness of the medication.

MODIFY THE PLAN OF CARE

Once it is determined that a plan of care is ineffective, the plan must be modified. The changes in the plan of care are based on new patient assessments, nursing diagnoses, goals, and/or nursing strategies that are designed to address the specific needs of the patient. The modified plan must then be implemented and the whole evaluation process begins again. The process of evaluation is continuous.

SAMPLE ITEM 5–39

A newly admitted patient was provided with a regular diet consisting of three traditional meals a day. After a week it was identified that the patient was eating only approximately 50 percent of the meals and was losing weight. What should the nurse do?

(1) Assist the patient until meals are completed

(2) Schedule several between-meal supplements

(3) Change the plan of care to provide five small meals daily

(4) Secure an order to increase the number of calories provided

This item is designed to test your ability to recognize that the nursing plan of care must be changed when care is ineffective. The new actions must be within the legal definition of nursing and address the specific needs of the patient.

Answers and Rationales for Sample Items in Chapter 5

An asterisk (*) is in front of the rationale that explains the correct answer.

ASSESSMENT

5–1 * ① An assessment must be made to determine if any intervention is necessary to stabilize an injured body part before moving a patient; moving an injured person could exacerbate an injury.

② Moving an injured patient before assessment and stabilization could exacerbate an injury.

③ Same as #2.

④ Reporting the incident would be done after the patient is safe; this does not address the need for an immediate assessment of the patient's condition.

5–2 * ① Nurses must always assess a patient before having the patient walk to ensure that the patient has the strength to ambulate safely.

② This is concerned with implementing care; assessment of the patient's strength is the priority.

③ Same as #2.

④ The patient's strength must be assessed before the transfer to the wheelchair; not all patients using a wheelchair need a vest restraint to maintain safety.

5–3 ① These are within the normal range.

② Same as #1.

③ Same as #1.

* ④ Twenty-eight breaths are outside the normal range; normal respirations are 14 to 20, effortless, and noiseless. This patient may be experiencing respiratory distress.

5–4 ① A nurse may permit an alert and capable patient to insert a rectal thermometer; however, if the patient has physical or cognitive deficits, this may not be possible.

② When taking a rectal temperature, the patient can be safely positioned on either the right or left side.

③ The use of an electronic thermometer is not always practical; electronic thermometers are usually not used in isolation because of the inconvenience related to the need to decontaminate equipment after use.

* ④ Lubricating a rectal thermometer is always done to facilitate entry into the rectum; a lubricant reduces resistance when inserting a thermometer past the anal sphincters.

5–5 * ① To calculate ideal body weight, the nurse needs to know the patient's height, age, and extent of bone structure.

② Daily intake reflects the amount of food the patient is ingesting; this information does not contribute to the calculation of ideal body weight.

③ Clothing size is determined by weight and inches reflecting circumference of the chest and waist; this information does not contribute to the calculation of ideal body weight.

④ Determining food preferences supports the patient's right to make choices about care; this information does not contribute to the calculation of ideal body weight.

5–6 ① Data are classified as objective or subjective, not primary. "Primary" refers to a source of data; a patient is the primary source of data.

② Objective data are measured or assessed by one of the senses.
* ③ Subjective data are collected when the patient shares feelings, perceptions, sensations, and thoughts.
④ Types of data are classified as objective or subjective, not secondary. "Secondary" refers to sources of data; a secondary source of data produces information from a source other than the patient.

5–7 ① The wife is a secondary source, not a primary source.
② The wife is a secondary source, not a tertiary source.
③ The wife is not a subjective source. "Subjective" refers to a type of data; subjective data are collected when the patient shares feelings, perceptions, sensations, and thoughts.
* ④ Family members are secondary sources. Secondary sources provide supplemental information about the patient.

5–8 ① A letter is considered verbal communication; words are written.
* ② Holding hands is nonverbal communication; a message is transmitted without using words.
③ Sounds may or may not communicate meaning; a sound that communicates a meaning is considered verbal communication.
④ A telephone message is verbal communication; words are generally spoken in a telephone message.

5–9 * ① Light yellow is the normal color of urine; this color indicates that a patient is receiving adequate fluid intake.
② Dark would indicate concentrated urine; reduced fluid intake will cause urine to be dark yellow.
③ A light amber color may reflect concentrated urine, an infection, or a small amount of blood in the urine.
④ A dark amber color may reflect very concentrated urine, an infection, or blood in the urine.

5–10 * ① The reading should be verified by retaking the blood pressure because the nurse may have made a mistake when originally taking the blood pressure.
② Taking the other vital signs is done once the initial blood pressure is verified; once one vital sign is identified as abnormal, all the vital signs should be assessed.
③ This may be done after the blood pressure is verified and all the vital signs are taken.
④ Same as #3.

5–11 * ① This is correct; nursing care should be documented immediately after it is provided. There are 30 cc in each ounce; therefore, the patient received 240 cc.
② This would be too early to evaluate the patient's response to fluid intake.
③ This would be too early to expect the patient to void.
④ Mouth care is usually not required after drinking fluid; mouth care is generally provided on awakening, after meals, and at bedtime.

ANALYSIS

5–12 ① Expressive aphasia is not associated with the data cluster presented in the stem. Expressive aphasia is an inability to communicate basic thoughts either in writing or verbally.

* ② This could contribute to a potential for aspiration; it is associated with the data identified in the stem and together they present a cluster of information that is significant.

③ An inability to perform ADLs is not associated with the data cluster identified in the stem; this is associated with the inability of the patient to provide for self-care.

④ Incontinence of urine and stool is not associated with the data cluster identified in the stem; this is associated with hygiene needs and supports the fact that the patient is at risk for altered skin integrity, not aspiration.

5–13 * ① Patients who are immobilized are subject to increased pressure over bony prominences with a subsequent decrease in circulation to tissues.

② This is unrelated to the development of pressure ulcers.

③ Same as #2.

④ Same as #2.

5–14 ① Acting-out behaviors commonly reflect anger.

② Refusing to believe or accept a situation, not depressive adaptations, are reflective of denial.

* ③ Depression is commonly exhibited by patients with adaptations, such as avoiding contact with others, withdrawing, loss of appetite (anorexia), and difficulty falling asleep (insomnia).

④ Acceptance is related to the final step of grieving; a patient reconciles and accepts the situation and is at peace.

5–15 ① The patient is seeking independence, not trying to be left alone.

② The primary motivation for this behavior is to feel independent, not to belong or be accepted.

* ③ This is correct; the patient is attempting to perform self-care to demonstrate the ability to be self-sufficient.

④ The patient is seeking independence, not trying to manipulate the staff.

5–16 * ① These patient adaptations are related to a decreased blood volume associated with postoperative hemorrhage.

② With this adaptation, the patient would more likely be hypertensive with a rapid pulse.

③ Same as #2.

④ Same as #2.

5–17 ① This statement is identifying a need, not a nursing diagnosis.

② This statement is a combination of an expected outcome and an intervention, not a nursing diagnosis.

③ This statement is an incorrectly worded nursing diagnosis; a stroke is not something a nurse can treat.

* ④ This statement is an appropriately worded nursing diagnosis that uses NANDA terminology; it contains a health problem appropriate for nursing interventions.

PLANNING

5–18 ① This is correct wording for a goal, but it is unrealistic; it takes 3 to 5 days for a new colostomy to function.

② This is a long-term goal, not a short-term goal.

③ This is the problem statement, the first part of a nursing diagnosis.

* ④ This is a short-term goal; it is patient centered, specific, and the word "remain" reflects the time frame.

5–19 * ① Providing for a patient's oxygenation is essential to maintain life and is always the priority.
② This is important; however, providing for a patent airway takes priority.
③ Same as #2.
④ Same as #2.

5–20 * ① Washing the hands with soap and water mechanically removes microorganisms from the skin; handwashing is the most effective way to prevent cross-contamination.
② Using contact precautions is unnecessary; this is only necessary when a patient has an extremely virulent microorganism.
③ Antibiotics are usually given not to prevent infection, but to treat it.
④ Although foot-operated linen hampers would contain and limit the spread of microorganisms, they are not the most effective intervention to prevent cross-contamination.

5–21 * ① An occupied bed is made for a patient on complete bed rest; this patient is not permitted out of bed.
② This is inappropriate; all the linens should be changed regularly and whenever necessary.
③ This is unnecessary; an occupied bed can be made without a mechanical lift just by turning the patient.
④ This is unsafe; a patient on bed rest is not allowed out of bed for any reason unless directed by a physician's order.

5–22 ① The patient can be transferred out of bed while the linen is changed.
② Same as #1.
③ Same as #1.
* ④ Patients on bed rest must remain in bed when the linens are changed; this is called "making an occupied bed."

5–23 * ① This statement contains an expected outcome. The phrase "50 percent of every meal" is a specific (measurable) outcome.
② This statement is the problem statement of a nursing diagnosis, not an expected outcome.
③ This statement is the nurse's goal, not an expected outcome.
④ This statement is a planned intervention, not an expected outcome.

5–24 * ① The nurse manager has an obligation to ensure that all patients' needs will be appropriately met; this is the only option that addresses this concept.
② This is inappropriate; all patients must have their needs met.
③ Providing only essential care does not ensure that appropriate care will be provided; this action will increase anxiety and cause patients to doubt the quality of care being provided.
④ Once the nurse assumes a course of duty, the nurse is responsible for the care that is delivered.

5–25 ① Giving care as quickly as possible will increase the demand on the patient's respiratory system. This increases activity, which in turn increases oxygen needs; rushing may cause the patient to become upset.

② This does not address the patient's respiratory needs; the patient may need a full bath.

* ③ Providing rest periods conserves energy; this reduces the strain of activity by decreasing the demand for oxygenation, which in turn decreases the rate and labor of respirations.

④ The patient's dyspnea cannot be ignored; the plan must be changed to allow for rest periods to reduce the physical demand for oxygen.

5–26 ① When a patient is unresponsive to common nursing interventions, the nurse needs to consult with an expert nurse, not a medical specialist.

② The physical therapist is a specialist in the area of assisting a patient to achieve or maintain physical mobility; the nurse needs to consult with an expert nurse, not a physical therapist.

③ The physician is responsible for the patient's medical care and is not an expert in providing nursing care.

* ④ The clinical nurse specialist is educated and prepared to provide expert assistance when other members of the health team seek solutions to difficult clinical nursing problems.

IMPLEMENTATION

5–27 ① The procedure should be explained after the order is verified.

② Equipment is gathered after the order is verified and the procedure is explained to the patient.

* ③ Inserting an indwelling urinary catheter is a dependent nursing intervention and requires a physician's order that must be verified by the nurse implementing the order.

④ Handwashing is done once the order is verified and the procedure is explained to the patient.

5–28 * ① Salt used to season meals contains sodium; sodium must be avoided when a patient is on a 2-gram sodium diet.

② Sugar is avoided when a patient is on a reduced-calorie or diabetic diet, not on a 2-gram sodium diet.

③ Fluids need to be avoided when the patient is on fluid restriction, not on a 2-gram sodium diet; however, the patient must be alert to avoid fluids that are high in sodium such as diet sodas.

④ Margarine is to be avoided when a patient is on a low-fat diet, not on a 2-gram sodium diet.

5–29 ① Positioning the head between the knees does not support or protect the vomiting patient.

② The high-Fowler's position does not facilitate the exit of vomitus from the mouth.

③ This is unsafe; vomiting takes energy and could cause the patient to become weak during the transfer.

* ④ Turning the patient on his or her side drains the mouth via gravity and reduces the risk of aspiration.

5–30 ① This is unnecessary; oral hygiene is sufficient every 8 hours and whenever necessary.

② Delaying meals is inappropriate; nausea may be a long-standing problem.

        * ③ An emesis basin provides physical and emotional comfort; the emesis basin collects vomitus rather than soiling the bed linens and reduces the patient's concern regarding soiling.

        ④ This action provides false reassurance; the nurse cannot predict when nausea will subside.

5–31 * ① Turning relieves pressure from body weight and permits circulation to return to the area; prolonged pressure can cause cell death from lack of oxygen and nutrients needed to sustain cellular metabolism.

        ② Although this should be done, relieving pressure is the main purpose of regularly turning and positioning a patient.

        ③ Same as #2.

        ④ Same as #2.

5–32 ① This is unsafe; the patient could be cognitively impaired.

        * ② Checking the identification band is the safest method to identify a patient; it is the most reliable because each patient on admission receives an identification bracelet with his or her name and an identification number.

        ③ Same as #1.

        ④ This will not verify the name of the person.

5–33 * ① This provides a clean surface for each stroke when washing; it avoids contaminating the meatus with soiled portions of the cloth.

        ② For some patients this can be irritating, contribute to the risk of impaired skin integrity, and it does not remove bacteria.

        ③ Same as #2.

        ④ Using a circular motion is unsafe; this would bring soiled matter into contact with the urinary meatus. Washing from the pubis toward the rectum using a clean portion of the cloth with each stroke, not circular motions, limits contamination of the meatus.

5–34 ① This is unnecessary; a nurse can delegate tasks to other qualified nursing staff members as long as delegated tasks are supervised and their delivery evaluated.

        ② It is inappropriate to refuse to implement delegated tasks as long as the tasks are within the legal definition of LPN practice and the LPN can safely implement the task; the question is asking which of the options is accurate in terms of the responsibility of the RN, not the LPN.

        ③ This is a true statement; however, the question is asking which of the options is accurate in terms of the responsibility of the RN, not the LPN.

        * ④ This is an accurate statement; the delegating nurse is responsible for supervising and evaluating the delivery of delegated tasks.

5–35 ① This care should be implemented when a patient is turned and positioned; however, the turning and positioning form only indicates that the patient was turned and positioned.

        * ② This indicates that turning and positioning were implemented as planned.

        ③ Same as #1.

        ④ A patient must actually be turned and positioned before the nurse signs the turning and positioning flow sheet; although a patient might be encouraged to turn, it does not mean that the patient was actually turned.

EVALUATION

5–36   ①   This might be done after it is determined that the patient has lost weight.

          ②   It is unnecessary to wait; the patient's nutritional status can be assessed immediately by comparing a current weight with the patient's weight history.

          ③   Same as #1.

      * ④   Measuring a patient's weight and comparing the weight with a previous weight is an easy and quick way to determine a patient's nutritional status.

5–37   ①   This has more sodium than fruit.

      * ②   Fruit has the least amount of sodium compared to the distractors.

          ③   Same as #1.

          ④   Same as #1.

5–38   ①   This would be inappropriate before collecting additional data associated with the present plan of care; this may be necessary later.

          ②   Same as #1.

      * ③   Determining compliance with the medical regimen is the priority; antibiotics must be taken routinely and consistently to maintain adequate blood levels of the drug.

          ④   Same as #1.

5–39   ①   Patients must not be forced to eat all their meals; the portions may be too large for an anorectic patient to ingest.

          ②   Adding between-meal supplements is a dependent intervention and requires a physician's order.

      * ③   Arranging for five small meals daily is an independent intervention and does not require a physician's order; small frequent feedings spread the meals throughout the day and provide a volume that is not as overwhelming as a full meal.

          ④   The problem is not the number of calories provided on the tray but the amount of food the patient is able to ingest at any one time.

Test-Taking Techniques

Performing well on multiple-choice questions requires both roots and wings. The previous chapters provided you with roots by giving you information about formulating a positive mental attitude, using critical thinking, and exploring a variety of study skills and an understanding of the multiple-choice question and the fundamentals of the nursing process. This chapter attempts to provide you with the wings necessary to "fly through" multiple-choice questions. Flying through multiple-choice questions has nothing to do with speed; it relates to being test-wise and able to navigate through complex information with ease.

Tests in nursing involve complex information that has depth and breadth. As well as having its own body of knowledge, nursing draws from a variety of disciplines, such as sociology, psychology, and anatomy and physiology. To perform well on a nursing examination, you must understand and integrate the subject matter. Nothing can replace effective study habits or knowledge about the subject being tested. However, being test-wise can maximize the application of the information you possess. Being test-wise entails specific techniques related to individual question analysis and general techniques related to conquering the challenge of an examination. One rationale for learning how to use these techniques is to provide you with skills that increase your command over the testing situation. If you are in control, you will maintain a positive attitude and increase your chances of selecting the correct answers. When you have knowledge and are test-wise, you should fly through a test by gliding and soaring, rather than by flapping and fluttering.

Specific Test-Taking Techniques

A specific test-taking technique is a strategy that uses skill and forethought to analyze a test item before selecting an answer. A technique is not a gimmick but a method of examining a question with consideration and thoughtfulness in the hope that the outcome will be the selection of the correct answer. When an item has four options, the chance of selecting the correct answer is one out of four, or 25 percent. When you eliminate one distractor, the chance of selecting the correct answer is one out of three, or 33.3 percent. If you are able to throw out two distractors, the chance of selecting the correct answer is one out of two, or 50 percent. Each time you successfully eliminate a distractor, you dramatically increase your chances of correctly answering the question.

Before you attempt to answer a question, break the question down into its components. First, read the stem. What is it actually asking? It may be helpful to paraphrase the stem to focus in on its content. Then, try to answer the question being asked in your own words before looking at the options. Hopefully, one of the options will be similar to your answer. Then examine the other options and try to identify the correct answer. If you know, understand, and can apply the information being tested, you can often recognize the correct answer. However, do not be tempted to select an option too quickly, without careful thought. An option may contain accurate information, but it may not be correct because it does not answer the question asked in the stem. Be careful. Each option deserves equal consideration.

Use test-taking techniques for every question. The use of test-taking techniques becomes necessary when you are unsure of the answer, because each distractor that you are able to eliminate will increase your chances of selecting the correct answer. Most nursing students are able to reduce the number of plausible answers to two. However, contrary to popular belief, multiple-choice questions in nursing have only one correct answer. Use everything in your arsenal to conquer the multiple-choice question test: effective studying, a positive mental attitude, and, last but not least, test-taking techniques.

The correct answers for the sample items in this chapter and the rationales for all the options are at the end of the chapter.

IDENTIFY KEY WORDS IN THE STEM THAT INDICATE NEGATIVE POLARITY

Read the stem slowly and carefully. Look for key words such as not, except, never, contraindicated, unacceptable, avoid, unrelated, violate, and least. These words indicate a negative polarity, and the question being asked is probably concerned with what is false. Some words that have a negative polarity are not as obvious as others. A negatively worded stem asks you to identify an exception, detect an error, or recognize nursing interventions that are unacceptable or contraindicated. If you read a stem and all the options appear correct, reread the stem because you may have missed a key negative word. These words are sometimes brought to your attention by an underline (not), italics (*except*), boldface (**never**), or capitals (VIOLATE). Many nursing examinations avoid questions with a negative polarity. However, examples of these items are included for your information.

SAMPLE ITEM 6–1

Which action would violate medical asepsis when making an occupied bed?

(1) Wearing gloves when changing the linen

(2) Returning unused linen to the linen closet

(3) Using the old top sheet for the new bottom sheet

(4) Tucking clean linen against the springs of the bed

The key term in this stem is *violate*. The stem is asking you to identify the option that does **not** follow correct medical aseptic technique. If you misread the stem and were looking for the answer that indicated correct medical aseptic technique, then there would be more than one correct answer. When this happens, reread the stem for a word with negative polarity. In this item you had to be particularly careful because the word *violate* is not emphasized for your attention.

SAMPLE ITEM 6-2

A patient is on a low-sodium diet. Before discharge, the patient should be taught to *avoid*:

(1) Stewed fruit

(2) Luncheon meats

(3) Whole-grain cereal

(4) Green leafy vegetables

The key word in this stem is *avoid.* The stem is asking you to select the food that a patient on a low-sodium diet should **not** eat. If you misread the question and were looking for foods that are permitted on a low-sodium diet, then there would be more than one correct answer. When there appears to be more than one correct answer, reread the stem for a key negative word that you may have missed.

SAMPLE ITEM 6-3

When rubbing a patient's back, the nurse should NEVER:

(1) Knead the skin

(2) Wipe off excess lotion

(3) Use a continuous firm stroke

(4) Put pressure over the vertebrae

The key in this stem is NEVER. The stem is asking you to identify which option is **not** an acceptable practice associated with a backrub. If you missed the word NEVER and were looking for what the nurse should do for a backrub, then there would be more than one correct answer. This should clue you to the fact that you may have missed a key negative word.

IDENTIFY KEY WORDS IN THE STEM THAT SET A PRIORITY

Read the stem carefully while looking for key words such as first, initially, best, priority, and most. These words modify what is being asked. This type of question requires you to put a value on each option and then place them in rank order. If the question asks what the nurse should do first, what the initial action by the nurse should be, or what the best response would be, then rank the options in order of importance from 1 to 4 with the most desirable option as number 1 and the least desirable option as number 4. The correct answer would be the option that you ranked number 1. If you are having difficulty ranking the options, eliminate the option that you believe is most wrong among all the options. Next, eliminate the option you believe is most wrong from among the remaining three options. At this point you are down to two options, and your chance of selecting the correct answer is 50 percent. When key words such as "most important" are used, frequently all of the options may be appropriate nursing care for the situation; how-ever, only one of the options is the **most** important. When all the options appear logical for the situation, reread the stem to identify a key word that asks you to place a priority on the options. These words are occasionally emphasized by an underline, *italics,* **boldface,** or CAPITALS.

SAMPLE ITEM 6–4

The nurse is assigned to care for a patient who is incontinent of urine and stool. What should the nurse apply to *best* protect this patient's skin?

(1) A petroleum-type jelly

(2) An incontinence pad

(3) Talcum powder

(4) Corn starch

The key term in this stem is *best*. Each of these options is something a nurse might do for the incontinent patient. The stem is asking you to place a value on each option and decide which nursing intervention **best** protects the skin when compared to the other options. If you are having difficulty ranking these options, eliminate the option that is most wrong. Although an incontinence pad absorbs urine and is often used for incontinent patients, it holds excreta next to the skin and actually promotes skin breakdown. Eliminate option 2. Continue to eliminate options you believe are wrong, and then make your final selection of the correct answer.

SAMPLE ITEM 6–5

What should be the nurse's <u>first</u> action before administering an enema?

(1) Verify the physician's order.

(2) Collect the appropriate equipment.

(3) Arrange for the bathroom to be empty.

(4) Inform the patient about the procedure.

The key word in this stem is <u>first.</u> Each of these options includes a step that is part of the procedure for administering an enema. You must decide which option is the first step among the four options presented. Before you can teach a patient, collect equipment, or actually administer the enema, you need to know the type of enema ordered. The type of enema will influence the other steps of the procedure. If option 1 were different, such as "Use medical asepsis to dispose of contaminated articles," then the correct answer among these four options would be option 4. You can choose the first step of a procedure only from among the options presented.

SAMPLE ITEM 6–6

A patient has significant short-term memory loss and does not remember the primary nurse from day to day. When the patient asks, "Who are you?" what would be the *most appropriate* response?

(1) "You know me. I take care of you every day."

(2) "Don't worry. I'm the same nurse you had yesterday."

(3) "My name is Sue Clark. I am the nurse caring for you."

(4) Say nothing, because it would probably upset the patient.

The key words in this stem are *most appropriate*. Potential responses by the nurse are the options in this question. You are asked to select the **best** or **most suitable** response from among the four options presented. You may dislike all of the statements. You may even think of a response that you personally prefer to the offered options. You cannot rewrite the question. You must select your answer from the options presented in the item. The words *most appropriate* are not highlighted in this item, and therefore you must be diligent when reading the stem.

IDENTIFY CLUES IN THE STEM

Generally the stem is short and contains only the information needed to make it clear and specific. Therefore, a word or phrase in the stem may provide a hint for choosing the correct answer. A clue is the intentional or unintentional use of a word or phrase that leads you to the correct answer. Most often a clue is a word or phrase that is important because of its relationship to another word or phrase in the stem (see Item 6–7). Sometimes a word or phrase in the stem is significant because it is similar to or a paraphrase of a word or phrase in the correct answer (see Item 6–8). Occasionally a word or phrase in the stem is identical to a word or phrase in the correct answer and is called a **clang association** (see Item 6–9). Every word in the stem is important, but some words are more significant than others. The identification of important words and the analysis of the significance of these words in relation to the stem and the options require critical thinking.

SAMPLE ITEM 6–7

To meet a patient's basic physiological need according to Maslow's hierarchy of needs, what should the nurse do?

    (1) Pull the curtain when the patient is on a bedpan.

    (2) Maintain the patient in functional alignment.

    (3) Respond to the call light immediately.

    (4) Raise both side rails on the bed.

An important word in the stem is *physiological*. It is an intentional use of a word to specifically limit consideration to one aspect of Maslow's theory.

SAMPLE ITEM 6–8

What should the nurse do to help meet a patient's self-esteem needs?

    (1) Encourage the patient to perform self-care when he or she can.

    (2) Suggest that the family visit the patient more often.

    (3) Anticipate needs before the patient requests help.

    (4) Assist the patient with bathing and grooming.

An important word in the stem is *self-esteem*. The word "self-esteem" is similar to the word "self-care." Thoughtfully examine option 1. An option that incorporates words that are similar to words in the stem is often the correct answer.

SAMPLE ITEM 6–9

What should the nurse do to meet a patient's basic physical needs?

    (1) Pull the curtain when providing care.

    (2) Answer the call bell immediately.

    (3) Administer physical hygiene.

    (4) Obtain vital signs.

An important word in the stem is *physical*. It is a clue that should provide a hint that option 3 is the correct answer. The use of the word "physical" in both the stem and the option is called a *clang association*. It is the repetitious use of a word. Examine option 3 because when a clang association occurs, it is often the correct answer.

IDENTIFY THE CENTRAL PERSON IN THE QUESTION

Test questions usually require the nurse to respond to the needs of a patient. When a stem is limited to just the patient and the nurse, the patient is almost always the central person in the question. However, some questions focus on the needs of others, such as a child, parent, spouse, or roommate. To select the correct option, you have to identify the central (significant) person in the stem. The significant person is the person who is to receive the care. Sometimes, in addition to the patient, a variety of people are included in the stem. The inclusion of others may set the stage for the question or test your ability to discriminate. These people may also distract you from who is actually the significant person in the stem. Therefore, to answer the question accurately, you must determine WHO is the central person in the question.

SAMPLE ITEM 6-10

A nurse will be going on vacation. To involve the patient in the excitement, what is the <u>best</u> thing the nurse should say?

(1) "Let me tell you about the plans for my vacation."

(2) "Tell me about some of your past vacations."

(3) "I'll bring the brochures for you to see."

(4) "What do you think about vacations?"

There are two people in this stem, the patient and the nurse. There are two clues in the stem. The first clue is "involve the patient." To involve the patient, the patient has to be active. Therefore, options 1 and 3 can be eliminated because they focus on the nurse, who is not the central person in the question. The second clue is the word <u>best.</u> The word <u>best</u> is asking you to set a priority. More than one option may include appropriate nursing care, but only one is the best action. Options 2 and 4 include appropriate nursing care. However, option 2 requires a more detailed response than option 4. Reminiscing involves more than just giving an opinion.

SAMPLE ITEM 6-11

A patient who has experienced the surgical removal of a breast (mastectomy) says to the nurse, "My husband can't look at my incision and hasn't suggested having sex since my surgery." What should be the initial action of the nurse?

(1) Arrange to speak with the husband about his concerns.

(2) Plan to teach the husband that the wife needs his support.

(3) Explore the patient's feelings about her husband's behavior.

(4) Make an appointment with Reach for Recovery for the patient.

There are three people in this stem: the patient, the husband, and the nurse. There are two clues in the stem. The first clue is the quoted statement by the patient about her husband's behavior. The second clue is the word *initial*. The word *initial* is asking you to set a priority. The situation may require one or more of these responses, but only one of them should be done first. The patient's statement reflects the patient's concern. Addressing the patient's concern should come first. The patient is the central person in this question, not the husband. Options 1 and 2 focus on the husband, who is not the central person in this question and can be eliminated. In option 4 the nurse uses a referral to sidestep the issues involved and avoid professional responsibility.

The nurse observes another nurse treating a patient in an abusive manner. The nurse's **initial** action should be to:

    (1) Tell the nurse in charge and write a report

    (2) Become a role model for the other nurse

    (3) Talk with the nurse about the incident

    (4) Reassure and calm the patient

    There are three people in this stem: the patient, the abusive nurse, and the nurse observer. There are two clues in the stem. The first clue is that a patient is being treated in an abusive manner. The second clue is the word **initial,** which is asking you to set a priority. These clues help you to identify that the patient is the significant person in the stem. The nurse must be the patient's advocate, and the patient is more important than the abusive nurse. Option 4 is the only option that puts the patient first and protects the patient.

IDENTIFY PATIENT-CENTERED OPTIONS

Nursing is a profession that is involved with providing both physical and emotional care to people. Therefore, the focus of the nurse's concern should be the patient. Items that test your ability to be patient centered tend to explore patient feelings, identify patient preferences, empower the patient, afford the patient choices, or in some other way put emphasis on the patient. Because the patient is the center of the health team, the patient is always the priority.

When assisting a patient who recently had an above-the-knee amputation to transfer into a chair, the patient starts to cry and says, "I am useless with only one leg." What would be the nurse's best response?

    (1) "You still have one good leg."

    (2) "Losing a leg must be very difficult."

    (3) "A prosthesis would make a big difference."

    (4) "You'll feel better when you can use crutches."

    Option 2 is patient centered. It focuses on the patient's feelings by using the interviewing technique of reflection. Option 1 denies the patient's feelings, and options 3 and 4 provide false reassurance. When a patient's feelings are ignored or minimized, the nurse is not being patient centered. To be patient centered, the nurse should concentrate on the patient's feelings or concerns.

An oriented patient states, "I always forget the questions I want to ask when my doctor visits me." What would be the nurse's best response?

    (1) Remind the patient of the doctor's next visit.

    (2) Suggest that a family member question the doctor.

    (3) Offer to stay with the patient when the doctor visits.

    (4) Give the patient paper and a pen to write down questions.

Option 4 is patient centered. It focuses on the patient's ability, fosters independence, and empowers the patient. Option 1 does not address the patient's concern, and options 2 and 3 promote dependence, which can lower self-esteem. Avoiding patient concerns and promoting dependence are actions that are not patient centered. To be patient centered, the nurse should encourage self-care.

SAMPLE ITEM 6–15

What should the nurse do first when combing a female patient's hair?

    (1) Moisten the hair with tap water

    (2) Apply a hair conditioner to the hair

    (3) Ask the patient how she prefers to wear her hair

    (4) Begin at the roots and comb with long, even strokes

Option 3 is patient centered. It allows choices and supports the person as an individual. Options 1, 2, and 4 do not take into consideration patient preferences. Option 4 is also wrong because combing should begin at the ends of the hair with combing progressively moving toward the roots as tangles are removed. A procedure that is begun before determining patient preferences or teaching the patient about the procedure is not patient centered. The Patient's Bill of Rights mandates that the patient has a right to considerate and respectful care and to receive information before the start of any procedure and/or treatment.

SAMPLE ITEM 6–16

A patient enjoys television programs about animals. After one of these programs the patient sadly talks about a beloved cat who died. What should be the nurse's initial response?

    (1) Tell the patient a story about a cat.

    (2) Ask the patient to share more about the cat.

    (3) Hang a picture of a cat in the patient's room.

    (4) Obtain a book about cats for the patient from the hospital library.

Option 2 is patient centered. It encourages the patient to communicate further. Options 1, 3, and 4 may eventually be done because they take into consideration the patient's interest in cats. However, they should not be the initial actions because they do not focus on the patient's feelings at this point in time. The nurse is being patient centered when encouraging additional communication and verbalization of feelings and concerns from the patient.

IDENTIFY SPECIFIC DETERMINERS IN OPTIONS

A specific determiner is a word or statement that conveys a thought or concept that has no exceptions. Words such as just, always, never, all, every, none, and only are absolute and easy to identify. They place limits on a statement that would generally be considered correct. Statements that use all-inclusive terms frequently represent broad generalizations that are usually false. Frequently these options are incorrect and can be eliminated. However, some absolutes, such as "all patients should be treated with respect," are correct. Because there are few absolutes in this world, options that contain specific determiners should be examined carefully. Be discriminating.

SAMPLE ITEM 6–17

How can the nurse best improve circulation when giving a patient a bath?

(1) Apply soap to the washcloth

(2) Keep the patient covered

(3) Use only hot water

(4) Use firm strokes

In option 3 the word *only* is a specific determiner. It allows for no exceptions. Hot water could burn the skin and would also be contraindicated for patients with sensitive skin such as children, elderly persons, and people with dermatologic problems. Because option 3 allows for no exceptions, it can be eliminated as a viable option.

SAMPLE ITEM 6–18

When providing perineal care for patients, by what action can nurses most appropriately protect themselves from microorganisms?

(1) Washing their hands before giving care

(2) Wearing clean gloves during perineal care

(3) Discarding the contaminated water in the toilet

(4) Encouraging patients to provide all of their own care

In option 4 the word *all* is a specific determiner. It is a word that obviously includes everything. Expecting patients to provide all of their own care is unreasonable, unrealistic, and could be unsafe. Option 4 can be eliminated. This raises your chances of choosing the correct answer because you have to choose from among only three options rather than four.

SAMPLE ITEM 6–19

What should the nurse do when a patient complains that the elastic straps of the oxygen face mask feel tight?

(1) Explain that the mask must always stay firmly in place.

(2) Replace the face mask with a nasal cannula.

(3) Pad the straps with gauze.

(4) Adjust the elastic straps.

In option 1 the word *always* is a specific determiner. It is an absolute term that places limits on a statement that might otherwise be true. This option can be eliminated. By deleting option 1, the chances of your selecting the correct answer become 33.3 rather than 25 percent.

IDENTIFY OPPOSITES IN OPTIONS

Sometimes an item contains two options that are the opposite of each other. They can be single words that reflect extremes on a continuum, or they can be statements that convey converse messages. When opposites appear in the options, they must be given serious consideration. One of them will be the correct answer, or they both can be eliminated from consideration. When one of the opposites is the correct answer, you are being asked to differentiate between two responses that incorporate extremes of a concept or principle. When the opposites are distractors, they are attempting to divert your attention from the correct answer. If you correctly evaluate opposite options, you can increase your chances of selecting the correct answer to 50 percent because you have reduced the plausible options to two.

SAMPLE ITEM 6–20

The progress of growth and development in all elderly people:

(1) Slips backward

(2) Moves forward

(3) Becomes slower

(4) Becomes stagnant

Options 1 and 2 are opposites. They need to be carefully considered in relation to each other and then in relation to the other options. These options are the reverse sides of a concept, movement in relation to growth and development. Options 3 and 4, although true for some individuals, are not true statements about *all* elderly people as indicated in the stem. You now must select between options 1 and 2. Option 2 is the correct answer. By focusing on options 1 and 2 and then progressively examining and deleting options 3 and 4, you have systematically scrutinized this item.

SAMPLE ITEM 6–21

The physician orders anti-embolism stockings for a patient. When should the anti-embolism stockings be put on?

(1) While the patient is still in bed

(2) When the patient complains of leg pain

(3) When the patient's feet become edematous

(4) After the patient gets out of bed in the morning

Options 1 and 4 are opposites. Examine these options first. They are contrary to each other in relation to before or after an event, getting out of bed. Now assess options 2 and 3. These options expect the nurse to apply anti-embolism stockings after a problem exists. The purpose of these stockings is to foster venous return, thereby preventing edema and discomfort. Options 2 and 3 can be omitted from further consideration. The final selection is between options 1 and 4. You have increased your chances of correctly answering the question from 25 to 50 percent. Because edema occurs when the feet are dependent, anti-embolism stockings should not be applied after the patient gets out of bed. You have arrived at the correct answer, option 1, using a methodical approach.

SAMPLE ITEM 6–22

When a patient is in bed, a wrist restraint should be tied to the:

(1) Side rails

(2) Footboard

(3) Bed frame

(4) Headboard

Options 2 and 4 are opposites. Consider these options first in relation to securing a restraint. These options are the opposite ends of a hospital bed. Neither option would be more appropriate than the other. They are probably both distractors. Now examine options 1 and 3. Side rails are movable, and a restraint must be applied to something that is stationary. Now consider option 3. The bed frame is immovable. Options 1, 2, and 4 can be eliminated, and option 3 is the correct answer. You have assessed these options in an orderly fashion, which has maximized your chances for successfully choosing the correct answer.

SAMPLE ITEM 6–23

In relation to extracellular body fluids, normal saline is:

(1) Hypertonic

(2) Hypotonic

(3) Isotonic

(4) Acidotic

Options 1 and 2 are opposites. Appraise these words in relation to each other and their relationship to body fluids and normal saline. They are extremes in the concentration of solutes. Because normal saline is equal to body fluids in the concentration of solutes, these options are probably distractors. Now examine options 3 and 4. Normal body fluids have a neutral pH (between 7.35 to 7.45). Acidosis, which is referred to in option 4, has a pH below 7.35. Option 4 can be deleted from consideration. By an efficient process of examination and elimination, you have arrived at the correct answer, option 3.

IDENTIFY EQUALLY PLAUSIBLE OR UNIQUE OPTIONS

Sometimes items contain two or more options that are similar. It is difficult to choose between two similar options because they are comparable. One option is no better or worse than the other option in relation to the statement presented in the stem. Usually equally plausible options are distractors and can be eliminated from consideration. You have now improved your chances of selecting the correct answer to 50 percent. If you find three equally plausible options when initially examining the options, the fourth option will probably be different from the others and appear unique. Children's activity books and a popular children's television program present a game based on this concept. Four pictures are presented, and the child is asked to pick out the one that is different. Which one of these is not like the others? Which one of these is not the same? For example, the picture contains three types of fruit and one vegetable, and the child is asked to identify which one is different. The correct answer to a test item can sometimes be identified by using this concept of similarities and differences.

SAMPLE ITEM 6–24

What should the nurse do to most effectively help meet a patient's basic physical safety and security needs?

(1) Serve adequate food

(2) Provide sufficient fluid

(3) Place the call bell near the patient

(4) Store the patient's valuables in the hospital safe

Options 1 and 2 are similar because they both provide nutrients. They are equally plausible when compared to each other and particularly when assessed in relation to the concepts of physical safety and security. These options are distractors and can be eliminated from consideration. By just having to choose between options 3 and 4, you have raised your chances of correctly answering the question to 50 percent.

SAMPLE ITEM 6–25

How can the nurse best promote circulation when providing a backrub?

(1) Place the patient in the prone position.

(2) Use moisturizing lotion.

(3) Apply baby powder.

(4) Knead the skin.

Options 2 and 3 use substances when performing the backrub. Because no specifics about the patient's adaptations—such as extent of perspiration or dryness of skin—are provided, these two options are comparable. Because equally plausible options are usually distractors, you can delete these options. Now evaluate the remaining options. One of them is the correct answer.

SAMPLE ITEM 6–26

What is the main reason why passive range-of-motion (PROM) exercises are performed?

(1) Increase endurance

(2) Prevent loss of mobility

(3) Strengthen muscle tone

(4) Maximize muscle atrophy

Options 1, 3, and 4 all improve something: endurance, muscle tone, and atrophy. They are alike. Option 2 is different. It prevents something from happening, loss of mobility. Option 2 is unique when compared to the presentation of the other options, and it should be given careful consideration. Even if you do not know the definition of "atrophy" and do not recognize that the loss of muscle mass should not be maximized, you can still use the test-taking technique of identifying similar and unique options. Which one of these is not like the others? Which one of these is not the same?

SAMPLE ITEM 6–27

Before performing any patient procedure, the nurse should first plan to:

(1) Shut the door

(2) Wash the hands

(3) Close the curtain

(4) Drape the patient

Options 1, 3, and 4 are similar in that they all somehow enclose the patient and provide for patient privacy. They are all plausible interventions when providing patient care. It is difficult to choose the most correct answer from among these three options. Option 2 is different. It relates to microbiological safety rather than emotional safety. Because this option is unique when compared to the other options, it should be thoroughly examined in relation to the stem because it is likely to be the correct answer.

IDENTIFY DUPLICATE FACTS AMONG THE OPTIONS

Sometimes items are designed so that each option contains two or more facts. Usually identical or similar facts appear in at least two of the four options. If you identify a fact as incorrect, you can eliminate all the options that contain this fact. By deleting distractors you increase your chances of selecting the correct answer.

SAMPLE ITEM 6-28

A patient has a vest restraint. While making this patient's occupied bed, what must the nurse do to promote patient safety?

    (1) Keep the vest restraint tied and lower both side rails.

    (2) Keep the vest restraint tied and lower one side rail.

    (3) Untie the vest restraint and lower both side rails.

    (4) Untie the vest restraint and lower one side rail.

This item is testing two concepts: whether a vest restraint should be tied or untied when providing direct care, and whether one or both side rails should be lowered when providing direct care. If you only know the fact that the side rail should be lowered just on the side on which you are working, then you can eliminate options 1 and 3. If you only know the fact that a vest restraint can be untied when the nurse is at the bedside providing direct care, then you can eliminate options 1 and 2. In either case you can eliminate two options as distractors, and you have raised your chances of selecting the correct answer from 25 to 50 percent.

SAMPLE ITEM 6-29

The physician orders a 2-gram sodium diet. Which group of nutrients would be most appropriate for this diet?

    (1) Fruit, vegetables, and bread

    (2) Hot dogs, mustard, and pickles

    (3) Hamburger, onions, and ketchup

    (4) Luncheon meats, rolls, and vegetables

This item is testing your knowledge about the sodium content of foods. If you recognize that hot dogs and luncheon meats are both processed foods that are high in sodium, then you can eliminate options 2 and 4. If you recognize that ketchup and mustard are both condiments that are high in sodium, then you can delete options 2 and 3. By knowing either fact, you can reduce the final selection to between two options. The similarities between these options are less clear than if the parts were identical, but the technique of identifying duplicate facts in options can still be used.

SAMPLE ITEM 6-30

When monitoring a patient who is at risk for hemorrhage, the nurse should assess the patient for:

    (1) Warm, dry skin; hypotension; bounding pulse

    (2) Hypertension; bounding pulse; cold clammy skin

    (3) Weak, thready pulse; hypertension; warm dry skin

    (4) Hypotension; cold clammy skin; weak, thready pulse

This item is testing your knowledge about patient adaptations associated with hemorrhage. Three patient adaptations are presented: the condition of the skin, the blood pressure, and the characteristic of the pulse. Even if you only know one of these facts about hemorrhage, you can reduce your final selection to between two options. If you know that hypotension is associated with hemorrhage, then you can eliminate options 2 and 3. If you know that cold clammy skin is related to hemorrhage, then you can delete options 1 and 3. If you know that a weak, thready pulse is associated with hemorrhage, then you can eliminate options 1 and 2. If you know only one or two of the facts presented, you can maximize the information you have in answering this type of item. Options that have three parts work to your advantage if you use the technique of identifying duplicate facts in options.

IDENTIFY OPTIONS THAT DENY PATIENT FEELINGS, CONCERNS, AND NEEDS

Because nurses are human and caring, and primarily want their patients to get well, they often assume the role of deliverer, champion, protector, or savior. However, by inappropriately adopting these roles, nurses often diminish patient concerns, provide false reassurance, and/or cut off further patient communication. To be a patient advocate, the nurse cannot always be a Pollyanna. Pollyanna, the heroine of stories by Eleanor Hodgman Porter, was a person of irrepressible optimism who found good in everything. Sometimes nurses must focus on the negative rather than the positive, acknowledge that everything may not have the desired outcome, and recognize patients' feelings as a priority. Options that imply everything will be all right deny patients' feelings, change the subject raised by the patient, encourage the patient to be cheerful, or abdicate nursing responsibility to other members of the health team are usually distractors and can be eliminated from consideration.

SAMPLE ITEM 6–31

The day before surgery for a hysterectomy, a patient says to the nurse, "I am worried that I might die tomorrow." What would be the most appropriate response?

(1) "It is really routine surgery."

(2) "You need to tell your doctor about this."

(3) "The thought of dying can be frightening."

(4) "Most people who have this surgery survive."

Options 1 and 4 minimize the patient's concerns because these messages imply that there is nothing to worry about; the surgery is routine and most patients survive. In option 2 the nurse avoids the opportunity to encourage further discussion of the patient's feelings and surrenders this responsibility to the physician. After collecting more information, the nurse may inform the physician of the patient's concern about death. Options 1, 2, and 4 deny the patient's feelings and can be eliminated because they are distractors. Option 3 is the correct answer because it encourages the patient to focus on the expressed feelings about death.

SAMPLE ITEM 6–32

After surgery, a patient complains of mild incisional pain while performing deep-breathing and coughing exercises. What would be the nurse's best response?

(1) "Each day it will hurt less and less."

(2) "This is an expected response after surgery."

(3) "With a pillow, apply pressure against the incision."

(4) "I will get the pain medication the physician ordered."

Option 1 is a Pollyanna-like response that provides false reassurance. The nurse does not know that the pain will get less and less for this patient. Option 1 can be deleted from consideration. Although option 2 is a true statement, it cuts off communication because it diminishes the patient's concern and does not explore a solution for minimizing the pain. Option 2 can be eliminated as a distractor. You now must choose between options 3 and 4. The stem indicates that the patient has pain when coughing; the pain is not continuous. Option 4 can be deleted because it would be inappropriate to administer an analgesic at this time. Mild pain should subside after the activity is completed. The correct answer is option 3 because it recognizes the mild pain and offers an intervention to help relieve the temporary discomfort. Each time you can eliminate an option that denies a patient's feelings, you raise your chances of selecting the correct answer.

SAMPLE ITEM 6–33

An elderly woman with a right-sided hemiplegia and tears in her eyes sadly states, "I used to brush my hair 100 strokes a day and now I have to rely on others to do it." What should be the initial response by the nurse?

(1) "It must be hard not to be able to do things for yourself."

(2) "With physical therapy you will be able to brush your own hair some day."

(3) "Let me brush your hair 100 strokes, and then I'll help you with breakfast."

(4) "That's true, but there are lots of other things you are capable of doing for yourself."

Option 3 changes the subject and cuts off communication. Option 2 is a Pollyanna-like response because it implies that everything will eventually be all right. Option 4 initially accepts the patient's statement but then attempts to refocus the patient on the positive before exploring the negative. Options 2, 3, and 4 in one way or another deny the patient's feelings, concerns, and/or needs. The correct answer is option 1 because it is an open-ended statement that focuses on the patient's feelings.

USE MULTIPLE TEST-TAKING TECHNIQUES

You have just been introduced to a variety of test-taking techniques. As you practice applying each of these techniques to test items, you will become more skillful at being test-wise. As you become better at applying test-taking techniques, you can further maximize success in choosing the correct option if you use more than one test-taking technique within an item.

SAMPLE ITEM 6–34

A patient's plan of care indicates that passive range-of-motion (PROM) exercises of the right leg are to be done every four hours while awake. What should the nurse do?

(1) Demonstrate how to perform PROM exercises

(2) Explain that all patients do PROM by themselves

(3) Move the patient's leg through PROM when indicated

(4) Take the patient to physical therapy for PROM exercises

Option 2 includes the specific determiner *all* and should be carefully evaluated. Some patients are able to perform PROM exercises themselves (e.g., a patient with a hemiplegia can perform PROM on the affected arm and hand with the extremity that is unaffected), whereas some patients are unable to perform PROM (e.g., a patient with quadriplegia). Because some patients cannot perform PROM exercises, there are exceptions to the statement in option 2. This option can be deleted from consideration by using the technique Identify Specific Determiners in Options. Option 4 abdicates the responsibility for care that the nurse is educated and licensed to provide. This option can be eliminated from consideration by using the technique Identify Options That Deny Patient Feelings, Concerns, and Needs. By using two test-taking techniques, you have eliminated options 2 and 4, reduced the number of options to two, and increased your chances of selecting the correct answer to 50 percent.

SAMPLE ITEM 6-35

Which patient adaptations are unexpected in response to the general adaptation syndrome?
- (1) Dilated pupils and bradycardia
- (2) Mental alertness and tachycardia
- (3) Increased blood glucose and tachycardia
- (4) Decreased blood glucose and bradycardia

By carefully reading the stem you should identify that the word *unexpected* is a significant word in this item. You have just used the test-taking technique Identify Key Words in the Stem That Indicate Negative Polarity. If you know that tachycardia is associated with the general adaptation syndrome, you can eliminate options 2 and 3. This reasoning uses the test-taking technique Identify Duplicate Facts Among Options. If you recognize that options 3 and 4 are opposites, you should give these options particular consideration. By seriously considering these options, you are using the test-taking technique Identify Opposites in Options. A variety of test-taking techniques can be applied to analyze and answer this item.

SAMPLE ITEM 6-36

When the nurse administers a backrub to reduce the physical discomfort of a backache, what patient needs are being met?
- (1) Safety needs
- (2) Security needs
- (3) Self-esteem needs
- (4) Physiological needs

By thoughtfully reading the stem you should identify that the important words are *reduce the physical discomfort of a backache.* When reviewing the options, you should recognize that the word "physiological" in option 4 is closely related to the word "physical" in the stem. Option 4 should be given serious consideration. This reasoning uses the test-taking technique Identify Clues in the Stem. Options 1 and 2 present the words "safety" and "security." They are comparable, and choosing between them would be difficult. They are distractors. This reasoning uses the test-taking technique Identify Equally Plausible or Unique Options. The use of multiple test-taking techniques in considering an item can facilitate the deletion of distractors and the selection of the correct answer.

General Test-Taking Techniques

A general test-taking technique is a strategy that is used to conquer the challenge of an examination. To be in command of the situation, you must be able to manage your internal and external domains. The test-taker who approaches a test with physical, mental, and emotional authority is in a position to regulate the testing situation, rather than to have the testing situation dominate.

FOLLOW YOUR REGULAR ROUTINE THE NIGHT BEFORE A TEST

Follow your normal routine the night before a test. This is not the time to make changes that may disrupt your equilibrium. If you do not normally eat pepperoni pizza, exercise, or study until 2 AM, do not start now. Go to bed at your usual time. Avoid the temptation to have an all-night cram session. Studies have demonstrated that sleep deprivation decreases reaction times and cognitive skills. An adequate night's sleep is necessary to produce a rested mind and body that provide the physical and emotional energy required to maximize performance on an examination.

ARRIVE ON TIME FOR THE EXAMINATION

Plan your schedule so that you arrive at the testing site approximately 15 to 30 minutes early. Arrange extra time for unexpected events associated with traveling. There may be a traffic jam, a road may have a detour, the car may not start, the train may be late, the bus could break down, or you may have to park in the farthest lot from the testing site. If the location of the testing site or classroom is unfamiliar to you, it would be wise to take a practice run and locate the room. On the day of the examination you should avoid getting lost or being late.

By arriving early, you have an opportunity to visit the rest room, survey the situation, and collect your thoughts. Because anxiety is associated with an autonomic nervous system response, you may have urgency, frequency, or increased intestinal peristalsis. Visit the rest room before the test to avoid using testing time to meet physical needs. The test may or may not be administered in the room in which the content is taught. Arriving early allows you to survey the situation and become more comfortable in the testing environment. Decide where you want to sit if seats are not assigned. Students have preferences such as sitting by a window, being in the back of the room, or surrounding themselves with friends. Selecting your own seat allows you to manipulate one aspect of your environment. In addition, this time before the test provides you with an opportunity to collect your thoughts. You may desire to review content on a flash card, perform relaxation exercises, or reinforce your positive mental attitude. However, avoid comparing notes with other students. They may have inaccurate information or be anxious. Remember, anxiety is contagious. If you are the type who is readily affected by the anxiety of other people, avoid these people until after the test.

BRING THE APPROPRIATE TOOLS

To perform a task, you need adequate tools. Pens, pencils, an eraser, and a watch are essential. A pen is usually required to complete the identifying information on the answer sheet. A pencil is usually necessary to record your answers on the answer sheet if it is a computer answer form. Use number 2 pencils because they have soft lead that facilitates the computer scoring of the answer sheet. Bring at least two pens and two or more pencils. Backup equipment is advisable because ink can run out and points can break. Sharpen all your pencils and/or bring a small, self-contained pencil sharpener if you prefer to work with a sharp point on your pencil. Have at least one eraser. You may decide to change an answer or need to erase extraneous marks that you make on the question book or the answer sheet. A watch is also a necessary tool for taking every test. Some proctors will announce time frames as the test progresses and others will not. Bringing your own watch provides you with a sense of independence and control. Depending on your individual needs, other tools might include eyeglasses, a hearing aid, or a calculator. Assemble all your equipment the night before the test, and be sure to take them with you to the testing site.

98

UNDERSTAND ALL THE DIRECTIONS FOR THE TEST BEFORE STARTING

It is essential to understand the instructions before beginning the test. On some tests you are responsible for independently reading the instructions, whereas on others the proctor verbally announces the instructions. However, more often than not you will have a written copy of the instructions while the proctor reads them aloud. In this instance do not read ahead of the proctor. The proctor may elaborate on the written instructions, and you do not want to miss any of the additional directions. If you do not understand a particular part of the instructions, immediately request that the proctor explain them again. You must completely understand the instructions before beginning the examination.

MANAGE THE ALLOTTED TIME TO YOUR ADVANTAGE

All tests have a time limit. Some tests have severe time restrictions in which most test-takers do not complete all the questions on the examination. These are known as "speed tests." Other tests have a generous time frame in which the majority of test-takers have ample time to answer every question on the examination. These are known as "power tests." The purpose of tests in nursing is to identify how much information the test-taker possesses about the nursing care of people. Most nursing examinations are power tests. Regardless of the type of test, you must use your time well.

To manage your time on an examination, you must determine how much time you have to answer each item while leaving some time for review at the end of the testing period. To figure out how much time you should allot for each item, divide the total time you have for the test by the number of items on the test. For example, if you have 90 minutes to take a test that has 50 items, divide 90 by 50. This allots 1 minute and 48 seconds for each item. If you actually allot $1^1/_2$ minutes per item, you will leave 15 minutes for a final review. Be aware of the time as you progress through a test. If you determine that you have approximately $1^1/_2$ minutes for each question, then by the time you have completed 10 items, 15 minutes should have passed. Pace yourself so that you do not spend more than $1^1/_2$ minutes on an item if possible. If you answer an item in less than $1^1/_2$ minutes, then you can use the extra time for another item that may take slightly longer than $1^1/_2$ minutes or add this time to the end for review. The allocation of time for test completion depends on the complexity of the content, the difficulty of the reading level, and the number of options presented in the items. Timed multiple-choice nursing examinations generally allot 1 minute per item when there are four options.

Use all the time allocated for the examination. The test constructors calculated that the time parameters for the test were appropriate for a thoughtful review of the items. Read the items slowly and carefully. If you process items too quickly, you may overlook important words, become careless, or arrive at impulsive conclusions. Work at your own pace. Do not be influenced by the actions of other test-takers. If other test-takers complete the examination early, ignore them and do not become concerned. Just because they finish early does not indicate that they will score well on the test. They may be imprudent speed demons. A cautious, discriminating, and judicious approach is to your advantage. Be your own person and remember that time can be your ally rather than your adversary.

Time allocation varies for tests taken on a computer. See Chapter 8, Computer Applications in Education and Evaluation, for more information.

CONCENTRATE ON THE SIMPLE BEFORE THE COMPLEX

Answer the easy questions before the difficult questions. This uses the basic teaching-learning principle of moving from the simple to the complex. By doing this, you can maximize your use of time and maintain a positive mental attitude. Begin answering questions. When you are confronted with a difficult item, have already used your allotted time to answer it, and still do not know the answer, skip over this item and move on to the next one. Make a notation on scrap paper, next to the item in the question booklet, and/or next to the number of the skipped item on the answer sheet so that you can return to this item later in the test. Making a mark on the answer sheet should prevent you from making the error of recording the next answer in the previous item's location on the answer sheet. These and any other extraneous marks must be erased from the answer sheet before handing it in to the proctor. Extraneous marks confuse the computer, and you will probably lose credit because the mark will be scored as an incorrect answer. When you reach the end of the test, return to those items that you reserved for the end. You should have time to spend on these items, and you may have accessed information from other items that can assist you in answering these questions. Concentrating on the simple before the complex permits you to answer the maximum number of items in the time allocated for the examination.

On computer-administered examinations this strategy may not be applicable. You may be required to enter an answer before the next item will appear on the screen.

MAKE EDUCATED GUESSES

An educated guess is the selection of an option based on partial knowledge, without knowing for certain that it is actually the correct answer. When you have reduced the final selection to two options, it is usually to your advantage to reassess these options in the context of the knowledge you do possess and make an educated guess. Making a wild guess by flipping a coin or choosing your favorite number should depend on whether or not the test has a penalty for guessing.

Some examinations assign credit when you select a correct answer and do not allocate credit when you select one of the distractors. The directions for these examinations may state that only correct answers will receive credit, that you should answer every question, that you should not leave any blanks, or that there are no penalties for guessing. In these tests it is to your advantage to answer every question. First, select answers based on knowledge. If you are unsure of the correct answer, reduce the number of options and then make an educated guess. If you have absolutely no idea what the answer can be, then make a wild guess because you will not be penalized for a wrong answer.

Some tests assign credit when you select a correct answer and subtract credit when you select a distractor. The instructions for these examinations may inform you not to guess, that credit will be subtracted for incorrect answers, or that there is a penalty for guessing. In these tests a statistical manipulation is performed to mathematically limit the advantage of guessing. When taking these tests, it is still to your advantage to make an educated guess if through knowledge you can reduce your final selection to two options. However, wild guessing is not to your advantage because you are penalized for guessing.

MAINTAIN A POSITIVE MENTAL ATTITUDE

It is important that you foster a positive mental attitude and a sense of relaxation. A little apprehension can be motivating, but too much can interfere with your attention, concentration, and problem-solving ability. Use the positive techniques you have practiced and that work for you to enhance relaxation and a positive mental attitude. For example, feel in control by skipping the difficult questions; enhance relaxation by employing diaphragmatic breathing for several deep breaths, rotating your shoulders, or flexing and extending your head; foster a positive mental attitude by telling yourself, "I am prepared to do this well!" or "I know I have studied hard and I will be successful!"

100   **CHECK YOUR ANSWERS AND ANSWER SHEET**

Most examinations incorporate time at the end of the testing period for review. Reassess your answers, particularly for those items in which you made an educated guess. Subsequent questions may contain content that is helpful in answering a previous question; you may access information you did not remember originally; or you may be less anxious at the end of the test and able to assess the question with more objectivity. Be aware of your success in changing answers on previous tests. Every time you review a test, evaluate your accuracy in changing answers. Keep score of how many answers you change from wrong to right and how many you change from right to wrong. If the number of items you changed from wrong to right is greater than the number of items you changed from right to wrong, then it would probably be to your advantage to change answers you ultimately believe you answered incorrectly. On the other hand, if you change more answers from right to wrong, then you should avoid changing your answers unless you are positive that your second choice is the correct choice. Make sure that you have answered every question, especially on tests that do not penalize for guessing.

Review your answer sheet for accuracy. Computer-scored tests usually use separate answer sheets in which each item has numbers or letters that represent the corresponding responses to each item in the test. Make sure that every mark is within the lines, heavy and full, and in the appropriate space. Erase any extraneous marks on the answer sheet. Additional pencil marks, inadequately erased answers, and marks outside the lines will confuse the computer and alter your score. An effective and thorough review should leave you with a feeling of control and a sense of closure at the end of the examination.

Answers and Rationales for Sample Items in Chapter 6

An asterisk (*) is in front of the rationale that explains the correct answer.

6–1   ① Used linens may be contaminated with body secretions; wearing gloves is part of universal (standard) precautions.

   *② These linens are considered soiled, and if returned, they would contaminate the linen room.

   ③ Reusing a top sheet for the bottom sheet is an acceptable practice if the sheet is not wet or soiled.

   ④ Tucking clean linen against the springs of the bed is an acceptable practice; the entire bed is washed with a disinfectant between patients.

6–2   ① Stewed fruit is low in sodium.

   *② Luncheon meats are generally processed with large amounts of sodium.

   ③ Whole-grain cereal is low in sodium.

   ④ Green leafy vegetables are low in sodium.

6–3   ① Kneading the skin increases circulation and should be part of a backrub unless contraindicated.

   ② Excess lotion can be an irritant to the skin and should be removed.

   ③ Using continuous, firm strokes is soothing and relieves muscle tension; this action is based on the gate-control theory of pain relief.

   *④ Putting pressure over the vertebrae should be avoided because it can cause unnecessary pressure over bony prominences; backrub strokes should massage muscle groups, not vertebrae.

6–4   *① Ointments and jellies have an oil base that provides a barrier; they also hold in moisture, which prevents drying and cracking of skin.

   ② Although incontinence pads are often used for patients who are incontinent, they tend to hold urine and feces against the skin, promoting maceration and skin breakdown.

   ③ Although talcum powder and corn starch are often used, when excessive amounts are mixed with urine and perspiration, this results in a paste that promotes the growth of microorganisms and can be an irritant.

   ④ Same as #3.

6–5   *① Verifying the physician's order should be done first. It is essential that the specific type of enema ordered be given; enemas have different solutions, volumes, and purposes.

   ② Collecting the appropriate equipment is done after the type of enema is verified; each type of enema has different requirements.

   ③ Arranging for an empty bathroom should be done once all the equipment and the patient are prepared and ready.

   ④ Explaining the procedure to the patient is implemented once the nurse verifies the type of enema ordered; the nurse's explanation depends on the type of enema being administered.

6–6   ① This statement is a demeaning response and does not answer the patient's question.

   ② This statement denies the patient's concern and does not answer the question.

   *③ This statement answers the question, which meets the patient's right to know; it is also a respectful response.

④ Not responding would make the patient more upset; the patient has a right to know who is providing care.

6–7   ① Pulling the curtain supports the patient's need for self-esteem; it provides privacy.

* ② Maintaining functional alignment supports a basic physiological need; this reduces physical strain and potential injury to joints, muscles, ligaments, and tendons and can prevent the formation of contractures.

③ Responding to the call light immediately supports the patient's need for security and safety; patients need to know that help is immediately available when needed.

④ Raising both side rails on the bed supports the patient's need for safety and security; bed rails prevent a patient from falling out of bed.

6–8   * ① Self-care encourages a patient's independence, which increases self-esteem.

② Family member visits would meet the patient's needs for love and belonging, not self-esteem.

③ When a person is dependent on another, such dependency often lowers self-esteem.

④ Same as #3.

6–9   ① Pulling a curtain when providing care supports the patient's self-esteem needs, not physical needs.

② Answering a call bell immediately meets the patient's safety needs, not physical needs.

* ③ Administering physical hygiene meets a patient's basic physiological need to be clean.

④ Vital signs are not a physiological need of the patient's, but an assessment done by the nurse to determine the patient's needs.

6–10   ① This response focuses on the nurse rather than the patient.

* ② This response directly involves the patient and invites the patient to relive a past vacation.

③ Same as #1

④ This question by the nurse asks for an opinion, which can be answered with a short response.

6–11   ① This might be done later. It is not the initial action.

② Same as #1.

* ③ The fact that the patient raised the issues about her husband indicates that she is concerned about his behavior. Her feelings need to be explored and her self-esteem supported.

④ Same as #1.

6–12   ① This would be done later; the nurse's first action is to support the patient.

② Same as #1.

③ Same as #1.

* ④ The patient is the priority at this point in time; once the patient is protected and safe, the actions of the abusive nurse must be addressed.

6–13   ① This statement denies the patient's feelings.

* ② This statement focuses on the patient's feelings by the use of reflection.

③ This statement offers false reassurance.

④ Same as #3.

6–14   ① Reminding the patient of the physician's next visit does not address the patient's concern; the patient forgets the questions to be asked, not when the physician will visit.

② This may foster feelings of dependence and could violate the patient's privacy if the questions to be asked are personal.

③ Same as #2.

* ④ Providing a paper and pen to write down questions promotes independence, self-esteem, and privacy.

6–15 ① This may be done after obtaining the patient's permission.

② Same as #1.

* ③ Seeking preferences promotes individualized care by allowing personal choices.

④ Combing from the roots is unsafe; combing should begin at the ends and progressively move toward the roots as tangles are removed.

6–16 ① Although this may eventually be done, the primary intervention should be exploring the patient's feelings.

* ② Asking the patient to share more encourages verbalization of feelings.

③ Same as #1.

④ Same as #1.

6–17 ① Soap lowers the surface tension of water, which promotes cleaning, not circulation.

② Keeping the patient covered prevents chilling, it does not improve local circulation.

③ Hot water can damage delicate tissue and should be avoided; bath water should be between 110 and 115°F.

* ④ Pressure and friction produce local heat, which dilates blood vessels, improving circulation.

6–18 ① Handwashing before care protects the patient from the nurse.

* ② Gloves are a barrier against body secretions and are used with universal (standard) precautions.

③ The nurse is still exposed to body secretions if not wearing gloves when discarding contaminated water.

④ Expecting patients to provide all of their own care is unreasonable and inappropriate; some patients need assistance with meeting their needs.

6–19 ① Straps and a mask that are firm against the skin can cause tissue trauma.

② Changing the method of oxygen delivery requires a physician's order.

③ Padding the straps with gauze without adjusting the straps would make the mask tighter against the face.

* ④ Loosening the elastic straps will reduce the pressure of the mask against the face; the elastic straps can be adjusted for comfort while keeping the edges of the mask gently against the skin.

6–20 ① This is untrue because aging is progressive and does not move backward.

* ② Aging, from conception to death, advances and moves onward.

③ Although this may be true for some elderly people, it is not true for all.

④ Same as #3.

6–21 * ① Dependent edema is minimal while the feet are still elevated; anti-embolism stockings should be applied before the legs are moved to a dependent position.

② The purpose of anti-embolism stockings is to promote venous return, not reduce pain.

③ This would cause tissue trauma because of the presence of fluid in the interstitial compartment; anti-embolism stockings are applied to prevent edema.

④ Anti-embolism stockings should be applied before the feet are moved to a dependent position.

6–22 ① Side rails do not provide a stable base of support. Injury can occur when the rails are lowered before the straps are removed.

② Tying a restraint to the footboard would require an excessively long strap in which the patient's legs could get entangled.

* ③ The bed frame is a stable base of support and is beyond the patient's reach.

④ Tying a restraint to the headboard could result in an uncomfortable line of pull with the arm above the head.

6–23 ① A solution is hypertonic when the total electrolyte content is 375 mEq/L or greater.

② A solution is hypotonic when the total electrolyte content is below 250 mEq/L.

* ③ A solution is isotonic when the total electrolyte content is approximately 310 mEq/L; normal saline (sodium chloride) is isotonic.

④ Acidotic refers to excessive levels of hydrogen ions in the blood affecting pH values.

6–24 ① Nutrients, such as food and fluids, meet basic physiological needs.

② Same as #1.

* ③ Being able to summon help when needed provides a sense of security and actual physical safety for the patient.

④ Storing a patient's valuables in the hospital safe provides emotional safety.

6–25 ① Placing the patient in the prone position exposes the entire area to permit a thorough backrub; it does not promote circulation.

② Lotion moisturizes the skin and makes it supple; it does not promote circulation.

③ Although baby powder may be used for backrubs to permit the hands to slide against the skin, it should not be used for patients who perspire because it can cause a pastelike substance that promotes skin breakdown.

* ④ Kneading causes friction and pressure against the skin that promotes localized heat, precipitates vessel dilation, and improves circulation.

6–26 ① Active range of motion (ROM), not passive range of motion (PROM), can increase endurance.

* ② PROM prevents shortening of muscles, ligaments, and tendons, which causes a joint to become fixed in one position.

③ Active, not passive, range of motion can strengthen muscle tone.

④ Maximizing muscle atrophy would never be a patient goal. Atrophy is the loss of muscle mass due to lack of muscle contraction. Active range of motion will minimize muscle atrophy.

6–27 ① Shutting the door provides privacy and prevents drafts, but if the nurse's hands are not clean, they will contaminate the door.

* ② Between patients and before providing care, the nurse must wash his or her hands to remove dirt and microorganisms; otherwise, equipment and the patient will be affected by cross-contamination. Medical asepsis is a priority.

③ Closing the curtain provides for privacy and prevents drafts, but if the nurse's hands are not clean, they will contaminate the curtain.

④ Draping the patient provides for privacy and prevents chilling, but if the nurse's hands are not clean, they will contaminate the linen and patient.

6–28 ① Both actions could injure the patient. The patient could fall out of bed on the side opposite the nurse; moving a restrained patient exerts stress on the patient's musculoskeletal system.

② Although one side rail can be lowered, moving a restrained patient could injure the patient.

③ Although the vest restraint can be untied while the nurse is at the bedside, lowering the rail on the side opposite to which the nurse is working could result in the patient's falling out of bed.

* ④ Untying a restraint permits free movement, which limits stress on the patient's musculoskeletal system. Lowering one side rail allows the nurse to provide direct care. Keeping the side rail raised on the side opposite to which the nurse is working provides a barrier to prevent the patient's falling out of bed.

6–29 * ① These foods contain the least amount of sodium as compared to the other options.

② These all contain a high level of sodium and should be avoided.

③ Ketchup is high in sodium and should be avoided.

④ Luncheon meats are processed foods that contain a high level of sodium and should be avoided.

6–30 ① With hemorrhage, the patient's skin would be cold and clammy, not warm and dry, and the pulse would be weak and thready, not bounding.

② Because of the reduced blood volume associated with hemorrhage, the patient's blood pressure would be decreased, not increased, and the pulse would be weak and thready, not bounding.

③ With hemorrhage, the patient's blood pressure would be decreased, not increased, and the skin would be cold and clammy, not warm and dry.

* ④ Because of the decreased blood volume associated with hemorrhage, there would be a reduced blood pressure and weak, thready pulse; because of the autonomic nervous system response and the constriction of peripheral blood vessels, the patient's skin would be cold and clammy.

6–31 ① This statement denies the patient's feelings about death and cuts off further communication.

② This statement abdicates the responsibility of the nurse (to explore the patient's feelings) to the physician; it cuts off communication and does not meet the patient's immediate need to discuss fears of death.

* ③ This statement uses reflective technique because it focuses on the underlying feeling expressed in the patient's statement.

④ Same as #1.

6–32 ① This is a Pollyanna-like response that provides false reassurance.

② Although this is a true statement, it cuts off communication and does not present an intervention to help limit the patient's temporary discomfort.

* ③ This response recognizes the mild pain and offers the patient an intervention to help limit the temporary discomfort.

④ This response would be inappropriate at this time. If more than mild pain is expected, analgesics should be administered before painful interventions are made.

6–33 * ① This response identifies the patient's concern and offers an opportunity to further discuss the topic.

② This is a Pollyanna-like response that provides false reassurance; the patient may never be able to brush her own hair.

③ This response offers a solution before allowing the patient to discuss concerns, thereby cutting off communication.

④ Once the patient's present feelings are explored, then pointing out the patient's abilities would be appropriate.

6–34 ① PROM exercises of a leg cannot be performed independently; this is appropriate for active ROM exercises.

② Some patients are not capable of performing PROM exercises, depending on the strength of the unaffected extremity and their physical, mental, and/or emotional status.

* ③ PROM exercises are interventions within the role of the nurse and meet the patient's need to prevent contractures.

④ Taking the patient to physical therapy abdicates the nurse's responsibility to other members of the health team.

6–35 ① Tachycardia, not bradycardia, is associated with the general adaptation syndrome (GAS); dilated pupils are expected.

② Both these adaptations are expected autonomic nervous system responses that occur during the alarm stage of the GAS.

③ Same as #2.

* ④ During the alarm stage of the GAS, both the blood glucose level and heart rate of the patient increase, not decrease.

6–36 ① Safety and security needs, the second level of needs according to Maslow, are met when the patient is protected from harm.

② Same as #1.

③ Self-esteem needs are met when the patient is treated with dignity and respect.

* ④ Being free from pain or discomfort is a basic physiological need; a backrub improves local circulation, reduces muscle tension, and limits pain.

Testing Formats Other Than Multiple-Choice Questions

Introduction

Teachers make many decisions that influence students. Some decisions are instructional decisions. What teaching strategies should be used to teach certain content? Some decisions are curricular decisions. What information should be included in a unit of instruction? The decisions teachers make that produce the most anxiety for most students are the measurement and evaluation decisions. What does the student know? What can the student do? To make these decisions, teachers use tests to appraise progress toward curricular goals, assess mastery of a skill, and evaluate knowledge of what was taught in a course. Three factors are involved in making measurement and evaluation decisions.

- *What knowledge or ability is to be measured?* Generally, that which is most important or relevant is measured. Examples include the range of normal vital signs in an adult, the principles of patient teaching, legal and ethical implications of health care delivery, and patient safety. You can usually identify what is most significant by the emphasis placed on the material. Content in a textbook that is highlighted, boldfaced, capitalized, or repeated several times is usually important. Information that appears in the textbook and is incorporated into the teacher's classroom instruction is also significant. Concepts that are introduced in the classroom setting and then applied in a classroom laboratory or clinical setting are critical concepts. You can often predict the content that will be on a test and therefore use your study time more efficiently.

- *How can the identified knowledge or ability be measured?* A set of operations must be devised to isolate and display the knowledge or ability that is to be measured. Examples include multiple-choice questions, true-false questions, completion items, matching columns, extended essay questions, and the performance of a procedure. To feel in control when taking tests, you should be familiar with the various testing formats. Dealing with a particular test format is a skill, and to develop a skill you must practice. Student workbooks that accompany required textbooks, practice questions at the end of chapters, and books devoted to testing usually contain practice questions. Practice answering these questions. Experience promotes learning and practice makes perfect!

- *How can the results of the devised operations be measured or expressed in quantitative terms?* In other words, the unit of measure that indicates a passing grade or an acceptable performance must be identified by the instructor. Examples of acceptable results include a grade within 10 percent of the average grade in the class, a grade of 80 percent, or the correct performance of previously identified steps (critical elements) of a procedure. When taking tests, you should be aware of the criteria for scoring the test. You should ask the following questions. What is the passing grade? How many points are allocated to each question? Can partial credit be received for an answer? Is there a penalty for guessing? What are the critical steps that must be performed to pass the test for each skill? Answers to these and other questions can help you make decisions such as how much time to devote to certain questions or whether or not to guess at an answer.

In previous chapters, the multiple-choice question was discussed in detail. In this chapter, testing formats other than multiple-choice questions are presented. Test questions can be classified as structured-response questions, restricted-response questions, extended essay questions, or performance appraisals. A **structured-response question** requires you to select the correct answer from among available alternatives. Multiple-choice, true-false, and matching items are examples of structured-response questions. A **restricted-response question** requires you to write a short answer. The response is expected to be a word, phrase, or sentence. Short-answer and completion items are examples of restricted-response questions. An **extended essay question** requires you to generate the answer, via a free-response format, in reply to a question or problem that is presented. A **performance appraisal** presents a structured situation and requires you to demonstrate a skill.

Structured-Response Questions

A structured-response item is one that asks a question and requires you to select an answer from among the options presented. These items include multiple-choice, true-false, and matching questions. This format is usually efficient, dependable, and objective. Because multiple-choice questions are discussed elsewhere in the book, just true-false and matching questions will be presented here.

TRUE-FALSE QUESTIONS

A true-false question is also known as an alternate-response item. A question is presented and only two options are given from which to select an answer. This item frequently is used to test knowledge of facts because the response must be absolutely true or false. It can be a demanding format because no frame of reference is provided. The question is usually constructed out of context, and the truth or falsity of the statement can be difficult to evaluate. However, true-false questions can work to your benefit because you have a 50 percent chance of getting the answer right. If you do not know the answer and there is no penalty for guessing, make an educated guess. Never leave a blank answer if there is no penalty for guessing.

The answers and rationales for all the sample items in this chapter are at the end of the chapter.

SAMPLE ITEM 7–1

Soap helps in cleaning because it lowers the surface tension of water.
True _____   False _____

SAMPLE ITEM 7–2

When transferring a patient from the bed to a wheelchair, the nurse should assume a broad stance.
True _____   False _____

SAMPLE ITEM 7–3

Exercising just before going to bed promotes sleep.
True _____   False _____

SAMPLE ITEM 7–4

Pulse pressure is the difference between the apical and radial pulse rates.
True _____   False _____

Variations of true-false items have been developed to simplify and clarify what is being asked. These questions may also obtain more information about what you know and limit guessing. **Highlighting a word or phrase in the question** is a simple variation that helps to reduce ambiguity and increase precision. This technique also can be used by you when answering true-false questions that are not highlighted. Underline key words, as well as words that modify key words, to focus your attention on the most important part of the statement.

SAMPLE ITEM 7–5

Palpation is the examination of the body using the sense of **touch.**
True _____   False _____

SAMPLE ITEM 7–6

The process in which solid, particulate matter in a fluid moves from an area of higher concentration to an area of lower concentration is known as osmosis.
True _____   False _____

Grouping short true-false items under a common question is a variation of the true-false question that attempts to arrange affiliated information together. It is an effective approach to assess knowledge about related categories, classifications, or characteristics. Each statement that is being evaluated must be considered in relation to the original question. This variation reduces the amount of reading and provides a greater frame of reference for evaluating each statement. This type of question increases specificity and clarity.

SAMPLE ITEM 7–7

Indicate if the following choices are true or false in relation to the introductory statement. Surgical asepsis is maintained when the nurse:

(1) Removes the drape from a sterile package by touching the outer 1 inch with ungloved hands.
True _____   False _____

(2) Holds the hands below the elbows during a surgical hand scrub.
True _____   False _____

(3) Dons the first sterile glove by touching just the inside of the glove.
True _____   False _____

(4) Holds a sterile object below waist level.
True _____   False _____

SAMPLE ITEM 7–8

Signify whether or not each procedure employs the principle of positive pressure.

(1) Mechanical ventilation
True _____   False _____

(2) Instillation of fluid into a nasogastric tube with a piston syringe
True _____   False _____

(3) Continuous bladder irrigation
True _____   False _____

(4) Chest tubes (water-seal drainage system)
True _____   False _____

Requiring the test-taker to correct false statements is another variation of the true-false question. With this type of question you are instructed to rewrite the question whenever you determine that the statement is false. This approach guarantees that you understand the information underlying a false statement. It also decreases guessing because you will receive credit only if able to revise the question to make it a correct statement. This variation is sometimes combined with the true-false variation that highlights a word or phrase in the original question.

SAMPLE ITEM 7–9

Mark your answer with an X in the space provided. If you identify the statement as false, revise the statement so that it is accurate. The normal range of the heart rate for an adult is 75 to 120 beats per minute.
True _____   False _____

SAMPLE ITEM 7–10

Indicate if the statement is true or false. Correct the underlined words if the statement is false. According to Erikson's developmental theory, the central task of <u>young adulthood</u> is identity versus role confusion.

True _____   False _____

True-false items can be asked in relation to specific stimulus material included with the question. This variation of the true-false question provides a frame of reference for the specific questions being asked within the item. Examples of stimulus material include a graph, map, chart, table, or picture. Memorization of information generally is not sufficient for answering these types of questions because they test more than the recall or regurgitation of facts. These questions test comprehension, interpretation, application, and reasoning, which are higher levels of cognitive ability.

SAMPLE ITEM 7–11

The vital signs sheet on page 112 reflects an adult patient's 7-day hospitalization. Determine if each statement is true or false in relation to the information plotted on the vital signs sheet.

(1) On June 7 at 10 PM the patient's temperature was 101.2°F.
   True _____   False _____

(2) During the last 3 days of the patient's hospitalization, the patient's temperature reflected a normal circadian rhythm.
   True _____   False _____

(3) During the first 4 days of the patient's hospitalization, the patient's blood pressure was consistent with a developing fluid volume deficit.
   True _____   False _____

(4) While hospitalized, the patient's pulse rate ranged from 76 to 110 beats per minute.
   True _____   False _____

(5) The patient's baseline pulse rate on admission to the hospital was within normal limits.
   True _____   False _____

(6) When the patient's temperature increased during the acute phase of the illness, the patient's respirations decreased.
   True _____   False _____

SAMPLE ITEM 7–12

A patient's daily intake and output (I&O) record for the 7 AM to 3 PM shift is illustrated on page 113. Identify if the following statements correctly or incorrectly reflect the information presented in the I&O record.

(1) If the intravenous solution infused at an equal volume per hour, then the hourly rate was 75 mL per hour.
   True _____   False _____

(2) If the patient had 4 oz of orange juice with breakfast at 8:30 AM, then the patient also drank another 10 oz of fluid with breakfast.
   True _____   False _____

(3) The patient's intake and output was equal at the completion of the 7 to 3 shift.
   True _____   False _____

(4) The additive to the patient's intravenous solution was 20 mg of vitamin K.
   True _____   False _____

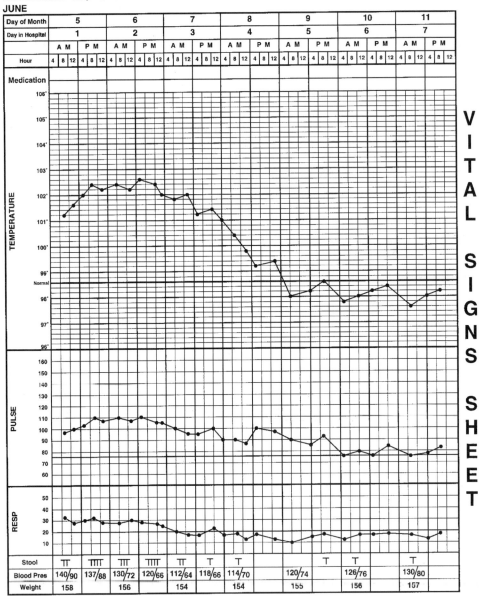

MATCHING QUESTIONS

A matching question begins by establishing a frame of reference for the question. It explains the topic of the question and the basis on which matches should be made. The item then divides into a double-column format. It presents a statement in column one and then requires you to select a corresponding, related, or companion statement from among a list of possible options in column two. Usually the question assesses information about related categories, classifications, or characteristics. Sometimes the items in the two columns are equal in number, and sometimes column one will have fewer statements than column two. When the columns are equal in length, the format can either work for you or work against you. If the columns have seven items each and you know six of the answers, then you will automatically get the last answer correct, whether or not you understand the content. On the other hand, if you make an incorrect choice,

DAILY INTAKE AND OUTPUT RECORD

DATE   JUNE 5

	INTAKE							OUTPUT			
	I.V. FLUIDS						ORAL	URINE	EMESIS	N.G. TUBE	HEMOVAC
Time	Bottle	Amount	Solution	Medication and Dosage	*ABS.	℔LIB					
8	1	1000	NS	20 mEq KCl				650			
8:30							360				
10:00							120				
11:30							240	150			
12:00									160		
1:40									90		60
2:15								250			
3:00						525	475					45
7-3 TOTAL		8-HR TOTAL			525	475	720	1050	250		105
3-11 TOTAL		8-HR TOTAL									
11-7 TOTAL		8-HR TOTAL									
24 HOUR TOTAL											

INTAKE GRAND TOTAL [   ]   OUTPUT GRAND TOTAL [   ]

* ABS. = amount absorbed   ℔ LIB = Left in bag

then you will automatically get two answers wrong. These problems are minimized if the response column (column two) has more options than the question column (column one).

You must first read the directions for the matching questions carefully because they specify the basis for the matching. In addition, they will tell you where to place the correct answer and the number of times an option can be selected. Next, match items that you are absolutely certain are correct matches. This eliminates the options that you have correctly matched, leaving a reduced list on which to focus. Now consider the remaining options, moving from the simple to the complex as determined by your frame of reference.

The matching question is a relatively superficial testing format that lends itself to factual information that usually is memorized. Therefore, another strategy would be to cover column two and for each item in column one attempt to recall the memorized information without being cued by the content in column two. Hopefully, the information you memorized will appear as an option in column two. By doing this you may become less confused or distracted by the list of options. If you do not know the answer and there is no penalty for guessing, make an educated guess.

SAMPLE ITEM 7–13

Column I contains terminology used to describe types of breathing exhibited by patients. Match each term to its correct description in Column II. Place the number you select from Column II on the line at the left of the term in Column I. Use each number only once.

Column I	Column II
_____ a. Bradypnea	1. Respirations that are increased in depth and rate
_____ b. Apnea	2. Difficulty breathing
_____ c. Hyperpnea	3. Respiratory rate less than 10 breaths per minute
_____ d. Tachypnea	4. Absence of breathing
_____ e. Eupnea	5. Respiratory rate greater than 20 breaths per minute
_____ f. Dyspnea	6. Normal breathing
	7. Shallow breathing interrupted by irregular periods of apnea

SAMPLE ITEM 7–14

Column I lists types of exercises. Match a type of exercise with its most therapeutic value or outcome. Indicate, in the space provided, the number from Column I that matches the letter in Column II. Options from Column I can be used more than once.

Column I—Exercises	Column II—Outcomes
1. Passive range of motion	a. Promote urinary continence ( )
2. Aerobic	b. Improve strength of pelvic floor muscles ( )
3. Isometric	c. Promote pulmonary functioning ( )
4. Kegel	d. Improve cardiovascular conditioning ( )
	e. Increase muscle mass, tone, and strength of an extremity in a cast ( )
	f. Maintain joint mobility ( )

Restricted-Response Questions

Restricted-response questions are also known as free-response items. Completion and short-answer questions are examples of restricted-response questions. These questions pose a simple question and expect you to furnish the answer. The response can be a word, a phrase, or even several sentences. Because these types of questions usually have an uncomplicated, direct format, they are most effective for assessing the understanding of simple concepts, the definition of terms, the knowledge of facts, or the ability to solve mathematical problems.

COMPLETION QUESTIONS

A completion question is generally a short statement with one or more blanks. You are required to furnish the word, words, or phrase that accurately completes the sentence. In a completion question the key word or words are the ones that are omitted. This forces you to focus on the important information reflected in the question rather than trivia. This type of question does not permit much flexibility or creativity in your response. The question anticipates a particular word or phrase that will produce an accurate statement.

SAMPLE ITEM 7–15

Flexion and fixation of a joint is called a _____.

SAMPLE ITEM 7–16

Postural drainage uses gravity to drain secretions from the _____.

SAMPLE ITEM 7–17

The normal respiratory rate for an adult is _____ to _____ breaths per minute.

The inclusion of two possible answers to fill in the blank is a simple variation of a completion question. This format resembles an alternate-response question because you are asked a question and two choices are presented from which to pick an answer. This type of question gives you an advantage because the words presented are clues. These words nudge your memory and, hopefully, the recall of information necessary to answer the question. When faced with a question that has only two possible options, the chance of selecting the correct answer is 50 percent.

SAMPLE ITEM 7–18

When describing "radiating pain," the nurse is referring to its (intensity/location).

SAMPLE ITEM 7–19

The feeling that a person needs to void immediately is called (frequency/urgency).

SHORT-ANSWER QUESTIONS

A short-answer question is a free-response item because it asks a question and expects you to compose an answer. It provides some flexibility and creativity because the response does not have to complete a sentence or fill in a blank. You usually can use anywhere from one word to several sentences to answer the question. A short-answer question that needs only a word or a phrase to answer the question is similar to a completion question, but the original question is a complete sentence rather than an incomplete sentence. A short-answer question that requires several sentences to answer the question goes beyond the standards or criteria of a completion question, but it still focuses on the knowledge of facts, terminology, simple concepts, or the ability to perform mathematical computations. The more relevant information you include in the response, the better you can demonstrate comprehension of the information being tested. Short-answer questions do not lend themselves to test-taking strategies. However, write as much as the format permits in the hope that what you include answers the question and contains the specific information expected by the teacher.

Short-answer and completion questions can be used interchangeably to address the same content. For example, compare Sample Items 7–15 through 7–17 with Sample Items 7–20 through 7–22, respectively.

SAMPLE ITEM 7–20

What is the definition of the word *contracture?*

SAMPLE ITEM 7–21

What is the purpose of postural drainage?

SAMPLE ITEM 7–22

What is the normal range of respirations per minute in an adult?

SAMPLE ITEM 7–23

The physician orders an intravenous solution of 1000 mL of D5W to be administered at 100 mL per hour. The drop factor of the intravenous administration set is 15 drops per mL. How many drops per minute should the patient receive?

Extended Essay Questions

An extended essay is a free-response question because the answer is drafted by you in reply to a question. It requires higher cognitive skills than just recall and comprehension. Essay questions expect you to select, arrange, organize, integrate, synthesize, compare, or contrast information. You must be able to use language constructively, be creative when solving problems, and employ critical thinking to manipulate complicated information. The extended essay is most suitable for evaluating mastery of complex material.

When writing responses to extended essay questions, it is wise to follow a three-part format when possible. First, begin with an introduction. The **introduction** should, in a general way, indicate what will be discussed. It introduces the topic and serves as a preface or prologue for what will follow. Next, present the central part or body of the answer. The **central part** of the answer should explore all the information that is being presented to answer the question. Organize this part of the answer by writing a topical outline. This blueprint promotes an orderly flow of information, prevents departure from your script, and ensures that significant material is included. Finally, complete the answer with a summary. The **summary** should recap what was discussed and come to several conclusions. It serves as a finale and brings closure to your answer.

Generally, instructors examine your writing from the viewpoint of **writing for evaluation.** Instructors measure your knowledge by evaluating an end product such as a written assignment or essay question on an examination. To answer an essay question, you must be able to put your thoughts on paper in a logical manner using correct spelling, grammar, and punctuation. There is no easy way to develop effective writing skills without practice. Most learning institutions today have writing centers that provide specialized faculty to assist you with writing activities. To maximize your success in formulating written assignments, you must view writing from the perspectives of **learning to write** and **writing to learn.**

LEARNING TO WRITE

When learning to write you are not looking at an end product that will be evaluated by the instructor, but rather focusing on the process of writing. Writing requires a basic understanding of the English language. For example, you need to have an adequate vocabulary, understand the rules of grammar and punctuation, and be able to spell. When learning to write, you also must focus on the organizational and analytical skills that help you to assess, advise, teach, argue a point of view, and challenge new and old theories. Critical thinking is an essential skill needed to process the information that is to be writen. Techniques that can be used to promote learning to write include brainstorming, setting priorities, and editing and revising previously written material.

Brainstorming is a method of exploring a topic by spontaneously listing thoughts or ideas. Making lists of words or phrases that relate to a topic allows you to explore a topic and your perspectives of the topic. For example, when students were asked to make a list of everything and anything relevant to patient progress notes, interesting insights developed. Some students were content oriented, in that they listed everything a health care provider should include in progress notes, such as vital signs, specific care provided, and patients' responses to care. Other students were process oriented, in that they stated that notes should be specific, legible, and comprehensive. Brainstorming not only helps you to learn to write but also to explore topics through writing. If you take the time to examine what you have written, it also may tell you a lot about yourself.

Setting priorities is an analytical skill that requires you to compare and contrast information and identify that which is most important or significant. Use a systematic method or theoretical base to make priority setting easier. Maslow's hierarchy of needs is an excellent framework because it also helps to organize information. Data can be clustered in each of the five levels or categories of needs. These needs are ranked according to how critical they are to survival. The physiological needs are the most basic and carry the highest priority; safety and security, love and belonging, self-esteem, and self-actualization follow. You can practice setting priorities each day just by ranking your activities for the day in order of importance.

Analyzing, editing, and revising previously written material are other ways to learn to write. Consider writing directly on a computer. On a computer it is easy to move words, phrases, and sentences around as you edit and revise your writing. Seeing your words in print helps to separate you from your own handwriting, making it easier to examine your writing. When you have the luxury of time, it is always to your advantage to write an assignment one day and then several days later review this first draft. Your analytical skills may improve, you may acquire new information since you first wrote the material, or your perspective may be different or clearer. Also, you will probably be more amenable to constructive criticism when it comes from within. Analyzing, editing, and revising your own written compositions are excellent ways to improve your writing abilities.

The hardest thing to overcome when engaging in learning-to-write activities is the feeling that because you may not have completed a project, you have not learned. Remember, learning takes place in the learner and it is a lifelong process.

WRITING TO LEARN

When writing to learn you are focusing on what you will eventually understand or remember, not on the process of writing. You learn content by the very act of writing because at least two cognitive domains are being integrated: cognitive (thinking) and psychomotor (writing).

You learn the course content you are writing about and discover what you know, what you need to know, and what you think about certain topics. When you are writing to learn, you are writing for yourself, and what you learn is the end product. Techniques that can be used to promote writing to learn include writing lists, writing journals, posing and answering questions, and note taking.

Writing a list can be a simple or complex task. A simple list would be repetitiously writing a phase or fact in an effort to reinforce learning. This requires a low-level thinking process that involves the recall of information. For example, writing common equivalents in the apothecaries' and metric systems (15 to 16 grains = 1 gram). A complex list might require the writer to discriminate between the commonalties and differences of content material. This requires higher levels of the thinking process and includes comprehension, application, and analysis. For example, making a list of nursing interventions that use the concept of gravity (IV infusion, urinary catheter, elevation of an extremity to promote venous return). To compile this list, you must comprehend a variety of concepts and be able to identify the commonalties among the applications of these concepts.

Writing a journal focuses on the use of words, the expression of ideas and feelings, and the documentation of activities; no consideration should be given to format, grammar, or punctuation. For 5 to 10 minutes each day, write a diary. It will improve your thinking and learning as well as document where you have been, where you are, and where you are going.

Posing and answering questions can lead to a better understanding of the content you are learning as well as improve your critical-thinking skills. Many textbooks have a companion study guide or workbook. Answering questions from these books and questions that you make up for yourself are excellent ways to reinforce the understanding of information. Putting your thoughts into concrete words and using the psychomotor skill of writing helps you to learn.

Note taking can be a simple or complex task. A simple note-taking strategy would be the rewriting of class notes. When you rewrite notes you revise information so that it is more organized and clear. A complex note-taking strategy would be to add relevant information from the textbook to your class notes. You can even add to your notes your own thoughts and reactions.

SAMPLE ITEM 7–24

Compare and contrast critical thinking and problem solving and include at least three characteristics of each.

Performance Appraisal

A performance appraisal evaluates the ability to complete a procedure. Psychomotor skills, the motor effects of mental processes, are most effectively assessed by performance appraisals. Obtaining a blood pressure, changing a sterile dressing, administering a tube feeding, and performing tracheal suctioning are examples of psychomotor skills. When evaluating these skills, the criteria for passing should be identified before you attempt the procedure. For example, the criteria in obtaining a blood pressure reading might be that you must obtain accurate systolic and diastolic readings. In another testing situation the criteria for passing might be previously identified steps of the procedure such as washes hands, checks functioning of equipment, evenly places cuff around the upper arm, places stethoscope over brachial artery, inflates cuff 20 mm Hg above palpated systolic reading, deflates cuff at 2 to 3 mm Hg per second, obtains accurate systolic reading, and obtains accurate diastolic reading.

Any step that must be accurately performed to receive a passing score is known as a *critical element*. Critical elements are very specific criteria. Other criteria may be more general. For example, when obtaining a temperature reading, you must maintain medical asepsis, provide for physical safety, and ensure privacy. These are less specific because there are numerous ways to meet each of these criteria. For example, physical safety can be provided by holding the thermometer while it is in place, taking a tympanic temperature when the patient is confused, or taking a rectal temperature because the patient is a mouth breather. Performance appraisals should be objective and the criteria for an acceptable performance identified. Clinical techniques and skills textbooks are helpful when practicing procedures and preparing for performance appraisals. A clinical skills checklist of step-by-step elements can be used by another student to assess your performance of a psychomotor skill in a laboratory setting. This is a nonthreatening way to practice, and it supports reciprocal study relationships. It also provides an opportunity to simulate a testing situation and helps with desensitization, which may give the student a feeling of control.

Summary

To promote success when challenged by an examination with a variety of testing formats, it is wise to be familiar with the various formats. Structured-response, restricted-response, extended essay, and performance appraisal formats have some commonalities, but each is unique. Pretests and post-tests that are presented within chapters in textbooks, student workbooks that accompany textbooks, and textbooks devoted to helping students prepare for examinations should be used to practice test-taking skills. Understanding the commonalities and differences in these formats and using a variety of test-taking techniques facilitates a feeling of control, which contributes to a positive mental attitude.

Answers and Rationales for Sample Items in Chapter 7

7–1   TRUE—The surface tension of water, the tendency of a liquid to minimize the area of its surface by contracting, is lowered in the presence of soap. This increases the ability of water to wet another surface.

7–2   TRUE—A broad stance widens the nurse's base of support, which promotes stability.

7–3   FALSE—Exercise is a stimulating activity that should be avoided before bedtime. Adequate exercise during the day promotes sleep later in the day.

7–4   FALSE—Pulse pressure is the difference between the systolic and diastolic blood pressures. Pulse deficit is the difference between the apical and radial pulse rates.

7–5   TRUE—Palpation is a technique in which the examiner applies the fingers or hands to the body to assess the texture, size, consistency, and location of body parts.

7–6   FALSE—The process in which solid, particulate matter in a fluid moves from an area of higher concentration to an area of lower concentration is known as diffusion. The process in which a pure solvent, such as water, moves through a semipermeable membrane from an area that has a lower solute concentration to one that has a higher solute concentration is known as osmosis.

7–7   ① TRUE—The outer border of a drape is considered contaminated. After sterile gloves are donned, the nurse can touch inside this border and still maintain sterility of the field.
         ② FALSE—During a surgical hand scrub the hands are held above the elbows; this allows water to flow downward by gravity without contaminating the nurse's hands. Handwashing associated with medical asepsis requires the hands to be held below the elbows.
         ③ TRUE—Because the hands are not sterile, the nurse avoids contaminating the sterile glove by touching only the inside of the glove. The second sterile glove is donned by touching just the outside of the glove with the hand that is already covered by the first sterile glove.
         ④ FALSE—Sterile objects held below the waist are not within the nurse's direct visual field and inadvertently may become contaminated.

7–8   ① TRUE—Mechanical ventilation employs positive pressure to push air and/or oxygen into the lungs during the inspiratory phase of the respiratory cycle. Positive pressure is pressure greater than that of the atmosphere.
         ② TRUE—Positive pressure is exerted when the plunger of a piston syringe is pushed toward its cone tip.
         ③ FALSE—A continuous bladder irrigation uses the principle of gravity to instill fluid into the bladder as well as to promote the flow of fluid out of the bladder through the triple-lumen indwelling urinary catheter. Gravity is the force that draws all masses in the earth's sphere toward the center of the earth.
         ④ FALSE—Chest tubes (water-seal drainage system) exert negative pressure to remove air and fluids from the pleural space. Negative pressure is pressure less than that of the atmosphere, and it is the opposite of positive pressure.

7–9   ① FALSE—This statement can be revised two different ways. The normal range of the heart rate for an adult is *60* to *100* beats per minute, or the normal range of the heart rate for a *6-year-old child* is 75 to 120 beats per minute. Either of these revisions would result in a correct statement.

7–10 ① FALSE—To revise this question as directed, the words *young adulthood* must be changed to *adolescence*. You would not receive credit for this question if *identity versus role confusion* were changed to *intimacy versus isolation*. Although this statement would be accurate, the instructions for revising the statement would not have been followed.

7–11 ① FALSE—The patient's temperature was 101.4°F. Each line above 101 is $^2/_{10}$ of a degree.
② TRUE—Body temperature varies throughout the day with the lowest temperature in the early morning and the highest temperature between 8 PM and midnight. A circadian rhythm (diurnal variation) is a pattern based on a 24-hour cycle.
③ TRUE—With fluid volume deficit the volume in the intravascular compartment decreases (hypovolemia), resulting in a decreased blood pressure (hypotension).
④ TRUE—This patient's pulse rate ranged from 76 to 110 beats per minute.
⑤ TRUE—A pulse rate of 96 is within the normal range of 60 to 100 beats per minute.
⑥ FALSE—During the acute phase of the illness the patient's temperature, pulse, and respirations were all elevated.

7–12 ① TRUE—The intravenous solution was hung at 8 AM and infused 525 mL over the next 7 hours. The total volume (525) divided by the number of hours (7) equals 75 mL per hour.
② FALSE—If each ounce is equal to 30 mL, then 4 ounces is equal to 120 mL. If you subtract 120 from the total volume of fluid taken at 8:30 AM (360), the amount of additional fluid consumed was 240 mL. If you divide 240 mL by 30 mL, it equals 8 ounces, not 10.
③ FALSE—The intake was 525 + 720 = 1245 mL. The output was 1050 + 250 + 105 = 1405 mL. The output exceeded the intake by 160 mL.
④ FALSE—The additive to the patient's intravenous solution was 20 mEq of potassium chloride.

7–13 a. **3** *Bradypnea* is abnormally slow breathing (less than 10 breaths per minute) with a regular rhythm.
b. **4** *Apnea* is the temporary cessation of breathing.
c. **1** *Hyperpnea* is deep, rapid, labored respirations; it is usually associated with strenuous exercise.
d. **5** *Tachypnea* is abnormally rapid breathing (more than 20 breaths per minute) with a regular rhythm.
e. **6** *Eupnea* is breathing that is normal in rate (12 to 20 breaths per minute) and depth (tidal volume of approximately 500 mL).
f. **2** *Dyspnea* is difficulty breathing characterized by an increased effort and use of accessory muscles.
"Shallow breathing interrupted by irregular periods of apnea" (option 7) was an extra option included in Column II that did not have a matching term in Column I.

7–14 a. **4** Kegel exercises consist of repetitive contractions of the muscles of the pelvic floor. These muscles facilitate voluntary control of urination.
b. **4** Kegel exercises, which are performed by voluntarily starting and stopping the urinary stream, tone the perineal muscles of the pelvic floor.
c. **2** Aerobic exercises involve activity that demands that oxygen be taken into the body at a rate greater than the amount the body usually requires, promoting respiratory functioning.
d. **2** Aerobic exercises involve sustained muscle movements that increase blood

flow, heart rate, and metabolic demand for oxygen over time, promoting cardiovascular functioning.

e. **3** Isometric exercises cause a change in muscle tension but no change in muscle length; no muscle or joint movement occurs.

f. **1** Passive range-of-motion exercises occur when another person moves each of the patient's joints through their full range of movement, maximally stretching all muscle groups within each plane over each joint.

7–15 *Contracture* is the only acceptable answer to this question. Contractures are permanent flexion deformities of joints caused by disuse, atrophy, and shortening of muscles.

7–16 *Respiratory passages* or *lung* would both be acceptable answers to this question. With postural drainage the patient is placed in various positions to promote the movement of secretions from smaller to larger pulmonary branches, where they can be removed by coughing or suctioning.

7–17 The correct answer for this question is *12 to 20*.

7–18 The correct answer is *location*. Radiating pain is a description that relates to where the pain is experienced in the body. It includes the initial site of the pain and its extension to other parts of the body. Intensity refers to the perceived severity of the pain; intensity can be measured on a scale of 0 (no pain) to 10 (severe pain).

7–19 The correct answer is *urgency*. Urgency is the feeling that the person must void whether or not there is much urine in the bladder. It is precipitated by psychological stress and/or irritation of the vesical trigone and/or urethra. Frequency is the increased incidence of voiding.

7–20 Acceptable answers include: permanent flexion and fixation of a joint; a contracture is an abnormal shortening of a muscle that results in limited range of motion of a joint and eventually ankylosis. Compare this item with Sample Item 7–15.

7–21 Acceptable answers include: mobilize respiratory secretions; loosen pulmonary secretions to facilitate their expectoration; and postural drainage promotes a clear airway by draining respiratory secretions toward the oral cavity. Compare this item with Sample Item 7–16.

7–22 Acceptable answers may include just stating the numbers 12 to 20. A more complex answer might state: The normal number of breaths per minute for an adult ranges from 12 to 20 with an average of 16. The normal respiratory rate in relation to the heart rate is usually 1 respiration to every 4 heart beats. The respiratory rate normally increases with exercise and decreases with rest or sleep. Compare this item with Sample Item 7–17.

7–23 To arrive at the correct answer of 25 drops per minute you would have to perform the following calculation.

$$\frac{\text{Volume to be infused} \times \text{drop factor}}{\text{Number of hours} \times 60 \text{ minutes}}$$

$$\frac{100 \times 15}{1 \times 60}$$

$$\frac{1500}{60} = 25 \text{ drops per minute}$$

7–24 To answer this question, use the three-part format.

INTRODUCTION: The introduction functions as a preface, preamble, or prologue for what information will follow.

Although there are many detailed definitions of the practice of nursing, in the simplest terms nursing consists of helping people meet needs. To do this, nurses must employ cognitive skills such as critical thinking and problem solving. The commonalities and differences of critical thinking and problem solving will be discussed.

CENTRAL PART: The central part of the answer presents and explores the information necessary to answer the question. Make a topical outline of the facts to be included, and then write a narrative that incorporates and elaborates on the information in the outline.

Definition of critical thinking
    Reasoning
    Goal directed
    Reaching conclusions from a new perspective

Definition of problem solving
    Identifies a problem
    Suggests solutions
    Implements interventions to resolve problems

Commonalities of critical thinking and problem solving
    Strong knowledge base
    Attitude of inquiry and intellectual humility
    Systematic process
    Identifies priorities

Differences of critical thinking
    Uses problem-solving techniques
    Proactive
    Focuses more on the positive
    Open-ended and focuses on continuous improvement

Differences of problem solving
    Uses critical thinking
    Reactive
    Focuses more on the negative
    Starts with a problem and ends with a solution

SUMMARY: The summary should briefly recap or review the general tone of the discussion and come to one or more conclusions. It serves to formally close the response to the essay question.

The nurse of today and especially of the future must be able to integrate critical thinking and problem solving to maximize human potential. The nurse must use critical thinking to effectively resolve problems, and the nurse must use problem-solving techniques to think critically. Although they have a common foundation, each mode of thinking is unique. Nurses should blend them into a repertoire of cognitive strategies.

Computer Applications in Education and Evaluation

We are members of an informational society where information is created, stored, retrieved, communicated, and manipulated. Exploding knowledge and technology, the emerging health care reform initiatives, and the intensified and diversified role of the nurse all add to the complexity of functioning within this informational society. To process information efficiently, effectively, and economically, computers are essential. They have become a reality in every aspect of our world and are used in private homes, educational settings, industry, and health care facilities. To prepare for a career in nursing, you must have the basic skills to use computers in a comfortable manner and be a willing learner to keep pace with rapidly advancing computer technology. Although computers are used in the practice of nursing, this chapter will focus on the use of computers only in relation to education and evaluation.

Computing across the curriculum is not new in the educational setting. Educators immediately identified the potential of interactive participation to facilitate learning. Programmed-instruction textbooks were the predecessors of computer programs. These textbooks present information within blocked narrative material. Each grouping of material is called a frame. Each frame requires a response from the learner before moving on to the next narrative frame. These textbooks require active involvement by the learner. Computers make this programmed approach more interactive by increasing the potential, richness, and variety of frame styles, which improve the effectiveness of the lesson. Computers also use graphics, color, and sound to facilitate learning in a way that programmed-instruction textbooks are unable to do because of the limitations of the written format.

Students generally enjoy using the computer to facilitate learning because the programs hold their attention, provide immediate feedback, and never become impatient. Also, they are accessible, challenging, and fun. Computer-based instruction is not designed to replace the more traditional forms of teaching but to augment them. Computers allow you to review difficult material at your own rate, increase critical thinking, experience simulated clinical situations, and assess your knowledge. The greatest advantage of computer-based instruction is that you become an active participant, not just a passive spectator.

To be an active participant, you should have a simple understanding of a few essential keyboard keys. Most programs are "user friendly" and include on-screen instructions or help menus. Generally, students do not have difficulty manipulating the keyboard or mouse (handheld device to move an on-screen directional arrow). However, some students have "computer anxiety." Only exposure to computers in a secure and positive learning environment can lessen computer anxiety and promote computer literacy.

The following are examples of how computers can be used in education and evaluation. The computer can enhance student learning by accessing professional resources, managing information, teaching, simulating clinical situations, and evaluating knowledge.

The Computer as a Resource Tool

The computer is a resource tool that can be used to obtain information for academic assignments. A computerized literature search that uses national databases or networks can provide rapid access to current literature in nursing and its related fields. A modem (a device that allows transmission of data between computers over a telephone line) connects you to the information retrieval system, and specific protocols may be required to gain entry to a database. These searches can usually be conducted in most libraries with the assistance of the research librarian. However, cost may be a factor, because telephone lines must be maintained to transmit and receive information. Most systems also have on-line connect charges for accessing the database as well as for the length of time the database is being used, and a fee may be charged for on-line or off-line printing. On-line printing provides an immediate hard copy of the desired information, whereas off-line printing provides a hard copy that is sent by mail at a later date. Sometimes the fees incurred are beyond the financial means of the average student. Literature searches on the computer save time and energy. Therefore, you must decide whether these activities are cost effective for you by measuring the time saved against the money spent.

The Computer as an Information Manager

The computer has revolutionized the way in which information is managed, not only outside the home but inside the home. Many people now compose written material immediately on the computer. This is possible because you no longer need to have strong keyboard skills or expend extensive time and energy to learn how to use software programs. Today, user-friendly software programs have on-screen commands and effective help menus. Touch, a stylus, or a mouse also help facilitate computer use. The personal computer can be used for word processing, setting up spreadsheets, data processing, graphing data, and so on. You can now manipulate data, words, and images to complete your academic assignments with ease.

The Computer as an Instructor

Computer-assisted instruction (CAI) is an excellent addition to the repertoire of strategies available to educators and nursing students to facilitate the learning process. In CAI information is communicated from the computer to the learner without direct interaction with the teacher. These instructional delivery systems can present principles and theory, enhance comprehension, promote creative problem solving, and provide immediate feedback to enrich independent learning.

Some computer programs display information in a textual format that has limited interaction between you and the computer. These programs really function as an automated textbook. Other tutorial approaches present new information in small steps or frames, then require you to make responses to demonstrate your comprehension of the material just delivered. Such programs function as an automated, programmed-instruction textbook.

These types of programs generally use a linear format that proceeds from the beginning of the program to the end of the program without deviation. They present information in a straight line, with one beginning and one end, and every student is exposed to the same information. Although valuable, these programs do not recognize the learner as an individual with specific needs, interests, and abilities.

With the advent of CD-ROM (Compact Disk–Read-Only Memory) technology and sophisticated software programs, the computer learning experience has become more individualized. Programs that use a branching format allow you to select a path that focuses on information relevant to your ability and interest. When programs meet individualized needs, learning is more effective, use of time is more efficient, and student motivation increases.

The Computer as a Simulator

The role of the nursing educator is to assist you to move beyond the mere memorization of facts to the application of information in clinical situations. To do this, you must use critical thinking to integrate information into a meaningful frame of reference. Computer simulations are designed to enhance your ability to use critical thinking and safely make sound judgments in a fabricated situation. These simulation programs provide a supportive environment because they usually produce less anxiety and are obviously safe for the "patient." Although computer simulation has long been used in aeronautics and flight training, it is in its infancy in simulating experiences within the health care professions.

Nursing simulations may present a patient database that requires you to input, sort, and retrieve data. Simulations may focus on the application of information processing skills, which assist you to select sources of data that are most appropriate, classify data, cluster and sequence data, and even evaluate data. Simulations may focus on components of critical thinking. A program addressing critical thinking may require you to identify relationships, recognize commonalities and differences, and use deductive and inductive reasoning to support inferences. Simulations may be designed to improve decision making by requiring you to recognize the nature of the problem, choose a course of action from multiple options, establish priorities, and evaluate the outcome of the final decision. Simulations can present clinical situations that would be difficult to present in a classroom setting or events that you may not have had the opportunity to experience in the clinical setting. Curricula cannot guarantee that each and every student will have an opportunity to experience each and every situation that may be important to learning. However, computer simulation may be able to fill this void.

The disadvantage of simulation programs in nursing is that they cannot include all the unpredictable variables that occur in real-life situations. However, interactive videodisc instruction (IVD, IVI), a sophisticated form of computer-assisted instruction, uses the newest computer technology to enrich the clinical situations presented and encourage the highest degree of interaction between you and the computer. Studies have demonstrated that there is a highly significant degree of student satisfaction with interactive videodisc instruction and that a positive mental attitude is significant to the learning process because of its influence on student motivation, learning rate, and retention and application of information.

The Computer as an Evaluator

Evaluation (test-taking) programs are designed to measure your knowledge, skills, and abilities in relation to the domain of nursing. They can be self-administered or administered by a person in authority. Programs devised to be self-administered generally contain both a learning mode and a self-evaluation mode. In the **learning mode** you are presented with a multiple-choice question with four options and are asked to select the correct answer. Once you select an option, the program provides immediate feedback regarding the correctness of the choice. Rationales for the correct and wrong answers may be provided, depending on how the program is designed. The learning mode that provides rationales for all the choices has the potential to promote new learning or reinforce previous learning. These types of programs are a form of computer-assisted instruction. The **evaluation mode** enables you to conduct an assessment of your test-taking abilities regarding a specific body of knowledge addressed in the program. The evaluation mode also allows you to experience a testing situation. Some programs provide rationales for all the options at the completion of the program. Other, more detailed, programs may supply an individualized analysis of your performance. This analysis may include information such as the questions you got wrong and why, the content areas that you need to study further, your performance in relation to other nursing students, or predictions for passing future examinations. Self-administered evaluation programs are particularly successful because they focus on competency and provide immediate feedback.

An evaluation program conducted by a person in authority may be administered to assess your ability to pass a course of study or to demonstrate your competency for certification or licensure. These programs use computer technology and replace paper-and-pencil tests. Some programs may use a format in which you and every other test-taker are confronted by the same exact questions. Other programs may use **computerized-adaptive testing** (CAT), a unique format in which your examination is assembled interactively as you answer each question. In a typical CAT format, all the questions in the test bank have a calculated level of difficulty. You are presented with a question. If you answer the question correctly, then you are presented with a slightly more difficult question. If you answer the question incorrectly, then you are presented with a slightly easier question. This process is repeated for each question until a pass-or-fail decision is made. Passing is determined by your demonstration of knowledge, skills, and abilities in relation to a standard of acceptable performance. The advantages of the CAT format are that it individualizes each test, provides for self-paced testing, reduces the amount of time needed to complete the test, and produces greater measurement precision. The disadvantages of the CAT format are that you cannot review the entire test before starting, difficult questions cannot be skipped and returned to at a later time, and you cannot go back and change an answer once it is selected and entered.

In 1994 the NCLEX-RN and the NCLEX-PN, the licensure examinations for registered nurse and practical nurse, respectively, changed from standard paper-and-pencil tests to examinations using computerized-adaptive testing. Although no prior computer experience is necessary to take a test using CAT, it is always better to be familiar with the particular testing format used. There are many commercial products available that use the CAT format. Practice can only improve your performance on future CAT examinations.

Summary

Computers are causing major changes in the traditional ways things are done in health care education and evaluation. In our informational society some certainties exist: we are on information overload; the manipulation of information has become more sophisticated than ever before; and computers will be used more extensively in education, evaluation, and practice in the future. You must become computer literate and be willing to learn about new computer technology as it emerges. The most important implication of computer applications in learning, evaluation, and practice is that you can use the computer to increase the efficiency of your work and study, thereby leaving more time to interact with instructors, peers, and clients.

Fundamentals of Nursing Practice Tests

9

Introduction to Practice Tests

Three practice tests have been provided so that you can measure your knowledge of nursing content and test-taking skills for the purpose of comparison over time. Each test has been designed to test items with comparable content, in similar proportions to those you may find on a fundamentals of nursing examination, and with a similar degree of difficulty. Use these tests in a planned way. Do not take them haphazardly. Take Practice Test A before reading any of the chapters in this book. This will assess your knowledge of the fundamentals of nursing content and your ability to take a test. This test functions as a pretest, and your score will provide a baseline for future comparison. Carefully read Chapters 1 through 8 at your own pace. Once you complete reading these chapters, take Practice Test B. This will provide an interim score regarding your test-taking performance. Now study the practice questions in Chapter 10. The questions in Chapter 10 are grouped within content areas. It would be most beneficial to review the items in these content areas after you have covered this content in your curriculum. Take Test C after you have completed Chapter 10. This final test will serve as a post-test. Hopefully, you should improve your score each time you take a subsequent practice test.

Simulated testing is designed to demonstrate growth and motivate you to continue with your efforts to succeed in testing situations. Although it has been suggested that you take Practice Tests A, B, and C in sequence, the order in which you take the tests does not matter. You can choose to take Practice Test C first and then B and A. The three tests have been designed so that the tests are equal in their level of difficulty. The average score for each test is approximately 76 percent. This was determined by a statistical analysis of field testing conducted with fundamental nursing students from a variety of nursing schools from across the country. If your score is greater than 76 percent on any of the tests, you will have scored higher than the average fundamental nursing student who participated in the field testing. If your score is less than 76 percent, you will have scored lower than the average fundamental nursing student who participated in the field testing.

When self-administering a practice test, set aside 40 minutes of uninterrupted time. To simulate a testing environment, you must sit at a table and select a time when you will not be disturbed. You are allotted 40 minutes to take one practice test. If you divide 40 minutes by 30 questions, you have approximately $1^{1}/_{3}$ minutes to consider each question. To leave 10 minutes at the end of the examination for review, permit yourself 1 minute to answer each question. If you spend less than 1 minute on a question, you can use this time for the questions you find more difficult or add it to the time you have reserved for your review at the end of the test. Use the full 40 minutes to complete each practice test. If your school allots more or less time than 1 minute per question, adjust your time accordingly. If your examinations are not timed, use all the time you need to complete the test.

When taking a practice test, use the answer sheet provided at the end of the book. To record your answers, use a number 2 pencil because the lead is soft enough to easily fill the spaces provided on the answer sheet. Carefully darken the enclosed space on the answer sheet that corresponds to the number of the question on the test. Be particularly careful if you want to skip over an item that is difficult and move on to the next item. When you record your next answer, make sure that you darken the appropriate place on the answer sheet. Students have been known to score poorly on an important test because they inadvertently placed an answer on the wrong line, causing each subsequent answer to be incorrectly recorded. Answer every question. If you do not know the answer to a question, attempt to eliminate as many options as you can using test-taking skills and then make an educated guess. If you are preparing for a computer-administered test, answer each question before moving on to the next question. Do not go back to answer or change a previous question.

After you complete a practice test, review the correct answer and the rationales for the correct and incorrect options. If your answer was wrong, analyze your reasons for having selected a distractor instead of the correct answer. Ask yourself, "Was I careless?" "Did I lack knowledge about the content?" "Did I miss an important word in the stem?" "Did I quickly jump to the wrong conclusion?" "Did I read into the question and make it more complicated?" "Did I misunderstand what the question was asking?" It is important to identify why you answered an item incorrectly so that you can implement some corrective action to improve your score the next time. As you review the practice test, note the content areas that you answered incorrectly. For example, if you had difficulty answering questions related to patient assessments or to hygiene, then you should direct your future study toward these areas of concern. Also analyze the results of every item in which you changed your initial answer. If, when you change an answer, you invariably get the item correct, you might continue to profit from changing your answers on succeeding tests. If, when you change an answer, you consistently get the item wrong, it may be to your advantage not to change your answers on subsequent tests. Also determine what it was that caused you to change your initial choice to the correct or incorrect answer. If you can identify patterns of errors in test taking, you may be able to institute strategies to eliminate them on future examinations. Practice tests are learning experiences because they permit the application of test-taking strategies, reinforce information you understand, identify content areas that need to be emphasized in future study, and build your test-taking endurance.

PRACTICE TEST A

1   A female patient has just been informed that she will be transferred to a nursing home because her son is unable to care for her at home. While receiving a bed bath, the patient yells at the nurse, "You don't know what you are doing." The nurse's *best* reaction would be to:
   ① Request that another nurse take care of the patient
   ② Accept the behavior and not take it personally
   ③ Discontinue the bath and resume it later
   ④ Explain that she is getting good care

2   A patient is wearing bilateral mitt restraints. The nurse should release the restraints and exercise the patient's hands and wrists every:
   ① Hour
   ② Shift
   ③ 2 hours
   ④ 4 hours

3   A patient is incontinent of stool and smears it on the bed linens and bed rails. The initial goal should be that the patient will:
   ① Become continent
   ② Stay clean and dry
   ③ Call for the bedpan
   ④ Stop smearing stool

4   The best action for the nurse to take to prevent the patient from falling out of bed when using a bedpan should be to:
   ① Reposition the patient to a semi-Fowler's position
   ② Lower the height of the bed to its lowest position
   ③ Place an overbed table in front of the patient
   ④ Raise the side rails on both sides of the bed

5   A patient who is often short of breath is afraid to be left alone. What should the nurse do to help reduce this fear?
   ① Position the patient in a wheelchair near the nurses' station.
   ② Encourage the patient to become friends with other patients.
   ③ Stay with the patient as much as possible.
   ④ Answer the patient's call bell immediately.

6   A patient has bilateral wrist restraints. To provide adequate fluid intake, the nurse should:
   ① Encourage extra fluids at each meal
   ② Position a glass of water within reach
   ③ Serve fluids frequently between meals
   ④ Provide a long straw to encourage drinking

7   Obese patients often have serious difficulty breathing when positioned in the:
   ① Supine position
   ② Contour position
   ③ Orthopneic position
   ④ Semi-Fowler's position

8 Which fact about ambulation is most important to document in the patient's medical record?
① When the patient is ambulated
② Where the patient is ambulated
③ The patient's response to ambulation
④ The length of time it took to ambulate the patient

9 Hospice care lies in which level of prevention?
① Secondary prevention
② Morbidity prevention
③ Tertiary prevention
④ Primary prevention

10 Which is a physical reaction to moderate pain?
① Crying
② Moaning
③ Increased heart rate
④ Complaints of suffering

11 Which statement is accurate?
① Daily baths are necessary for homeostasis.
② Bathing decreases pathogens on the skin.
③ Patients want to be clean and neat.
④ A bath is ineffective without soap.

12 The nurse makes a work assignment for the nursing assistant at the beginning of the shift. An acceptable expectation of the nurse is that the nursing assistant will:
① Work without supervision by the nurse
② Be friends with other health team members
③ Complete everything that has been assigned
④ Perform within the role of the nursing assistant

13 A patient is cognitively impaired and confused. When assisting the patient with a meal, the nurse should say:
① "What would you like to eat first?"
② "It is good for you to eat all your food."
③ "This is your meat. Please eat your meat."
④ "If you finish your meat, you can have dessert."

14 Which patient would require a rectal temperature rather than an oral temperature?
① A confused patient
② An 8-year-old patient
③ A patient with no teeth
④ An elderly patient with dentures

15 A patient with an indwelling urinary catheter (Foley) is to be transferred to a wheelchair. To prevent reflux of urine into the bladder, the nurse should plan to:
① Hang it on the chair below the patient's hip
② Attach the bag to the arm of the wheelchair
③ Place it on the floor under the wheelchair
④ Place the bag in the patient's lap

16 The patient at the highest risk for developing a pressure (decubitus) ulcer is the patient with:
① Paraplegia

② Hypotension
③ Memory loss
④ Heart failure

17 Which is the most effective method to prevent the spread of microorganisms to all the patients in a hospital?
① Medical asepsis
② Surgical asepsis
③ Isolation precautions
④ The use of antibiotics

18 After an intramuscular (IM) injection, a drop of blood appears at the injection site. What should the nurse do?
① Massage the area gently.
② Take the patient's vital signs.
③ Apply pressure with the antiseptic swab.
④ Document this reaction in the nurse's notes.

19 Which food should be measured when a patient is on intake and output (I&O)?
① Yogurt
② Ice cream
③ Applesauce
④ Pureed peaches

20 A patient who is incontinent of feces says to the nurse, "This is disgusting. How can you stand this?" The nurse's best response would be:
① "You sound upset."
② "This is disgusting?"
③ "I am used to this by now."
④ "It's not as bad as you think."

21 The abdominal thrust (Heimlich maneuver) attempts to:
① Force air out of the lungs
② Increase systemic circulation
③ Induce emptying of the stomach
④ Put pressure on the apex of the heart

22 Before discharge, an elderly patient complains of cold feet. To best keep the feet warm, the nurse should teach the patient to:
① Submerge them in warm water
② Wrap a blanket around them
③ Place them on a heating pad
④ Wear a pair of cotton socks

23 To clean an indwelling urinary catheter (Foley) when providing perineal care, the nurse should:
① Scrub up and down the tube with soap and water
② Wear a gown and gloves throughout the procedure
③ Wash the tubing before washing the urinary meatus
④ Bathe around the catheter moving away from the meatus

24 Growth and development progress at a rate that can be described as:
① Fast
② Slow

③ Smooth
④ Irregular

25 When a fire is discovered in a dirty utility room, the nurse's FIRST action should be to:
① Close the fire doors on the unit
② Move patients toward the stairs
③ Attempt to put out the fire
④ Pull the fire alarm

26 When moving from a lying to a sitting position on the side of the bed, a patient complains of dizziness. The initial response of the nurse should be to:
① Position the patient's head between the knees
② Transfer the patient to a bedside chair quickly
③ Instruct the patient to sit on the side of the bed
④ Tell the patient to stand at the bedside for a few minutes

27 Which adaptation would indicate a toxic effect of an anticoagulant?
① Bradycardia
② Hematuria
③ Jaundice
④ Diarrhea

28 The patient has black, tarry-colored stools. The nurse recognizes that this is related to:
① Overproduction of bile
② Gastrointestinal bleeding
③ Decreased absorption of fat
④ Deficient pancreatic enzymes

29 When taking a patient's blood pressure, the nurse opens the pressure valve knob and the mercury drops quickly. The nurse should:
① Remove the cuff and send the sphygmomanometer for repair
② Squeeze the air out of the cuff and try again
③ Wait 2 minutes before pumping up the cuff
④ Check the tubing and cuff for air leaks

30 The most common reason why patients have a nasogastric tube in place after abdominal surgery is for the purpose of:
① Decompression
② Instillation
③ Lavage
④ Gavage

Answers and Rationales for Practice Test A

An asterisk (*) is in front of the rationale that explains the correct answer.

1   ① Having another nurse care for the patient might send a message to the patient that could precipitate feelings of guilt or imply to the patient that the nurse no longer wanted to provide care.

   * ② Anger is a defense or response to loss; the nurse must recognize that the patient is using displacement to deal with emotional pain.

    ③ Discontinuing the bath would abandon the patient at a time when the patient should be given an opportunity to verbalize feelings.

    ④ This is a defensive response that focuses on the nurse rather than the patient.

2   ① Range-of-motion (ROM) exercises are unnecessary every hour unless the patient had a concomitant neuromusculoskeletal problem.

    ② This is too long a period of time between the release of restraints and performing ROM and could result in contractures.

   * ③ Under usual circumstances, every 2 hours is often enough to perform ROM exercises to prevent contractures.

    ④ Same as #2.

3   ① The patient may not have the physical, mental, or emotional ability to achieve this goal; the patient should be clean first.

   * ② A patient's basic physical needs should be given first priority.

    ③ Same as #1.

    ④ Same as #1.

4   ① Repositioning could increase the risk of falling out of bed.

    ② Although this decreases the sensation of being up high, it does not provide a barrier to prevent a fall.

    ③ An overbed table is a movable object that would not provide a stable barrier.

   * ④ Side rails provide a barrier that prevents the patient from falling out of bed; they also provide a handhold for turning or maintaining balance.

5   ① This is impractical; the patient cannot sit at the nurses' station all the time.

    ② Patients should not be responsible for each other.

    ③ This is impractical; the nurse also must care for other patients.

   * ④ This reduces anxiety because the patient knows that someone will come immediately if help is needed.

6   ① Fluids given only three times a day would not be adequate.

    ② This is useless because the patient is restrained.

   * ③ The patient is dependent on the nurse because of the inability to be self-sufficient; frequent small amounts of fluid are more desirable than larger amounts of fluid given less frequently.

    ④ Using a long straw is unrealistic.

7   * ① The weight of the chest and pressure of the abdominal organs against the diaphragm limit thoracic excursion, causing dyspnea.

    ② This position allows the abdominal organs to drop via gravity, allowing the diaphragm to effectively contract and promoting full expansion of the lungs.

    ③ Same as #2.

    ④ Same as #2.

8 ① Although this would be documented, the patient's response to care is the most important fact.
② Same as #1.
* ③ This is most important because the patient's response will indicate if the care given was appropriate and effective and if future care should be altered.
④ Same as #1.

9 ① Secondary prevention refers to strategies for people in whom disease is present. The goal is to halt or reverse the disease process.
② There is no category called morbidity prevention. The word "morbidity" refers to illness; "mortality" refers to death.
* ③ Tertiary prevention uses strategies to assist people to adapt physically, psychologically, and socially to permanent disabilities.
④ Primary prevention refers to strategies used to prevent illness in people who are considered free from disease.

10 ① This is an emotional-behavioral response to pain.
② Same as #1.
* ③ An increased heart rate is part of the fight-or-flight response, which is controlled by the autonomic nervous system; it is a physical attempt to prepare for an emergency.
④ Same as #1.

11 ① Daily baths can remove protective oils and cause drying of the skin, which could compromise homeostasis.
* ② The use of soap and water with friction followed by rinsing the skin with water removes microorganisms on the skin.
③ These are not values held by all individuals.
④ Although soap reduces the surface tension of water, which facilitates cleaning, it is water and friction that primarily remove microorganisms and dirt from the skin. Not all patients can tolerate soap.

12 ① Although nursing assistants can be self-directed within their role, nursing assistants must work under the direct supervision of a nurse.
② Health team members must have a professional relationship with mutual respect; they do not have to be friends.
③ Nursing assistants can refuse to perform tasks that are outside the parameters of their role and job responsibilities.
* ④ Nursing assistants should perform only those tasks that are within the nursing assistant role, that have been learned, and that have been assigned. The responsibilities and job description of the nursing assistant must be clear to all members of the health team.

13 ① Decision making is difficult for patients who are cognitively impaired and confused.
② Cognitively impaired patients may have difficulty comprehending the concepts of *good* and *all*.
* ③ Simple direct statements are more easily understood by patients who are cognitively impaired and confused.
④ Cognitively impaired and confused patients have difficulty understanding the concept of *cause and effect*.

14   * ① A confused patient may not be able to follow directions and bite down on the thermometer, causing injury.
　　② An 8-year-old child is old enough to follow directions so that the nurse can safely obtain an accurate oral temperature.
　　③ The lips still can form an effective seal around the thermometer to result in an accurate reading.
　　④ Same as #3.

15   * ① The urinary collection bag of an indwelling urinary catheter (retention catheter, Foley) should be below the patient's bladder, and urine should flow by gravity; hanging it on the chair below the patient's hip and keeping it off the floor supports medical asepsis.
　　② This is unsafe. The bag and tubing would be at or above the level of the patient's bladder; urine could flow backward into the bladder, resulting in a urinary tract infection.
　　③ Placing it on the floor is unsafe. The urinary collection bag would become contaminated; this is a violation of medical asepsis.
　　④ Same as #2.

16   * ① Paralysis of the lower extremities results in reduced mobility; maintaining one position compresses the capillary beds, which causes tissue hypoxia resulting in pressure (decubitus) ulcers.
　　② A patient with hypotension is at risk for falls, not pressure ulcers, because hypotension can cause dizziness.
　　③ A patient with memory loss may have emotional or safety-related problems.
　　④ A patient with heart failure is at risk for a dysrhythmia, not a pressure ulcer.

17   * ① All patients in a hospital require care that employs medical aseptic techniques; procedures that break the chain of infection help control the transmission of microorganisms.
　　② Not all patients require care that necessitates this specific intervention.
　　③ Same as #2.
　　④ Same as #2.

18   　① Massaging may be traumatic and could cause further bleeding.
　　② Taking vital signs is unnecessary; the loss of a drop of blood would not influence vital signs.
　　* ③ Pressure constricts blood vessels, which limits bleeding.
　　④ Documentation of this event is unnecessary; although this is not an expected therapeutic response, it does occasionally occur because the needle may pierce a tiny blood vessel.

19   　① This is a solid.
　　* ② At room temperature ice cream melts, changing it from a solid to a liquid.
　　③ Same as #1.
　　④ Same as #1.

20   * ① This statement is an example of reflective technique; it focuses on the patient's feelings and encourages verbalization.
　　② Although this statement may encourage the patient to talk more, it focuses on the content of what the patient said rather than the emotional theme.
　　③ This statement denies the patient's feelings.
　　④ Same as #3.

21   * ① The rise in intra-abdominal and intrathoracic pressure and the abrupt jolt to the diaphragm uses air within the bronchial tree behind the obstruction to force out whatever is causing the obstruction in the trachea.

       ② This occurs during cardiac compression associated with cardiopulmonary resuscitation (CPR).

       ③ The obstruction is in the trachea of the respiratory system, not the stomach of the gastrointestinal system.

       ④ Same as #2.

22   ① This is impractical; it should be done to bathe the feet, not warm them. With decreased peripheral perception, it could cause injury if the water were too warm.

       ② The pressure of a blanket on the toes and feet could produce footdrop.

       ③ A heating pad could cause a burn, particularly in elderly people who tend to have decreased peripheral perception.

     * ④ Socks trap body heat, which keeps the feet warm; cotton socks absorb moisture and allow foot mobility.

23   ① This would move contaminated material toward the urinary meatus, which could result in an infection.

       ② Although gloves are appropriate for universal (standard) precautions, a gown is unnecessary.

       ③ Same as #1.

     * ④ This action supports the concept of cleansing from a clean area (urinary meatus) toward a contaminated area (down the catheter and away from the meatus).

24   ① Growth and development are not continuously fast, although infants and adolescents experience growth spurts.

       ② Growth and development are not continuously slow, although adults and the elderly may experience slower periods of growth.

       ③ Growth and development reflect change, and change is rarely smooth.

     * ④ Growth and development as a whole are uneven; some stages are faster than others and people move through the stages at their own pace. However, the commonalities of growth and development are somewhat predictable.

25   ① This may eventually be done, but it is not the priority.

       ② Same as #1.

       ③ Same as #1.

     * ④ Of the options presented, this would be the nurse's first action; this alerts other health team members and the fire department that help is needed.

26   ① Positioning the patient's head between his or her knees moves the patient's center of gravity forward and the patient could fall.

       ② This is unsafe; this would not permit time for the patient's vasomotor response to compensate for the change in position and the patient could fall.

     * ③ Sitting on the side of the bed for a few minutes gives the body time to adjust. Orthostatic or postural hypotension occurs because the ability of the autonomic nervous system to equalize the blood supply is diminished with lying in bed. Rising causes blood to pool in the lower extremities until the sympathetic nervous system causes peripheral vasoconstriction.

       ④ Same as #2.

27 ① Bradycardia is an abnormally slow heart rate; it is not a toxic effect of an anti-coagulant.
   * ② Hematuria is red blood cells in the urine. Bleeding can be caused by too high a dose of an anticoagulant because its action interferes with thrombus formation.
   ③ Jaundice is an yellowish coloring of the skin, eyeballs, and urine in response to an increase in bile pigments in the blood. Jaundice is caused by biliary disease, not anticoagulant therapy.
   ④ Diarrhea is an increase in the frequency of loose stool and is unrelated to antico-agulant therapy.

28 ① Bile pigments color the stool brown; in the absence of bile pigments, stool has a clay color.
   * ② Digestive acids and enzymes act on blood in the gastrointestinal system, causing the stool to become black or tarry in color.
   ③ In the absence of pancreatic enzymes there is a decreased absorption of fat, re-sulting in stool that contains white globules of fat and is foul smelling.
   ④ Same as #3.

29 ① This should be unnecessary because the sphygmomanometer should have been checked for proper functioning before being applied to the patient's arm.
   ② This is unsafe; pumping the cuff too soon traps excess blood in the extremity, re-sulting in an inaccurate reading and possible discomfort.
   * ③ This allows for venous return and prevents falsely elevated results.
   ④ Same as #1.

30 * ① Negative pressure exerted through a tube inserted in the stomach removes secre-tions and gaseous substances from the stomach, preventing abdominal distention.
   ② This is not the most common purpose of a nasogastric tube after surgery; instilla-tions in a nasogastric tube following surgery are done when necessary to promote patency.
   ③ This is not the most common purpose of a nasogastric tube after surgery; lavage following surgery may be done to promote hemostasis in the presence of gastric bleeding.
   ④ This would be contraindicated after abdominal surgery until peristalsis returns.

PRACTICE TEST B

1 A patient had a cerebrovascular accident (stroke) and is paralyzed on the right side (hemiplegia). When undressing the patient, the nurse should:
① Take the gown off the right side first
② Get assistance when undressing the patient
③ Sit the patient up to make undressing less stressful
④ Remove the gown from the left side before the right

2 To foster a patient's self-esteem needs, the nurse's best intervention would be to:
① Encourage the patient to make choices
② Answer the patient's call light immediately
③ Place an identification band on the patient's wrist
④ Give a compliment about the patient's appearance

3 When a patient is having a seizure while out of bed, the nurse's initial action should be to:
① Move the patient back to bed
② Get an airway and portable oxygen
③ Hold the patient's arms and legs securely
④ Move objects away from around the patient

4 What should the nurse teach patients to best promote healthy teeth?
① Drink milk daily
② Eat a high-calcium diet
③ Visit the dentist every year
④ Brush the teeth after eating

5 The factor that *most* upsets adults who are incontinent is the feeling of:
① Dependence
② Regression
③ Loneliness
④ Wetness

6 A patient is at risk for dehydration and has an "Encourage Fluids" order from the physician. To increase the patient's intake of fluid, the nurse should:
① Provide drinks that the patient likes
② Measure all the patient's fluid intake and urine output
③ Require the patient to drink 4 ounces of fluid every hour
④ Explain to the patient that a feeding tube may have to be used

7 The patient MOST likely to become constipated is the patient who:
① Leads a sedentary lifestyle
② Is on a low-sodium diet
③ Works sitting at a desk
④ Eats pears and peas

8 One factor common to all communication is the:
① Direction of the message being sent
② Fact that there is a message
③ Transmission route
④ Use of words

9 Which measurement should be assessed further?
① A rectal temperature of 99.8°F
② A pulse rate that is 68 and regular

③ A blood pressure measurement of 120/88
④ A respiratory rate of 28 breaths per minute

10 When people are on complete bed rest, their hair tends to become:
① Dry
② Oily
③ Sparse
④ Matted

11 A patient is disoriented to time and place and has impaired cognitive ability because of extensive brain damage after a motor vehicle accident. When administering care, the nurse should:
① Offer basic choices
② Explain the care in detail
③ Provide simple directions
④ Teach activities of daily living

12 An elderly patient says, "I am now 1 inch shorter than when I was young." The nurse should:
① Explain that people do not usually lose height
② Recognize this as part of growth and development
③ Understand that this could be the sign of a problem
④ Identify that the patient is worried about losing height

13 When a patient does not sleep well at night, the most effective nursing intervention would be to:
① Fix the patient a cup of tea before bedtime
② Encourage the patient to avoid daytime naps
③ Tell the patient to take a long walk before bedtime
④ Obtain a physician's order for a sleeping medication

14 A patient with a terminal illness says to the nurse, "Do you believe in life after death?" The nurse's most therapeutic response would be:
① "I don't know."
② "What do you think?"
③ "Why are you asking?"
④ "That's a difficult question."

15 An immobile patient is on a turning and positioning schedule. When turning the patient, the nurse identifies a small red area on the coccyx. The nurse's initial intervention should be to:
① Apply a warm soak to the area
② Expose the area to a heat lamp
③ Order an air mattress for the bed
④ Massage around the area with skin lotion

16 A patient has a small infected pressure (decubitus) ulcer and is on contact isolation (precautions). When providing a bed bath, what should the nurse wear in addition to gloves?
① A clean gown
② A face shield
③ A respiratory mask
④ A pair of eyeglasses

17 A semi-Fowler's position is used to:
① Minimize flexion contractures of the hip
② Relieve pressure on the ischial tuberosities
③ Prevent aspiration during a nasogastric tube feeding
④ Reduce the development of pressure (decubitus) ulcers

18 The major difference between acute and chronic pain is that chronic pain is usually:
① Severe
② Relentless
③ Unbearable
④ Predictable

19 The patient is on a therapeutic diet that includes liquid supplements. When should these supplements be served?
① Between meals
② When they arrive on the unit
③ Whenever the patient is hungry
④ If the patient eats less than half of a meal

20 A patient who has a below-the-knee amputation says, "It is easier for me to put on the prosthesis while sitting in a chair." The nurse should:
① Explain that it is unsafe to transfer with one leg
② Teach the patient to put the prosthesis on while lying in bed
③ Compromise and attach the leg while the patient sits on the bed
④ Communicate this preference to other members of the health team

21 To effectively put out a fire, the nurse should direct the spray from the fire extinguisher across the:
① Middle of the flames
② Edge of the flames
③ Base of the flames
④ Top of the flames

22 Which intervention is an example of primary disease prevention?
① Postmastectomy exercise program
② Immunization against the flu
③ Blood pressure screening
④ Breast self-examination

23 A patient's vital signs are oral temperature 99°F, pulse 84 with a regular rhythm, respirations 16 and deep, and blood pressure 180/110. The sign that should cause the most concern for the nurse would be the:
① Pulse
② Temperature
③ Respirations
④ Blood pressure

24 When providing perineal care to a female patient, the nurse should NEVER:
① Wash the vaginal area before the buttocks
② Let the patient bathe herself
③ Rub the area dry
④ Use soap

25 When inserting a vaginal cream, the nurse's initial action should be to:
① Apply a lubricant to the applicator
② Put on sterile gloves for the procedure
③ Perform perineal care with soap and water
④ Place the patient in the left-side-lying position

26 A patient has an order for morphine sulfate q4h for pain following abdominal surgery. The nurse would recognize that the morphine was effective when the patient:
① Does not ask for another injection for pain
② Is able to cough with minimal discomfort
③ Requests another injection in 3 hours
④ Has a decrease in respiratory rate

27 When transferring a patient who is weak on the right side from the bed to a chair, what should the nurse do?
① Place the feet of the patient close together
② Plan to use a mechanical lift for the transfer
③ Instruct the patient to bear weight equally on both legs
④ Put the right arm of the chair against the left side of the bed

28 Which adaptation associated with skin color is unrelated to hypoxia?
① Cyanosis
② Jaundice
③ Pallor
④ Dusky

29 When being given an enema, a patient complains of abdominal cramping. What should the nurse do?
① Lower the fluid container several inches
② Stop the fluid until the cramping subsides
③ Turn the patient to the right lateral position
④ Have the patient flex the knees toward the abdomen

30 When assessing a patient's respiratory status during recovery from general anesthesia, it is of primary importance for the nurse to evaluate the patient's ability to:
① Inhale voluntarily
② Breathe deeply
③ Swallow
④ Speak

144 Answers and Rationales for Practice Test B

An asterisk (*) is in front of the rationale that explains the correct answer.

1   ① Taking the gown off on the affected side first exerts excessive stress on the body.
② The patient needs assistance with undressing, and this activity can be safely performed by one nurse.
③ This is irrelevant; the gown should be removed from the left side first whether the patient is standing, sitting, or lying down.
* ④ This exerts less stress on the affected side; the unaffected side can better tolerate the tension or positioning required to remove the gown.

2   * ① This intervention promotes self-control, dignity, and individuality, which all support self-esteem; it provides independence which is a form of internal reinforcement of worth. Internal reinforcement of worth is usually more beneficial than external reinforcement.
② This meets needs associated with safety and security.
③ Same as #2.
④ Compliments provide external, rather than internal, reinforcement of self-esteem.

3   ① This is unsafe; restriction of movement or manipulation of limbs during the tonic-clonic phase of a seizure could result in fractures or tissue damage.
② Physical safety is the priority at this time; the patient will not breathe until the convulsive phase of the seizure is over, at which time this may be done.
③ Same as #1.
* ④ Physical safety is the priority; the patient's uncontrolled movements could result in injury if environmental obstacles are not removed from the patient's immediate vicinity.

4   ① Although this provides calcium, it will not prevent dental caries or gingivitis.
② Same as #1.
③ Although visits to the dentist are helpful, dentists usually limit problems rather than prevent them.
* ④ Oral hygiene several times daily, including brushing and flossing, is the best measure for promoting healthy teeth; friction removes food particles and other debris that cause dental caries and gingivitis.

5   ① Not all people who are incontinent are dependent on others; many people are capable of cleaning themselves.
* ② Incontinence is often associated with childlike behavior; most cultures value control over one's bodily functions, which is usually accomplished early in life.
③ Although incontinence is embarrassing, which may result in social isolation and loneliness, it is the feeling of being like a child that causes the most concern.
④ Although being wet and soiled are uncomfortable, it is the feelings associated with regression that are most upsetting.

6   * ① Providing for patient preferences increases the likelihood of the patient accepting the fluid; encouragement and support are motivating, which may increase fluid intake.
② This will document the patient's intake and output, but it will do nothing to promote intake.

③ This is a form of force and is unacceptable; the patient has a right to refuse. The patient should be taught the importance of fluid intake.

④ This is a threat, and the nurse could be held accountable for assault.

7 * ① People who are inactive have decreased peristalsis, which increases water reabsorption in the large intestine and promotes constipation.

② A low-sodium diet is unrelated to constipation.

③ Although this could reduce peristalsis, it does not address the patient's entire lifestyle; a patient with a job that does not require physical activity can exercise at other times.

④ These contain fiber, which increases intestinal peristalsis and promotes defecation.

8 ① Messages go in a variety of directions (e.g., from the nurse to the patient, from the patient to the nurse).

* ② Communication is the transfer of information from one person to another; in communication there is always a message.

③ A message can be transmitted via a variety of routes (e.g., verbal, nonverbal).

④ Communication can be nonverbal (e.g., touch, a smile).

9 ① This is within the normal range of 97.6 to 99.8°F for a rectal temperature, indicating no abnormalities.

② This is within the normal range of 60 to 100 beats per minute, and the rhythm is regular, indicating no abnormalities.

③ This is within the normal range of 100 to 140 mm Hg for the systolic reading and 60 to 90 mm Hg for the diastolic reading, indicating no abnormalities.

* ④ This is above the normal range of 14 to 20 breaths per minute and is abnormal.

10 ① Dry hair is caused by nutrition and endocrine problems, not bed rest; brushing will help disperse natural secretions down the shaft of the hair.

② Oily hair is caused by lack of washing the hair, not bed rest.

③ Sparse hair is caused by nutrition, endocrine, and genetic factors, not bed rest.

* ④ Pressure and friction of the hair against the pillow results in matted, tangled hair.

11 ① This is too challenging a task for a person with extensive brain damage.

② Patients with extensive brain damage lack the cognitive ability to integrate details or comprehend *cause and effect.*

* ③ Simple, short statements with a single message are the easiest to intellectually integrate.

④ Same as #1.

12 ① This is untrue; people do get shorter as they age.

* ② Compression of the vertebral column causes people to get slightly shorter as they age.

③ This is untrue; losing height is an expected response to aging.

④ Nothing in the patient's statement indicates anxiety; it is a declarative statement.

13 ① This is contraindicated; tea contains caffeine, which is a stimulant that will interfere with the ability to fall asleep.

* ② Naps rest and restore the body, reducing the need to sleep longer at night; an active routine throughout the day requires energy that promotes a need for sleep at night.

③ Exercise increases the basal metabolic rate, which would interfere with sleep if done immediately before bedtime; exercise should be performed earlier in the day.

④ Other measures such as avoiding daytime naps, exercising during the day, drinking milk (which contains L-tryptophan), and performing usual bedtime routines should be attempted before medication.

14
① Although this is a direct response to the patient's question, it does not focus on the patient's concern.

* ② This response focuses on the patient's concern and provides an opportunity to verbalize further.

③ A question asking "why" is too confrontational and may cut off communication.

④ This response sidesteps the patient's question and may or may not promote further dialogue.

15
① This requires a physician's order.

② Same as #1.

③ An air mattress may be ordered later; while the area is exposed, the nurse should massage around the area with lotion to promote circulation.

* ④ Friction increases blood, oxygen, and nutrients to the area, which promote healing.

16
* ① A gown protects the nurse's uniform from contact with contaminated material; it acts as a barrier and interrupts the chain of infection.

② A face shield is unnecessary; this is used when activities are likely to cause splashes of blood, body fluids, secretions, or excretions.

③ A mask is unnecessary; this is used for respiratory isolation (airborne or droplet precautions) when microorganisms are transmitted by respiratory secretions.

④ A pair of eyeglasses is unnecessary in this situation; a protective eyeshield may be used when treating a large wound with extensive drainage, a situation in which splattering is likely to occur.

17
① The semi-Fowler's position can cause hip flexion contractures if the patient's position is unchanged for prolonged periods of time.

② This position increases pressure over the sacrum, posterior iliac crests, and ischial tuberosities.

* ③ Raising the head of the bed keeps the nasogastric tube feeding in the stomach via the principle of gravity.

④ Same as #2.

18
① Both acute and chronic pain can have this characteristic.

* ② Chronic pain lasts over a prolonged period of time; acute pain usually has a short duration.

③ Same as #1.

④ Same as #1.

19
* ① Supplements imply *in addition to* and therefore should be supplied between meals.

② Supplements may be sent to the unit long before the time they should be offered, particularly if they are canned commercial formulas. Supplements should be offered between meals or when specifically ordered.

③ Offering supplements whenever the patient is hungry could interfere with the intake of the patient's ordered diet.

④ The patient should be encouraged to eat the entire meal; formulas should supplement, not substitute for, the diet.

20
① This is untrue; if all the principles of body mechanics are followed, a safe transfer can be performed on one leg.

② This negates the patient's right to individualized care.
③ Same as #2.
* ④ The patient has the right to individualized care; communicating patient preferences promotes continuity of care.

21 ① This is unsafe; this could scatter the burning debris, which would intensify the fire.
② Same as #1.
* ③ The source of the fire is at its base, where the fuel (e.g., linens, paper, flammable liquids) is burning.
④ This is ineffective; the top of the flames is too far from the source of the burning material.

22 ① A postmastectomy exercise program is related to the tertiary level of disease prevention, not primary. Tertiary prevention is associated with attempts to reduce the extent and severity of a health problem/disease in an effort to limit disability and restore, maintain, or maximize function and/or quality of life.
* ② This is correct. Primary prevention is associated with health teaching and actions that relate to specific protection and prevention of disease or injury. Primary prevention activities precede disease or dysfunction; this includes actions generally applied to a healthy population.
③ This action is related to the secondary level of disease prevention, not the primary level. Secondary prevention activities are associated with early detection and encouragement of treatment when actions may control or eliminate an already present risk factor, illness, or disease.
④ Same as #3.

23 ① A pulse of 84 is within the normal range of 60 to 100 beats per minute, and the rhythm is regular.
② A temperature of 99°F is within the normal range of 97.6 to 99.6°F for an oral temperature.
③ A respiratory rate of 16 is within the normal range of 12 to 20 breaths per minute.
* ④ A blood pressure of 180/110 is above the normal range of 90 to 140 mm Hg for the systolic measurement and 60 to 90 mm Hg for the diastolic measurement and should cause the most concern of the options presented.

24 ① This supports the principle of washing from clean to contaminated.
② Self-care supports the patient's privacy and promotes dignity and independence.
* ③ This is unsafe; rubbing could damage the delicate perineal tissue. The area should be patted dry.
④ Soap lowers the surface tension of water, which promotes cleaning of the perineal area.

25 ① This is unnecessary because a portion of the vaginal cream is ejected at the top of the applicator just before and during insertion, which lubricates the applicator.
② Sterile gloves are unnecessary because this is not a sterile procedure. Clean gloves are adequate.
* ③ Vaginal creams are usually administered to treat vaginal infections or discharges; the area must be bathed to remove secretions and microorganisms immediately before the administration of medication.
④ The dorsal recumbent position is used for vaginal insertions.

26 ① Some people are stoics and/or do not request medication for pain. Patients' pain should be assessed and pain medication offered if necessary.

    * ② The main purpose of pain relief medication is to enable the patient to engage comfortably in necessary activity.

    ③ The patient is experiencing pain before the next scheduled dose; this indicates that the patient is in pain and the intervention was ineffective.

    ④ This could indicate an overdose; opiates decrease respiration by depressing the respiratory center in the brainstem. This is a side effect, not a therapeutic effect.

27   ① Keeping the feet close together eliminates a wide base of support and raises the center of gravity, which promotes falls.

    ② A mechanical lift is unnecessary; a patient with hemiparesis is capable of transferring with assistance. A mechanical lift promotes dependency and eliminates an opportunity to strengthen the unaffected leg.

    ③ This is unrealistic and unsafe; the side with the hemiparesis cannot bear as much weight as the unaffected side.

  * ④ The patient with a hemiparesis should get out of bed by leading with the unaffected side; this allows the stronger arm and leg to lead the movement into a chair. A patient with a right hemiparesis should get out of the left side of the bed.

28   ① Cyanosis is a blue discoloration of the skin and mucous membranes caused by deoxygenated hemoglobin in the capillaries; it is a late sign of hypoxia.

  * ② Jaundice is a yellow-orange discoloration of the skin, mucous membranes, and sclera caused by elevated blood levels of bilirubin, which deposits bile pigments into tissues.

    ③ Pallor is an unnatural paleness or decreased color in the skin caused by reduced amounts of oxyhemoglobin.

    ④ Duskiness is a grayish discoloration of the skin, which frequently indicates deoxygenated hemoglobin in the capillaries in people with dark skin.

29   ① Lowering the container would still allow fluid to enter the colon, continuing the problem of abdominal cramping.

  * ② This interrupts the flow of the fluid, which is distending and irritating the bowel; it reduces intestinal pressure and allows the intestinal cramping to subside.

    ③ Movement raises intra-abdominal pressure, which may precipitate evacuation of the enema fluid from the bowel.

    ④ Same as #3.

30   ① A voluntary inhalation is a conscious action in response to a command or desire to take a breath. When recovering from anesthesia in the postanesthesia care unit, the unconscious patient usually breathes spontaneously.

    ② After the patient recovers from anesthesia, coughing and deep breathing become important to prevent atelectasis and pneumonia.

    ③ Although the patient would be monitored for a return of the gag reflex, monitoring for a patent airway takes priority.

  * ④ Impaired speaking or an inability to speak may indicate trauma to the vocal cords; the inflammatory response can cause a partial or total airway obstruction.

PRACTICE TEST C

1 What should the nurse do to help prevent injury to a patient with bone demineralization?
① Apply emollients to the skin every day.
② Have the patient walk in the hall once daily.
③ Encourage the patient to drink 2500 mL of fluid daily.
④ Support the patient's joints when turning and moving.

2 The nurse should brush a patient's hair daily to prevent:
① Pediculosis
② Dandruff
③ Alopecia
④ Tangles

3 A patient has a progressive, debilitating disease. Although usually pleasant, the patient begins to complain that the doctor is incompetent, the nurses are uncaring, the room is too cold, and the food is terrible. The patient is coping by using the defense mechanism of:
① Displacement
② Projection
③ Denial
④ Anger

4 What should the nurse do first when an assessment reveals a change in a patient's blood pressure?
① Report the change to the charge nurse.
② Document the observed change.
③ Obtain the other vital signs.
④ Notify the physician.

5 Which action by a patient should be reported to the physician because the patient may need a restraint?
① Climbing off the end of the bed at night
② Wandering into other patients' rooms
③ Picking at clothing and bed linens
④ Pulling out an IV line

6 A comatose patient begins to vomit while lying in bed. The nurse's initial response should be to position the patient in the:
① Supine position
② Lateral position
③ Fowler's position
④ Dorsal recumbent position

7 A patient whose spouse recently died begins to cry. The nurse's best response would be to:
① Arrange for grief counseling
② Explain that being sad is normal
③ Look away when the patient cries
④ Sit down and touch the patient's hand

8 The nurse should recognize that an adequate night's sleep was attained when the patient:
① Is able to remember dreams
② Demonstrates renewed strength

③ Sleeps at night without waking
④ Slept a minimum of 7 hours

9 Ethics is specifically concerned with:
① Preventing a crime
② Protecting civil law
③ Determining right or wrong
④ Potentially negligent actions

10 When feeding a patient with left-sided hemiparesis because of a stroke, the nurse should:
① Position the patient in a low-Fowler's position
② Offer fluids to assist with swallowing food
③ Place food on the strong side of the mouth
④ Position a towel under the patient's chin

11 A patient has a left-sided hemiplegia as the result of a cerebrovascular accident. While being dressed, the patient states in a disgusted tone of voice, "I feel like a 2-year-old. I can't even get dressed by myself." The nurse's BEST response would be:
① "It must be hard to feel dependent on others."
② "Most people who have had a stroke feel this way."
③ "It must be terrible not being able to move your arm."
④ "You are feeling down today, but things will get better."

12 A newly admitted patient complains of not having had a good bowel movement in 10 days. Which question asked by the nurse would identify symptoms of a fecal impaction?
① "Have you had small amounts of liquid stool?"
② "What types of food with fiber do you eat?"
③ "Do you notice a bad odor to your breath?"
④ "Are you having any nausea and vomiting?"

13 The <u>most</u> effective way to reduce the transmission of microorganisms at meal times for patients who are on droplet/airborne precautions is by:
① Washing and rinsing the dishes with hot water
② Having patients wash their hands after eating
③ Isolating used trays in the dirty utility room
④ Using disposable dishes and utensils

14 Which action uses inappropriate body mechanics?
① Holding clean equipment close to the body when walking
② Flexing the knees when lifting an object from the floor
③ Placing the feet apart when transferring a patient
④ Bending from the waist when making a bed

15 Which intervention is an example of primary disease prevention?
① Testicular self-examinations
② Mammography screening
③ Use of a bicycle helmet
④ Testing of well water

16 When giving a complete bed bath which of the following body parts should the nurse wash last?
① Legs
② Feet
③ Axilla
④ Rectum

17 To reduce pressure to the sacral area, the nurse should position the patient in the:
① Dorsal recumbent position
② Semi-Fowler's position
③ Lateral position
④ Supine position

18 When instilling ear drops into the ear of a young child, the nurse should:
① Hyperextend the child's head before instilling the drops
② Apply pressure to the tragus of the ear while instilling the drops
③ Pull the pinna of the ear downward and backward while instilling the drops
④ Maintain the child in the side-lying position with the affected ear down after instilling the drops

19 The bed of a patient with an indwelling urinary catheter (Foley) is found wet with urine. What should the nurse do?
① Insert a larger-size catheter
② Provide perineal care whenever necessary
③ Position a waterproof pad under the patient's buttocks
④ Tell the patient to use the bedpan when there is an urge to void

20 The location and characteristics of pain are important for the nurse to explore when determining its:
① Duration
② Etiology
③ Intensity
④ Threshold

21 A Class A fire extinguisher can put out a fire in a:
① Toaster oven
② Wastepaper basket
③ Stove in the pantry
④ Maintenance closet

22 What should the nurse do when providing mouth care for an unconscious patient?
① Apply Vaseline™ to the tongue and lips
② Explain to the patient what will be done and why
③ Use glycerine and lemon swabs to cleanse the mouth
④ Position the patient in the dorsal recumbent position

23 Across the spectrum of wellness and illness, *most* elderly people view themselves as:
① Frail
② Tired
③ Healthy
④ Dependent

24 A patient's therapeutic serum level for gentamicin should be between 4 to 10 mcg/mL (micrograms per milliliter). What is the implication of a peak level of 12 mcg/mL?
① The drug dose is safe.
② The drug dose is subtherapeutic.
③ The patient would be at risk for drug accumulation.
④ The patient's next dose should be administered over 1 hour rather than 30 minutes.

25 A patient with kidney failure is placed on fluid restrictions of 1000 mL of fluid in 24 hours. The nurse should:
① Eliminate liquids between meal times
② Divide the fluids equally among the three shifts
③ Indicate "just clear liquids" in the restriction plan
④ Give proportionally more fluids during the day than during the night

26 Which patient assessment made by the nurse would require immediate intervention?
① 10 respirations per minute by a sleeping patient
② Rattling sounds in the pharynx of an unconscious patient
③ Coughing and expectorating large amounts of thick mucus
④ Slight shortness of breath after returning from the bathroom

27 Which action by the nurse would support a patient's right to privacy?
① Leaving a crying patient alone
② Addressing a patient by the last name
③ Providing information about patient care
④ Pulling a curtain when interviewing the patient

28 When obtaining an oral temperature with an electronic thermometer, the nurse must:
① Use the red probe
② Take the temperature before breakfast
③ Use a new probe cover for each patient
④ Wipe the probe with alcohol after each use

29 When washing the penis of an uncircumcised patient, the nurse should:
① Wash down the shaft toward the meatus
② Retract the foreskin completely
③ Employ a very light touch
④ Use a rubbing motion

30 To prevent pulmonary complications postoperatively, the patient should be instructed to perform:
① Incisional splinting
② Progressive ambulation
③ Diaphragmatic breathing
④ Range-of-motion exercises

Answers and Rationales for Practice Test C

An asterisk (*) is in front of the rationale that explains the correct answer.

1 ① Emollients hold moisture in the skin, making it supple; they do not prevent bone injury.

② Weight bearing helps limit bone demineralization, but it will not prevent bone injury.

③ An intake of 2500 mL of fluid daily flushes the kidneys and limits calculi formation, which can occur because of the high level of calcium salts in the urine as a result of demineralization. It does not prevent bone injury.

* ④ Bone demineralization (osteoporosis) causes the bones to become weak, brittle, and fragile; supporting joints when turning or moving limits the stress that could cause a fracture.

2 ① Pediculosis is caused by direct contact with lice or their eggs (nits); brushing the hair will not prevent head lice.

② Shampooing the hair and rubbing the scalp help to limit dandruff.

③ Loss of hair can be caused by nutritional, emotional, iatrogenic, and genetic factors; it is not prevented by brushing.

* ④ Brushing separates tangles and evenly distributes secretions and oils down the hair shafts.

3 * ① The patient is anxious and is reducing the anxiety by transferring emotions from something stressful to substitutes that are less anxiety producing.

② Projection is the attribution of unacceptable thoughts or actions to another.

③ Denial is a defense mechanism used by the patient to avoid emotional conflicts and to refuse to deal with unpleasant realities by keeping them out of conscious awareness.

④ Anger is a behavior that is an adaptive response; it defends the individual, but is not known as a defense mechanism.

4 ① This may be done after the other vital signs are obtained; additional data should be collected.

② Same as #1.

* ③ Because of the interrelationships among the circulatory system, respiratory system, and the basal metabolic rate, all the vital signs should be obtained for an accurate assessment.

④ Same as #1.

5 ① Climbing off the end of the bed could result in self-harm, a factor indicating the need for nursing interventions other than a restraint.

② Wandering should be controlled by observation, not a restraint.

③ Picking at the gown and bed linens is not unsafe behavior that requires application of a restraint.

* ④ Physical or chemical restraints may be necessary to protect the patient from self-harm. Pulling out an IV can cause tissue injury and will interrupt medical therapy.

6 ① This position is contraindicated because it promotes aspiration by allowing vomitus to flow to the posterior oral pharynx and enter the trachea.

* ② The lateral position prevents aspiration because it allows vomitus to drain out of the mouth via gravity.

③ A high-Fowler's position provides inadequate support for an unconscious patient. A low- or semi-Fowler's position is a back-lying position that can contribute to aspiration.

④ Same as #1.

7 ① Grief counseling may be done later; the patient needs immediate support.

② Although feeling sad is a common response to a loss, the nurse is making an assumption the patient is sad without knowing the patient-spouse relationship; the tears may indicate other feelings such as relief or joy.

③ Avoiding eye contact may give the patient the message that it is not acceptable to cry.

*④ Sitting down and touching the patient's hand communicates acceptance and caring.

8 ① Remembering dreams is unrelated to adequate sleep; actually most dreams occur during REM sleep and are forgotten.

*② The purpose of sleep is to rest and restore the body, which would be evidenced by renewed strength.

③ Although a person sleeps at night without waking, the length of the sleep or the length of REM sleep may be insufficient to restore or renew the body.

④ Seven hours may or may not be enough sleep because each person has unique needs and a biological clock for determining sleeping intervals.

9 ① Criminal law is concerned with crimes.

② Civil law is concerned with wrongs committed by one person against another.

*③ Ethics is concerned with value judgments, such as what is right or wrong and behavior that is acceptable or unacceptable.

④ Negligence is concerned with a careless act of commission or omission that results in injury to another.

10 ① A low-Fowler's position could promote aspiration; the patient should be placed in a high-Fowler's position to allow gravity to facilitate swallowing.

② Offering fluids to assist with swallowing would promote aspiration and is contraindicated. Fluids should be taken after a mouthful of food is swallowed.

*③ Placing food on the strong side of the mouth allows the unaffected muscles to control chewing, moves the bolus of food to the posterior oral cavity, and facilitates swallowing.

④ This should be avoided because it has the same implication as a bib; the patient may feel childlike. The use of a napkin would be appropriate.

11 *① This statement identifies the patient's feelings and provides an opportunity for further discussion.

② This statement is a generalization that may not be true; it also cuts off communication.

③ This statement focuses on the inability to move rather than feelings of helplessness, dependence, and regression.

④ This statement is false reassurance because the nurse does not know if things will get better.

12 *① A fecal impaction is an obstruction in the large intestine; peristalsis behind the obstruction initially increases in an attempt to move the mass, causing liquid stool to pass around the area of the impaction.

② This question is not significant at this time; foods with fiber promote intestinal peristalsis, which prevents constipation.

③ A bad odor to the breath is unrelated to a fecal impaction; it may be related to a small bowel obstruction.

④ People with a fecal impaction may experience rectal pressure, bloating, and nausea, but rarely do they vomit; nausea and vomiting occur more frequently with small bowel obstructions.

13 ① Washing and rinsing are ineffective; boiling for 15 minutes will achieve disinfection.

② The hands should be washed before eating.

③ Used trays from an isolation room would contaminate the dirty utility room.

* ④ Contaminated disposable articles can be bagged and discarded, which prevents the spread of microorganisms to others.

14 ① This is desirable because the weight is being carried close to the center of gravity, which helps maintain balance.

② This is desirable because the strong muscles of the legs carry the load, which helps prevent back strain.

③ The wider the base of support and the lower the center of gravity, the greater the stability of the nurse.

* ④ Bending from the waist puts too much stress on the vertebrae and muscles of the back because it does not distribute the work among the largest and strongest muscle groups of the legs.

15 ① This action is associated with secondary disease prevention, not primary prevention. Secondary prevention activities are associated with early detection and encouragement of treatment, when actions may contribute to control or elimination of an already present risk factor, illness, or disease.

② Same as #1.

* ③ This is correct. This action is a primary-level disease prevention intervention. Primary prevention is associated with health teaching and actions that relate to specific protection and prevention of disease or injury. Primary prevention activities precede disease or dysfunction and include actions generally applied to a healthy population.

④ Same as #1.

16 ① This area is cleaner than the perianal area, and if washed last, would become more contaminated from microorganisms and fecal material from the rectum.

② Same as #1.

③ Same as #1.

* ④ The perianal area has fecal material and microorganisms that would contaminate other parts of the body; therefore, the perianal area should be washed last.

17 ① When in this position, pressure would still be on the sacrum because it is a back-lying position.

② In the semi-Fowler's position, pressure would still be on the sacrum, and with the head elevated, shearing force could occur if the patient were to slide down in bed.

* ③ In the lateral position, the iliac crest and greater trochanter, not the sacrum, bear the body's weight.

④ Same as #1.

18
① Hyperextension of the head is done for the instillation of nose drops, not ear drops.
② Applying pressure to the tragus of the ear would prevent the drops from entering the ear canal.
* ③ This is done to straighten the ear canal in a young child, which provides direct access to the deeper external ear structures; in an adult the ear is pulled back and upward because the canal is straighter in adults.
④ This is contraindicated; this position would allow the ear drops to flow out of the ear by gravity. The affected ear should be on the upper side for a minimum of 3 minutes to allow complete distribution of the medication.

19
* ① Urine is leaking around the Foley catheter and a larger-size catheter is required; once the physician orders a Foley catheter, it is within the role of the nurse to select the appropriate size and perform the catheter insertion.
② With a Foley catheter in place, the patient should not be wet with urine because it is a closed system from the bladder to the collection bag.
③ A waterproof pad should be unnecessary because with an adequate-size catheter there should be no leaking of urine.
④ The presence of a Foley catheter negates the need to void.

20
① The length of time of the pain is not as significant as its location and characteristics in determining its etiology.
* ② The location of pain is often related to the underlying disease or illness; the quality or subjective characteristics of pain often have common descriptions related to specific illness, such as burning epigastric pain associated with gastric ulcers and crushing chest pain associated with myocardial infarctions.
③ This is totally individual and unreliable for determining relationships among characteristics, location, or etiology of pain.
④ Same as #3.

21
① A Class A fire extinguisher contains water and is contraindicated in an electrical fire because water conducts electricity.
* ② A Class A fire extinguisher contains water, which safely and effectively puts out fires burning wood, paper, or cloth.
③ Water should not be used because it causes grease to spatter; also the stove might be an electric stove.
④ A maintenance closet usually contains flammable materials; water is contraindicated because it dilutes flammable liquids, which spreads the fire.

22
① A petrolatum-based lubricant is for external, not internal, use.
* ② Hearing is the last sense to deteriorate, and the patient may hear the nurse; all patients have a right to know what will be done and why.
③ Glycerine and lemon swabs should be applied after the mouth is cleansed.
④ This position would promote aspiration and is contraindicated. A side-lying position would be appropriate.

23
① This is untrue; the majority of elderly people are or perceive themselves as being independent, healthy, and active even if they have several chronic illnesses.
② Although people lead more sedentary lifestyles as they age, they are still active; most elderly people do not view themselves as tired.
* ③ Studies demonstrate that most elderly people perceive themselves as healthy because they measure their health in relation to how well they function rather than by the absence or presence of disease.
④ Same as #1.

24 ① The drug dose is too high, as indicated by a peak serum level higher that the therapeutic serum level range.
    ② The drug dose is too high, not too low.
  * ③ 12 mcg/mL is 2 mcg/mL higher than is necessary to be effective and will contribute to drug accumulation and toxicity if this continues for 3 to 5 days.
    ④ This is unsafe. The dose is too high and should be reduced, not just administered at a slower rate.

25 ① Liquid intake should be dispersed over the hours when the patient is awake and not just ingested with meals.
    ② This is inappropriate; patients should have more fluids during the day and evening than at night, when they are usually asleep.
    ③ Fluid restriction is concerned with limiting the volume of fluid, not the type of fluid.
  * ④ The patient and nurse should make a fluid schedule, taking into consideration factors such as periods of wakefulness, number of meals, oral medications, personal preferences, and so on. An appropriate schedule might be half the fluid volume between 8 AM and 4 PM (500 mL), $^2/_5$ of the fluid volume between 4 PM and 11 PM (400 mL), and the remainder of the fluid (100 mL) during the night.

26 ① Immediate intervention is unnecessary. While a person is awake, normal respiratory rates are usually between 12 and 20 per minute; when a person is asleep, the need for oxygen declines, resulting in a decrease in the respiratory rate and an increase in the depth of respirations.
  * ② This indicates mucus is in the airway; suctioning may be necessary to maintain a patent airway because an unconscious patient cannot cough voluntarily.
    ③ Immediate intervention is not necessary because coughing and expectorating are actions that maintain a patent airway.
    ④ This is an expected response to activity.

27 ① Leaving would abandon the patient and is not an acceptable intervention; a crying patient needs support, not isolation.
    ② Calling the patient by name supports the patient's need for identity, dignity, and respect, not privacy.
    ③ Providing information supports the patient's right to know what is going to be done and why, not privacy.
  * ④ Pulling a curtain provides a personal, secluded environment for a confidential discussion.

28 ① The red probe is used for a rectal temperature.
    ② This is unnecessary; however, daily temperatures should be taken at the same time for comparison purposes. Temperatures usually are lowest in the early morning and highest between 5 and 7 PM.
  * ③ Because an electronic thermometer is used for multiple patients, a probe cover is a medical aseptic technique used to prevent the spread of microorganisms. It provides a barrier between the patient and the machine.
    ④ This is unnecessary; a new disposable probe cover should be used for each patient to control the transmission of microorganisms.

29 ① Washing should be done in the other direction because it moves secretions and debris away from the urinary meatus, preventing infection.
  * ② Smegma collects under the foreskin, which must be retracted to permit thorough cleaning.

③ A light touch may be too stimulating; a gentle but firm touch is more effective.

④ A rubbing motion could injure delicate perineal tissue and be too stimulating.

30

① This limits incisional pain and prevents dehiscence.

② Although ambulation increases the respiratory rate, its primary purpose is to prevent circulatory complications such as thrombosis.

* ③ Diaphragmatic breathing helps promote alveolar expansion and facilitate oxygen–carbon dioxide exchange.

④ Range-of-motion exercises prevent contractures and circulatory complications.

Practice Questions With Answers and Rationales

Chapter 10 contains 14 categories of basic nursing practice. Each category contains 35 test items. These items provide an opportunity for applying the test-taking techniques that were presented in Chapter 6. A test-taking technique is a strategy that uses skill and forethought to analyze a test item before selecting an answer. Every test item should be examined to determine if any of the test-taking techniques apply. When it is appropriate to use a test-taking technique, a **Test-Taking Tip** will follow the item. Some items will not have a **Test-Taking Tip** because test-taking techniques do not pertain to every item. The **Test-Taking Tip** will cue you to one or more of the nine different strategies that can assist you in arriving at the correct answer. Use the **Test-Taking Tip** to examine the question with consideration and thoughtfulness. The rationales for items are at the end of each category and address:

- An application of the **Test-Taking Tip**
- The identification of the correct answer
- The rationale for why the correct answer is correct
- The rationale for why each of the distractors is incorrect

The World of the Patient and Nurse

This section includes factors that influence the role of the nurse and the delivery of health care. Questions address ethics, legal aspects of nursing practice, the nursing process, the responsibilities associated with the management of nursing practice, meeting spiritual needs of patients, patients' rights, the difference between dependent and independent roles of the nurse, supervising the practice of subordinate staff members, the standards of nursing practice, trends in health care, and agencies that provide structure for the delivery of health care.

Questions

1 A patient tells the nurse, "My new bathrobe is missing." The nurse's MOST appropriate response would be to:
① Determine if the patient is angry
② Initiate a search for the patient's bathrobe
③ Provide an isolation gown that can be used as a robe
④ State that it must have gone down with the soiled linen

TEST-TAKING TIP ● Identify the key word in the stem that sets a priority.

2 Which activity is a dependent function of the nurse?
① Documenting perioperative nursing care
② Changing a sterile dressing when soiled
③ Assisting with selection of choices on the menu
④ Administering oxygen for acute shortness of breath

TEST-TAKING TIP ● Identify the clue in the stem.

3 The *most* important reason why the nurse must understand the scientific rationale for the actions that constitute a procedure is that the nurse should be able to:
① Implement the procedure safely
② Formulate the nursing care plan
③ Document the nursing care given
④ Explain the required nursing care to the patient

TEST-TAKING TIP ● Identify the key word in the stem that sets a priority. Identify the unique option.

4 The nurse observes a patient going into another patient's room without permission, which upsets the other patient. When responding to the wandering patient's behavior, the nurse should initially:
① Help the patient to the correct room
② Place the patient in restraints temporarily
③ Determine the motivation for the patient's behavior
④ Share the observation about the patient with the health team

TEST-TAKING TIP ● Identify the key word in the stem that sets a priority. Identify the patient-centered options.

5 A voluntary agency is classified as such because it is:
① A health maintenance organization (HMO)
② Supported by volunteer services
③ Privately owned and operated
④ A nonprofit organization

TEST-TAKING TIP ● Identify the clue in the stem.

6 On the third day of hospitalization a patient communicates a preference to shower at night. To best promote continuity of care, the nurse should:
① Explain that AM care is given in the morning
② Orally inform the other health team members
③ Indicate this preference on the patient's plan of care
④ Encourage a modification of personal routines while hospitalized

TEST-TAKING TIP ● Identify the key word in the stem that sets a priority. Identify the clue in the stem. Identify options that deny patient needs. Identify patient-centered options.

7 Which task(s) should the nurse include when formulating an assignment for the nursing assistant?
① Monitoring patients' tube feedings
② Ambulating patients outside their rooms
③ Regulating patients' intravenous solutions
④ Assisting patients with taking medication

TEST-TAKING TIP ● Identify the option that is unique.

8 The nurse in charge directs a nurse to do something that is outside the legal role of the nurse. The nurse should:
① Complete the task and express a grievance later
② Notify the supervisor immediately
③ Inform the union representative
④ Decline to do the assigned task

TEST-TAKING TIP ● Identify opposites in options.

9 After a month in the hospital a Jewish patient says, "I miss lighting candles on Friday night." The <u>most</u> therapeutic response would be:
① "It must be difficult to change old habits."
② "I am sorry but that's against the fire code."
③ "Religious traditions have a peaceful effect."
④ "I will try to arrange it so you can light your candles."

TEST-TAKING TIP ● Identify the key word in the stem that sets a priority. Identify equally plausible options. Identify opposites in options. Identify the option that denies the patient's feelings.

10 Which action by the nurse would violate patient confidentiality and privacy?
① Interviewing a patient in the presence of others
② Writing patient statements in the progress notes
③ Sharing data about a patient at change of shift report
④ Presenting the patient's problems at a team conference

TEST-TAKING TIP ● Identify the key word in the stem that indicates negative polarity.

11 When a patient dies, the nurse should begin postmortem care:
① Only after the attending physician has been notified
② Once the nursing supervisor has been informed
③ After significant others have left
④ As soon as death is pronounced

TEST-TAKING TIP ● Identify the option with a specific determiner.

12 A patient is angry about not being able to perform the activities of daily living without help. To best reduce the patient's anger, the nurse should:
① Disregard angry behavior
② Offer choices about care

③ Gently set limits on angry behavior
④ Encourage recognition of limitations
TEST-TAKING TIP ● Identify the key word in the stem that sets a priority. Identify opposites in options.

13 Which is a "right" of patients in a hospital?
① Being able to smoke in their rooms
② Requesting meals at the times they prefer
③ Refusing treatment ordered by their physicians
④ Demanding that they be moved to private rooms
TEST-TAKING TIP ● Identify the unique option.

14 Which is an example of a goal?
① The patient will be assisted with meals.
② The patient will be at risk for weight loss.
③ The patient will need small, frequent feedings.
④ The patient will maintain a weight of 140 pounds.

15 The first task to be completed by the nurse when arriving on the unit for work is to:
① Count controlled drugs with the nurse going off shift
② Prioritize care to be completed during the shift
③ Make rounds and check the safety of patients
④ Receive a report on the status of patients
TEST-TAKING TIP ● Identify the key word in the stem that sets a priority. Identify the clue in the stem.

16 The nurse breaks a patient's dentures because of carelessness. What specific legal term applies to this action?
① Battery
② Assault
③ Negligence
④ Malpractice

17 A patient is often argumentative and demanding. When planning care, the nurse's **best** intervention would be to:
① Bring another staff member as a witness
② Involve the patient in decision making
③ Accept the behavior as probably a lifelong pattern
④ Explain that the staff would appreciate the patient's cooperation
TEST-TAKING TIP ● Identify the key word in the stem that sets a priority. Identify opposites in options. Identify the patient-centered option.

18 The American Nurses' Association (ANA) Standards of Nursing Practice are:
① Legal statutes guiding nursing practice
② Step-by-step actions for a nursing procedure
③ The requirements for registered nurse licensure
④ Policy statements defining the obligations of nurses

19 A patient with dementia needs assistance with hygiene, grooming, eating, and toileting. On discharge from the hospital the agency that would best meet this patient's needs would be:
① A nursing home
② A psychiatric institution
③ An adult daycare program
④ An outpatient care facility
TEST-TAKING TIP ● Identify the key word in the stem that sets a priority.

20 When a registered nurse stops at the scene of an accident, the nurse is:
① Given legal immunity by the Good Samaritan Law
② Held responsible for the care provided at the scene
③ Meeting the legal trust that accompanies an RN license
④ Immune from prosecution because a contract does not exist
TEST-TAKING TIPS ● Identify opposites in options. Identify equally plausible options.

21 A nurse says to a patient, "You should get a second opinion because your physician is not the best." The nurse could be sued for:
① Libel
② Assault
③ Slander
④ Negligence

22 A nurse's signature on an informed consent for surgery indicates that the:
① Surgeon described the procedure and its risks
② Patient is informed about expected outcomes
③ Patient actually signed the consent form
④ Surgeon is protected from being sued
TEST-TAKING TIP ● Identify equally plausible options.

23 The trend in health care that received the most attention in the 1990s was:
① Tertiary care
② Early diagnosis
③ Health promotion
④ Restorative rehabilitation
TEST-TAKING TIP ● Identify the key word in the stem that sets a priority. Identify the clue in the stem.

24 The purpose of the *National Council Licensure Examination for Registered Nurses* (NCLEX-RN) is to:
① Verify graduation
② Control nursing education
③ Accredit schools of nursing
④ Identify minimal safe practice
TEST-TAKING TIP ● Identify equally plausible options.

25 When obtaining a health history, the nurse identifies that a patient has gained 10 pounds in the last week. When the nurse communicates this information to the physician, the nurse is performing which step in the nursing process?
① Planning
② Analysis
③ Evaluation
④ Assessment

26 The nurse assigns a nurse aide to a patient who transfers to a chair with a mechanical lift. It has been a long time since the nurse aide has used the lift. To ensure the safety of the patient, the nurse should:
① Assign the patient to another nurse aide
② Explain to the nurse aide how to use the lift
③ Ask the nurse aide to demonstrate how to use the lift
④ Request another caregiver to assist with the transfer
TEST-TAKING TIP ● Identify the equally plausible options.

27 When the nurse formulates a nurse aide assignment, the nurse recognizes that the nurse aide job description generally includes which activities?
① Ensuring that patients swallow their medication
② Reporting unusual gross symptoms to the nurse
③ Orienting a new nurse aide to the unit
④ Teaching patients basic self-care

28 Which is the most appropriate activity for a nurse aide?
① Assessing vital signs
② Monitoring tube-feeding machines
③ Providing patients with physical hygiene
④ Assisting postoperative patients with their first ambulation
TEST-TAKING TIP ● Identify the word in the stem that sets a priority.

29 Nurses are required by law to:
① Stop at the scene of an accident to give care
② Report situations concerning any form of rape
③ Notify authorities about instances of child abuse
④ Obtain parental consent if a 16-year-old seeks an abortion

30 A male patient has dementia. He is verbally and physically abusive and paranoid. When providing care the nurse should always:
① Administer care as quickly as possible
② Tell him what he wants to hear
③ Explain what care is to be done
④ Tell him how nice he looks
TEST-TAKING TIP ● Identify equally plausible options.

31 The nurse would have to obtain a consent for surgery from the next of kin when the patient is:
① An illiterate 48-year-old man
② An extremely elderly woman
③ A 16-year-old married woman
④ A very depressed 55-year-old man

32 A patient says, "I don't like anyone to go into my closet or drawers." When returning hygiene equipment, the nurse should:
① Store the equipment on the bedside stand
② Allow the patient to put the equipment away
③ Explain the safety hazard of not putting equipment away
④ Provide reassurance that personal things will not be taken

TEST-TAKING TIP ● Identify the patient-centered option.

33 As an agency, Alcoholics Anonymous is classified in which category?
① Proprietary
② Voluntary
③ Official
④ Private

34 When identifying an excoriated perineal area in the patient with diarrhea, which step of the nursing process has the nurse performed?
① Analysis
② Evaluation
③ Assessment
④ Implementation

TEST-TAKING TIP ● Identify the clue in the stem.

35 Which is an example of a patient goal?
① The patient will establish regular bowel habits.
② The patient needs a commode when toileting.
③ The patient has perceived constipation.
④ The patient will be toileted q 4 h.

166 Rationales

1 **TEST-TAKING TIP** ● The word MOST in the stem sets a priority.
  ① Determining if the patient is angry does not address the problem of the missing bathrobe, although the nurse should recognize the patient's right to be angry in this situation.
  * ② Patients have a right to expect that efforts will be implemented to ensure security for their belongings.
  ③ Although this may be done, it does not address the problem of the missing bathrobe.
  ④ Explaining what may have happened does not address the feeling of loss, nor is it an attempt to find the robe.

2 **TEST-TAKING TIP** ● The word "dependent" is a clue in the stem.
  ① Documenting nursing care is an independent function of the nurse and does not require a physician's order.
  * ② Dependent activities of the nurse are those activities that require a physician's order; changing a sterile dressing requires a physician's order.
  ③ Selecting among choices of foods offered within a diet is an independent function and does not require a physician's order; however, the type of diet is a dependent function.
  ④ In an emergency, the nurse may administer oxygen to a patient experiencing acute shortness of breath until a physician's order can be obtained.

3 **TEST-TAKING TIP** ● The word *most* in the stem sets a priority. Option 1 is unique because it is the only option that does not use the words "nursing care."
  * ① The safety of the patient always takes priority; the nurse must perform only those skills that he or she understands and has practiced.
  ② Patient safety takes priority; however, nurses also need to understand scientific rationales to appropriately plan care.
  ③ Patient safety takes priority. Knowledge of the scientific rationale for care given is not necessary for the act of documentation.
  ④ Although it is important to explain all care to the patient, safety takes priority.

4 **TEST-TAKING TIP** ● The word "initially" in the stem sets a priority. Options 1 and 2 are patient centered and focus on the patient who is the victim. However, option 1 is correct because initially the patient who is upset must be protected.
  * ① Patients have a right to privacy and security for themselves and their belongings; helping the patient to the correct room protects the other patient.
  ② Restraining patients for any reason other than their own physical safety and without a physician's order is illegal.
  ③ First the patient needs to be removed from the other patient's room and then the nurse can explore the motivation for the behavior.
  ④ This does not address the immediate need to remove the patient from the room of another; once the behavior is addressed, it can be communicated.

5 **TEST-TAKING TIP** ● The word "voluntary" in the stem is a clue.
  ① A health maintenance organization (HMO) is a form of health care delivery and does not reflect how the organization is funded. An HMO can be voluntary (nonprofit), proprietary (for profit), and with emerging health care reform some may be official agencies (supported by government funds).
  ② Although volunteers serve as helpers at and supporters of voluntary agencies, this is not the reason for the classification; voluntary agencies are nonprofit organizations.

③ This would be a proprietary agency.

* ④ Voluntary agencies may not make a profit; any money made must be applied to operating expenses and provision of services.

6 **TEST-TAKING TIP** ● The word "best" is the key word in the stem that sets a priority. The word "continuity" in the stem is a clue that must be considered when selecting the correct option. Options 1 and 4 deny the patient's needs. Options 2 and 3 are patient centered.

① Hygiene care is not done only in the morning; care should be individualized.

② This would not provide a written plan of care for nurses to refer to when implementing nursing care.

* ③ This provides a written plan of care of what should be done for the patient; it supports communication among health team members, contributes to continuity, and individualizes care.

④ This is not necessary; care should be individualized and communicated via a care plan.

7 **TEST-TAKING TIP** ● Options 1, 3, and 4 all are associated with the intake of a substance. Option 2 is not like the others because it deals with an activity of daily living.

① This is the legal responsibility of the nurse, not the nursing assistant.

* ② Nursing assistants are responsible for meeting patients' basic activities of daily living (ADL) needs under the supervision of the nurse.

③ Same as #1.

④ Same as #1.

8 **TEST-TAKING TIP** ● Options 1 and 4 are opposites.

① Nurses should perform only those tasks that they are licensed to perform.

② The first action should be to respectfully decline to do the task; the nurse should notify the supervisor if the nurse in charge continues to insist that the task be performed.

③ Informing a union representative is unnecessary. The union representative may be notified if the nurse is threatened with repercussions for not following the order. Not all agencies are unionized.

* ④ Performing a task that is outside the legal definition of the nurse is illegal; a nurse has the responsibility to refuse to follow an order that is illegal.

9 **TEST-TAKING TIP** ● The word <u>most</u> in the stem sets a priority. Options 1 and 3 are equally plausible. Options 2 and 4 are opposites. Option 2 denies the patient's feelings.

① This response fails to recognize the religious significance of lighting candles and does not support the patient's need to perform this religious activity.

② This response is not true; if performed under supervision, the lighting of candles can be done safely.

③ This ignores the patient's need to experience the spiritual activity of lighting the candles.

* ④ Religious rituals, such as lighting Friday night candles (*Shabbes licht*), support spiritual and emotional needs and should be encouraged when they comfort the patient.

10 **TEST-TAKING TIP** ● The word "violate" in the stem indicates negative polarity.

* ① Interviewing a patient in the presence of others violates confidentiality; others may overhear information that should be kept confidential.

② Documenting statements in the patient's chart is an acceptable practice; the purpose of progress notes is to share and communicate data about the patient.

③ Sharing information at report notifies nursing team members of the patient's changing status and is an appropriate practice.

④ A team conference enables professionals to share important information about patients and is an acceptable practice.

11 TEST-TAKING TIP ● Option 1 contains the word "only," which is a specific determiner.

① Postmortem care should not begin until after death is pronounced and the family has an opportunity to make a last visit.

② Same as #1.

* ③ This allows the family members time to make a last visit before the body is prepared for transfer to a mortuary.

④ This does not recognize the right of the family to see the deceased one last time before postmortem care.

12 TEST-TAKING TIP ● The word "best" in the stem sets a priority. Options 1 and 3 are opposites.

① Behavior should not be disregarded or ignored; all behavior has meaning and requires recognition.

* ② Making decisions places the patient in control and supports feelings of independence.

③ Setting limits will only make the patient more angry because it is a controlling intervention.

④ Pointing out limitations only intensify the patient's feelings of dependence.

13 TEST-TAKING TIP ● Option 3 is unique because it has a negative connotation; it relates to an action of refusal. Options 1, 2, and 4 are statements from the positive perspective and are therefore alike.

① Patients are not permitted to smoke in their rooms. The Joint Commission on Accreditation of Healthcare Organizations, the agency responsible for accrediting hospitals, requires that accredited facilities be "smoke free." However, some facilities still provide limited, designated smoking areas.

② Meals are generally scheduled during regular meal times. It is impractical to serve meals any time a patient prefers; however, if a special need arises, the nurse generally should attempt to individualize care.

* ③ The patient has a right to refuse care against medical advice; the physician needs to explain to the patient the risks involved in lack of treatment.

④ A private room is generally a privilege, not a right, that is provided for at extra expense; it is not automatically provided on demand. However, a patient requiring isolation may be transferred to a private room.

14 ① This is an intervention, not a goal.

② This is part of a problem statement, not a goal.

③ This statement identifies a need or an intervention in response to an identified problem, not a goal.

* ④ This is a goal statement that is specific, measurable, and contains a time frame; *maintain* implies continuously.

15 TEST-TAKING TIP ● The word "first" is the key word in the stem that sets a priority. The word "arriving" in the stem establishes a time frame and is therefore an important clue.

① Controlled drugs can be counted after report. Communicating about the status of patients should be the nurse's first order of business on arrival on the unit.

② Before the nurse can prioritize care, the nurse must first receive a report to know about each patient's status.

③ Rounds are implemented after report. The nurse first needs to know the status of the patients; report provides baseline data about patients that are needed before additional assessments can be planned. Some institutions have walking rounds in which report and assessment of patients are simultaneously conducted.

* ④ Before care can be planned and implemented, the nurse needs to know the condition and immediate needs of patients.

16 ① Battery is the purposeful, angry, or negligent touching of a patient without consent.

② Assault is an act intended to provoke fear in a patient.

* ③ Negligence occurs when the nurse's actions do not meet appropriate standards and result in injury to another; negligence can occur with acts of omission or commission.

④ Malpractice is misconduct performed in professional practice that results in harm to another.

17 **TEST-TAKING TIP** ● The word **best** in the stem sets a priority. Options 3 and 4 are opposites. Option 2 is patient centered.

① This is a defensive response. All behavior has meaning; the nurse should initially involve the patient and identify the reason for the behavior.

* ② The patient is the center of the health team and has a right to be involved in the decision making concerning care; this individualizes care and promotes self-esteem, which often prevents argumentative and demanding behavior.

③ This is an assumption; many people cope with anxiety by being argumentative and demanding. This behavior may be an attempt to gain control in a situation in which the individual feels out of control.

④ This is judgmental and takes away the patient's coping mechanism.

18 ① Legal statutes are laws created by elected legislative bodies; they are not nursing standards.

② This step-by-step action is a procedure or protocol, not a standard of practice.

③ Requirements for licensure and the ANA Standards of Nursing Practice are unrelated. Most state licensing acts require a specified level of education and the passing of a special examination.

* ④ The ANA has general resolutions that recommend the responsibilities and obligations of nurses; these standards help determine if a nurse has acted as any prudent, reasonable nurse would given similar education, experiential background, and environment.

19 **TEST-TAKING TIP** ● The word "best" in the stem sets a priority.

* ① This patient needs long-term nursing care as well as 24-hour supervision.

② A psychiatric institution would be inappropriate for this patient; patients with dementia need supportive care for the rest of their lives. Psychiatric settings today provide acute care services for mentally ill patients.

③ There are no data that indicate the support of a family or the ability to provide self-care when not at the daycare center; many daycare programs function 5 days a week from 8 AM until 6 PM to assist working family members.

④ Outpatient care facilities usually provide acute care services, not long-term nursing care or 24-hour supervision.

20 **TEST-TAKING TIP** ● Options 2 and 4 are opposites. Options 1 and 4 are equally plausible.

① The Good Samaritan Law does not provide legal immunity; the nurse can still be held accountable for gross departure from acceptable standards of practice or willful wrongdoing.

   * ②   Nurses are responsible for their own actions, and the care provided must be what any reasonably prudent nurse would do under similar circumstances.

   ③   Assistance at the scene of an accident is an ethical, not a legal, duty.

   ④   A contract does not have to exist for a nurse to commit negligence.

21 ①   Libel is defamation of character via print, writing, or pictures, not spoken words.

   ②   Assault is an attempt or threat to touch another person unjustifiably.

   * ③   Slander is defamation of character by spoken words.

   ④   Negligence is the omission to do something a reasonably prudent nurse would do under similar circumstances or the commission of an act that a reasonably prudent nurse would not do under similar circumstances.

22   **TEST-TAKING TIP** ● Options 1 and 2 are equally plausible.

   ①   The nurse's signature does not document that the physician described the procedure and its risks; the patient's signature documents that the procedure and its risks are understood.

   ②   The nurse's signature does not document that the patient was properly informed about expected outcomes. The nurse only witnesses the patient's signature and examines the document for the correct date and time.

   * ③   The nurse only witnesses the patient's signature.

   ④   This is untrue; reasonably prudent practice protects the surgeon from being sued.

23   **TEST-TAKING TIP** ● The word "most" is the key word in the stem that sets a priority. The clue in the stem is "1990s."

   ①   *Tertiary care* involves helping patients adapt to limitations caused by illness; historically, this has always been a focus of health care.

   ②   *Secondary care* includes early diagnosis and treatment to prevent complications of illness; historically, this has always been a focus of health care.

   * ③   *Primary care* includes health promotion activities, such as exercise programs and low-cholesterol diets, that assist patients to maintain their present levels of health or enhance their health in the future. Primary care received increased importance in the 1990s.

   ④   *Tertiary care* includes rehabilitation services; historically, this has always been a focus of health care.

24   **TEST-TAKING TIP** ● Options 2 and 3 are equally plausible.

   ①   A degree or diploma verifies that the student has met the criteria for graduation from the granting institution, not NCLEX-RN.

   ②   This is not the purpose of NCLEX-RN.

   ③   Same as #2.

   * ④   The NCLEX-RN examination is designed to identify whether a candidate has met a minimum level of performance to safely practice as a licensed registered nurse.

25 ①   Planning is involved with setting goals, establishing priorities, identifying expected outcomes, identifying interventions designed to achieve goals and outcomes, modifying the plan as necessary, and collaborating with other health team members to ensure that care is coordinated. Planning does not include the communication of data collected during assessment.

   ②   Analysis is involved with the interpretation of data, collection of additional data, identification and communication of nursing diagnoses, and the assurance that the patient's health care needs are appropriately met. Analysis does not include the communication of data collected during the assessment phase of the nursing process.

③ Evaluation is involved with identifying a patient's response to care, comparing a patient's actual responses to the expected outcomes, analyzing factors that affected the actual outcomes for the purpose of drawing conclusions about the success or failure of specific nursing activities, and modifying the plan of care when necessary; evaluation does not include the communication of data collected during the assessment phase.

* ④ Communicating important assessment data to other health team members is a component of the assessment phase of the nursing process.

26 TEST-TAKING TIP ● Options 1 and 4 are equally plausible and can be eliminated.

① This does not address the nursing assistant's need to know how to move a patient safely with a mechanical lift.

② This is unsafe. This teaching method does not take into consideration the need for the nurse aide to practice the psychomotor skills associated with this task. Explaining is not enough. A demonstration and return demonstration meeting all the critical elements regarding principles of mechanical lift transfer should be reviewed before a nurse aide can use a mechanical lift.

* ③ Demonstration is the safest way to assess whether the nurse aide has the knowledge and skill to safely transfer a patient using a mechanical lift.

④ Another nurse aide should not be held accountable for the care assigned another staff member. The nurse is directly responsible for ensuring that delegated care is safely delivered to patients.

27 ① This is a legal responsibility of the nurse; it is illegal for the nurse aide to give drugs, even if under the supervision of the nurse.

* ② The nurse aide is trained to identify major abnormal signs and symptoms and to notify the nurse when a sign is outside the normal range or is changed from the patient's baseline; the nurse then completes a professional assessment of the patient's condition.

③ A nurse aide should always work under the direct guidance and supervision of a nurse, not another nurse aide.

④ Teaching requires a strong scientific knowledge base and an ability to use scientific teaching-learning principles when planning and implementing an educational plan; the nurse aide is not prepared for this responsibility.

28 TEST-TAKING TIP ● The word "most" sets a priority.

① This requires professional nursing judgment. The nurse is educationally prepared to determine the significance of vital sign measurements, not the nurse aide.

② It is not legal for a nurse aide to monitor tube feedings; this action is within the legal practice of nursing, not nurse aide practice.

* ③ Nurse aides are trained to provide basic hygiene measures under the direction of a nurse.

④ Nurses should ambulate postoperative patients for the first time; nurses have the knowledge to analyze a patient's response to ambulating postoperatively; the nurse aide can ambulate patients with simple, noncomplex needs.

29 ① This is an ethical responsibility, not a legal requirement.

② It is the responsibility of the injured person to report an incident of rape.

* ③ The law requires professionals, such as teachers, certain health care professionals, and social workers, to report suspicions of child abuse to the authorities.

④ In June 1992 the Supreme Court of the United States upheld the constitutional right of a woman to control her own body to the extent that she can abort a fetus in the early stages of pregnancy. However, the decision stipulated that each state may legislate its own reasonable restrictions. It is likely that some states will require parental notification if the woman seeking an abortion is a minor. Notification should not be confused with consent. Also, the question does not indicate that the daughter is a minor.

30 **TEST-TAKING TIP** ● Options 3 and 4 are equally plausible because neither option is better than the other.
 ① This does not address the right of the patient to know what is being done and why; rushing may increase the patient's anxiety.
 ② This is patronizing; when patients feel they are being humored, trust deteriorates.
 * ③ This supports every patient's right to know what care is being given and why.
 ④ This may not be true; trust is based on honesty.

31 ① A patient who is illiterate can sign by making a mark on the consent form; the nurse is a witness to attest that the mark was made by the patient.
 ② The ability to understand the surgery and its implications and alternatives is related to emotional and mental stability, not age.
 ③ A person under legal age with a valid marriage certificate can sign a surgical consent form.
 * ④ A patient must be mentally and emotionally competent to sign a surgical consent form; depression can interfere with cognitive processes and comprehension.

32 **TEST-TAKING TIP** ● Option 2 gives the patient control and is therefore the most patient-centered option.
 ① This does not support the patient's need to be in control of the immediate environment; equipment should be stored appropriately to protect it from pathogens in the environment.
 * ② This supports the patient's right to control personal space.
 ③ Logic generally does not reduce a patient's concern; the patient needs to feel in control, and this action does not support this need.
 ④ Same as #3.

33 ① Proprietary agencies are privately owned and operated to make a profit.
 * ② Alcoholics Anonymous (AA) is a voluntary organization. Voluntary agencies are not for profit and rely on professional and lay volunteers, in addition to a paid staff, to meet a specific health need on the local, state, or national level.
 ③ Official health agencies are supported by local, state, and national taxes and are designed to meet a specific health need on the local, state, or national level.
 ④ Same as #1.

34 **TEST-TAKING TIP** ● The word "identifying" in the stem is closely associated with the word "assessment" in option 3.
 ① In the analysis step of the nursing process the nurse interprets data, determines the significance of data, and formulates a nursing diagnosis.
 ② Evaluation involves determining patient responses to nursing interventions, identifying if goals and outcomes are met, and revising the plan of care when necessary.
 * ③ Observation of human responses is part of the assessment phase of the nursing process; assessment involves collecting, verifying, clustering, and communicating objective and subjective data.
 ④ Implementation involves carrying out the plan of care and documenting the care provided.

35* ① This is a goal because it identifies a desired patient outcome or change in patient behavior.

② This is not a goal. This is a patient need that directly influences the planned intervention.

③ This is not a goal. This is the problem statement part of a nursing diagnosis; it is the phrase that precedes the words "related to" in a nursing diagnosis.

④ This is not a goal. This is a planned intervention.

174 Common Theories Related to Meeting Patients' Basic Human Needs

This section includes questions related to the work of theorists such as Maslow, Selye, and Erikson. It also includes questions related to principles of teaching, growth and development, types of stresses, and the definition of health.

Questions

1 Of the human needs identified by Maslow's hierarchy of needs, which is the *most* basic?
   ① Physiological needs
   ② Belonging needs
   ③ Security needs
   ④ Safety needs
   TEST-TAKING TIP ● Identify the key word in the stem that sets a priority. Identify the equally plausible options.

2 To ensure that a patient understands the content of a teaching session, the nurse should:
   ① Use simple vocabulary and sentence structure
   ② Speak slowly when talking with the patient
   ③ Speak distinctly when giving directions
   ④ Ask the patient what was learned
   TEST-TAKING TIP ● Identify the option that is unique. Identify the patient-centered option.

3 A developmental task of elderly people, according to Erikson, is:
   ① Establishing trust
   ② Becoming dependent
   ③ Reconciling one's life
   ④ Assisting grown children
   TEST-TAKING TIP ● Identify the clue in the stem.

4 A mentally disadvantaged (retarded) adult patient is learning self-care. To increase learning, the nurse should:
   ① Verbally recognize when goals are met
   ② Set a variety of short-term goals to be met
   ③ Use candy as a reward when goals are met
   ④ Disregard the behavior when goals are not met
   TEST-TAKING TIP ● Identify opposites in options.

5 Which action would meet a patient's basic physiological needs?
   ① Raising the side rails
   ② Providing a bed bath
   ③ Explaining procedures
   ④ Conversing with the patient
   TEST-TAKING TIP ● Identify the clue in the stem.

6 Which is most relevant when predicting success of a teaching program regarding the learning of a skill?
   ① The learner's cognitive ability
   ② The amount of reinforcement

③ The extent of family support
④ The interest of the learner

TEST-TAKING TIP ● Identify the key word in the stem that sets a priority. Identify options that are patient centered.

7 In relation to Erikson's developmental theory, a question that could be asked that relates to the task of the school-age child is:
① "Who am I?"
② "What can I do?"
③ "Who can I trust?"
④ "What have I done?"

TEST-TAKING TIP ● Identify the clue in the stem. Identify opposites in options.

8 Patients draw pictures and sometimes hang them in their rooms. According to Maslow's hierarchy of needs, the specific human need being met is:
① Physiological
② Self-esteem
③ Security
④ Love

TEST-TAKING TIP ● Identify the key word in the stem that sets a priority.

9 Growth and development follows a pattern that:
① Is uncertain
② Is unpredictable
③ Is based on motivation
④ Is influenced by the previous step

TEST-TAKING TIP ● Identify equally plausible options.

10 According to Erikson's developmental theory, a statement that can be associated with the task of generativity versus stagnation is:
① "I want to do it myself."
② "I will be getting married next week."
③ "I enjoy mentoring the new employees."
④ "I am pleased with the decisions I have made."

TEST-TAKING TIP ● Identify the clue in the stem.

11 The sun is considered a:
① Physical stress
② Chemical stress
③ Physiological stress
④ Microbiological stress

12 According to Erikson, an event that would support the developmental tasks associated with the stage of middle adulthood would be:
① Getting married
② Retiring from work
③ Becoming a parent
④ Experiencing menopause

TEST-TAKING TIP ● Identify the clue in the stem.

13 An activity that would promote successful completion of the struggle associated with young adulthood would be:
① Going on a date
② Raising children
③ Promoting a cause
④ Sharing knowledge
TEST-TAKING TIP ● Identify the the clue in the stem.

14 When planning to teach colostomy care to a young adult male who has just had a temporary colostomy, the nurse should *initially:*
① Establish goals for the teaching plan
② Follow the patient's usual bowel habits
③ Identify the patient's interest in self-care
④ Reinforce that the colostomy is only temporary
TEST-TAKING TIP ● Identify the key word in the stem that sets a priority. Identify the unique option. Identify the specific determiner in an option. Identify the patient-centered options.

15 According to Maslow's hierarchy of needs, when planning care for several patients, the nurse should **first** assist the patient who needs to:
① Talk
② Void
③ Walk
④ Know
TEST-TAKING TIP ● Identify the key word in the stem that sets a priority.

16 An activity that supports the developmental task of the adolescent would be:
① Reading a book
② Learning how to use a computer
③ Helping parents with household chores
④ Attending a high school basketball game
TEST-TAKING TIP ● Identify the clue in the stem.

17 The process of growth and development within an individual can generally be described as:
① Plodding
② Unique
③ Simple
④ Even

18 Which word best describes the feelings associated with an infant in Erikson's stage of Trust versus Mistrust?
① Me
② We
③ You
④ They
TEST-TAKING TIP ● Identify the key word in the stem that sets a priority.

19 Considering theories about stress, which event generally precipitates the highest degree of stress?
① Retirement
② Relocation

③ Pregnancy
④ Marriage

TEST-TAKING TIP ● Identify the key word in the stem that sets a priority.

20 When collecting information to prepare a teaching plan in the cognitive domain, the nurse asks a patient with diabetes:
① "How do you inspect your feet each day?"
② "Can you measure a serum glucose level?"
③ "What do you know about diabetes mellitus?"
④ "Are you able to perform a subcutaneous injection?"

TEST-TAKING TIP ● Identify the clue in the stem. Identify the option that is unique.

21 The most effective approach to use in teaching a patient about self-injection with insulin would be through a:
① Book
② Video
③ Discussion
④ Demonstration

TEST-TAKING TIP ● Identify the key word in the stem that sets a priority.

22 According to Maslow's hierarchy of needs, which need takes priority?
① Security
② Belonging
③ Self-esteem
④ Self-actualization

TEST-TAKING TIP ● Identify the key word in the stem that sets a priority.

23 An adult has a sense of inadequacy and inferiority at work. One could say that this person had the most difficulty resolving the conflict associated with which developmental age?
① Birth to 1 year
② 4 to 8 years
③ 8 to 12 years
④ 13 to 20 years

TEST-TAKING TIP ● Identify the word in the stem that sets a priority. Identify the clue in the stem.

24 The stress of air pollution caused by wood-burning fireplaces in the home can be classified as a:
① Physical stress
② Chemical stress
③ Physiological stress
④ Microbiological stress

25 When defining health, one concept that is basic to most definitions is that health is:
① A progressive state
② The absence of disease
③ Relative to one's value system
④ An extreme of the wellness-illness continuum

TEST-TAKING TIP ● Identify the clue in the stem. Identify the patient-centered option. Identify equally plausible options.

178

26 A patient is terminally ill. Which is an unexpected behavior associated with the usual process of grieving?
① Talking about the illness
② Becoming angry with people
③ Attempting to commit suicide
④ Seeking alternative therapies
TEST-TAKING TIP ● Identify the polarity in the stem.

27 Psychosocial development is most influenced by:
① Food
② Society
③ Alcohol
④ Genetics
TEST-TAKING TIP ● Identify a key word in the stem that is close to a clang association.

28 Infants have very light yellow urine because they:
① Ingest just fluids
② Cannot control urination
③ Are unable to concentrate urine
④ Always urinate more frequently than adults
TEST-TAKING TIP ● Identify specific determiners in the options.

29 According to Maslow's hierarchy of needs, which would most clearly demonstrate physiological needs as a priority?
① Trauma
② Puberty
③ Restraints
④ Menopause

30 Which word best reflects the type of play associated with Erikson's stage of initiative versus guilt?
① Us
② Me
③ You
④ Them
TEST-TAKING TIP ● Identify the unique option.

31 Elderly persons tend to have higher blood pressures because older people have:
① Thicker blood
② Aging hearts
③ Lifestyle changes
④ Less elastic vessels

32 In relation to the general adaptation syndrome, the nurse recognizes that all patients who are exposed to a stressful event will:
① Adapt in a unique way
② Experience an iatrogenic stress
③ Eventually achieve homeostasis
④ Have an autonomic nervous system response
TEST-TAKING TIP ● Identify the option that has a specific determiner.

33 The most effective teaching strategy that can be used in the cognitive domain is:
① Explanation
② Demonstration
③ Group discussion
④ Individual practice
TEST-TAKING TIP ● Identify the options that are opposites.

34 A school-age child will be hospitalized for several months. To enhance achievement of the developmental task associated with this age group, the nurse should encourage the parents to:
① Bring a favorite stuffed animal from home
② Have siblings visit several times a week
③ Arrange for homework to be brought to the hospital
④ Contract for the television to be turned on in the room
TEST-TAKING TIP ● Identify the clue in the stem.

35 According to the Health-Belief Model, what factor would *directly* influence the likelihood of a smoker to use a nicotine patch to stop smoking?
① Perceived susceptibility to lung cancer
② Perceived benefit of the intervention
③ Perceived seriousness of the disease
④ Perceived self-efficacy
TEST-TAKING TIP ● Identify the clue in the stem.

180 Rationales

1 **TEST-TAKING TIP** ● The word *most* in the stem sets a priority. Options 3 and 4 are equally plausible.
* ① Physiological needs are most basic; oxygen, food, fluid, rest, sleep, and elimination are basic for life.
 ② Belonging needs are ranked third, after physiological and safety-security needs and before self-actualization.
 ③ Security and safety needs are ranked second, after physiological needs and before love and belonging.
 ④ Same as #3.

2 **TEST-TAKING TIP** ● Option 4 is unique and patient centered because it is the only one that seeks feedback from the patient. Options 1, 2, and 3, are similar because they all are concerned with how to send information to the patient.
 ① This action helps to send a clearer message, but it does not inform the sender whether the receiver understood the message.
 ② Same as #1.
 ③ Same as #1.
* ④ Seeking feedback enables the caregiver to know whether or not the message was understood as intended.

3 **TEST-TAKING TIP** ● The word "elderly" in the stem is a clue.
 ① An infant needs to develop trust; this is the major task of an infant, not an elderly person.
 ② Dependency is not a task for which one strives; dependency results if an 8- to 12-year-old is unable to resolve the conflict of industry versus inferiority.
* ③ Elderly people need to come to terms with the fact that the end of life is near; reviewing one's life is a step in this process.
 ④ Middle-aged adults may help grown children. This is usually a task of this age group.

4 **TEST-TAKING TIP** ● Options 1 and 4 are opposites.
* ① Recognizing goals supports feelings of self-esteem and independence; it provides external reinforcement and promotes internal reinforcement.
 ② A mentally disadvantaged person generally can focus on only one goal at a time; several goals may be overwhelming.
 ③ The routine ingestion of candy is not healthy; praise is a more acceptable reward.
 ④ A patient's behavior should never be disregarded; all behavior should be addressed in a nonjudgmental and supportive manner.

5 **TEST-TAKING TIP** ● The word "physiological" is a clue in the stem.
 ① Raising side rails relates to the patient's need for safety and security, the second level in Maslow's hierarchy of needs.
* ② A bed bath supports the patient's physiological need to be clean and is related to the first level, physiological needs, in Maslow's hierarchy of needs.
 ③ Explaining procedures relates to the patient's need for safety and security; patients have a right to know what is happening to them and why.
 ④ Conversing with a patient relates to the need for love and belonging, the third level in Maslow's hierarchy of needs.

6 TEST-TAKING TIP ● The word "most" in the stem is a key word that sets a priority. Options 1 and 4 are patient centered.
① Although a teaching program must be designed within the patient's developmental and cognitive abilities, it is useless unless the patient recognizes the value of what is to be learned and has a desire to learn.
② Although reinforcement is important, self-motivation is the most significant factor in learning.
③ Although family support is important, the patient's interest and readiness to learn are the priorities for the successful learning of a skill; some patients do not have a family support system.
* ④ The motivation of the learner to acquire new attitudes, information, or skills is the most important component for successful learning; motivation exists when the learner recognizes the future benefits of learning.

7 TEST-TAKING TIP ● The word "school-age" is a clue in the stem. Options 2 and 4 are opposites.
① "Who am I?" relates to the conflict of identity versus role confusion; the person aged 13 to 20 years seeks to develop peer relationships, defines goals, selects a vocation, gains independence, and seeks identity.
* ② "What can I do?" relates to the conflict of industry versus inferiority; the child of 6 to 12 years is developing a sense of competence and perseverance.
③ "Who can I trust?" relates to the conflict of trust versus mistrust. During the first year the infant depends on others to meet his or her basic needs; the infant develops trust if these needs are met in a comfortable and predictable manner.
④ "What have I done?" relates to the conflict of integrity versus despair; the person aged 60 years or more struggles to feel a sense of worth about past experiences and goals achieved and seeks a sense of integrity.

8 TEST-TAKING TIP ● The word "specific" is the key word in the stem that sets a priority.
① "Physiological" relates to meeting basic physical needs, such as the needs for oxygen, food, water, rest, sleep, and elimination, not self-esteem needs.
* ② The situation illustrated in the stem meets self-esteem needs; control, self-respect, and competence are reflected when a person hangs self-made pictures in a room for the enjoyment of self and others.
③ "Security" refers to shelter, clothing, and the need to feel comfortable with the rules of the society, community, and hospital.
④ "Love" refers to the need for bonds of affection and a sense of belonging.

9 TEST-TAKING TIP ● Option 1 and 2 are equally plausible.
① Although growth and development progress through some stages slower or faster than others, they still follow a certain predictable pattern.
② Same as #1.
③ Motivation may influence the achievement of tasks in some stages of growth and development; however, growth and development do not rely on motivation.
* ④ Success or failure of task achievement in one stage of development influences succeeding stages; failure to resolve a crisis at one stage damages the ego, which makes the resolution of the following stages more difficult.

10 TEST-TAKING TIP ● The words "generativity versus stagnation" provide a clue in the stem.
① This statement relates to stage two; this is the conflict of autonomy versus shame and doubt. The 2- to 4-year-old seeks a balance between independence and dependence and attempts to achieve autonomy.

    ② This statement relates to stage six; this is the conflict of intimacy and solidarity versus isolation. The young adult 20 to 30 years old seeks to select a partner for a life relationship.

* ③ This statement relates to stage seven; this is the conflict of generativity versus stagnation. The person 30 to 60 years old is interested in guiding younger individuals.

    ④ This statement relates to stage eight; this is the conflict of integrity versus despair. The person aged 60 years or more struggles to feel a sense of worth about past experiences and goals achieved and seeks a sense of integrity.

11* ① Physical stresses are stresses from outside the body and include light, environmental temperature, sound, pressure, motion, gravity, and electricity.

    ② Chemical stresses relate to toxic substances such as acids, alkalies, drugs, and exogenous hormones.

    ③ Physiological stresses are disturbances in structure or function of any tissue, organ, or system within the body.

    ④ Microbiological stresses are organisms such as bacteria, viruses, molds, or parasites that can cause disease.

12 TEST-TAKING TIP ● The words "middle adulthood" provide a clue in the stem.

    ① Getting married is most often associated with young adulthood, intimacy versus isolation.

    ② Retiring from work is most often associated with the older adult, integrity versus despair.

* ③ Concerns for the family and next generation are associated with middle adulthood, generativity versus stagnation.

    ④ Menopause is not associated with any developmental task according to Erikson; Erikson's theory is a psychosocial developmental theory based on the process of socialization, not physiological events.

13 TEST-TAKING TIP ● The words "young adulthood" provide a clue in the stem.

* ① The development task of the young adult is the establishment of intimacy with a relationship partner.

    ② This activity is related to the developmental task of generativity versus stagnation associated with middle adulthood.

    ③ Same as #2.

    ④ Same as #2.

14 TEST-TAKING TIP ● The word *initially* is the key word in the stem that sets a priority. Option 3 is unique because it is the only option that addresses assessment, the first step in the nursing process. The word "only" in option 4 is a specific determiner. Options 2 and 3 are patient centered.

    ① This would be done after a readiness for learning is established. Words such as "follow" and "establish" are action words that are more appropriately related to planning or intervention than assessment.

    ② Same as #1.

* ③ Determining the patient's readiness for learning and point of reference are the priorities. Assessment is the first step in the nursing process.

    ④ Although the colostomy may be only temporary, the patient still needs to be taught self-care. Focusing on the "only temporary" nature of the colostomy may offer false reassurance. A colostomy may become permanent if the patient's condition does not improve as expected.

15 TEST-TAKING TIP ● The word **first** in the stem is a key word that sets a priority.
   ① Although important, basic physiological needs should be met first.
 * ② Elimination is a basic physiological need. When setting priorities, the most basic physiological needs should be met first.
   ③ Same as #1.
   ④ Same as #1.

16 TEST-TAKING TIP ● The word "adolescent" in the stem is a clue.
   ① Middle childhood (6 to 12 years), not adolescence, is concerned with developing fundamental skills in reading, writing, calculating, and using a computer; the school-age child is very industrious.
   ② Same as #1.
   ③ The childhood years, not adolescence, are related to helping behaviors; 3- to 5-year-olds like to imitate parents and 6- to 12-year-olds are developing appropriate social roles.
 * ④ Adolescents are concerned with developing new and more mature relationships with their peers; adolescents tend to associate with their peers rather than parents.

17 ① Some stages are faster and some are slower.
 * ② Although a general pattern is followed, each individual grows and develops at a different rate or extent and is therefore unique.
   ③ Growth and development is an extremely complex process based on many influencing variables.
   ④ Some stages of growth and development are faster and some are slower, not even, depending on the stage and the individual.

18 TEST-TAKING TIP ● The word "best" is a key word in the stem that sets a priority.
 * ① The infant is egocentric and unaware of boundaries between the self and others; the infant is concerned with his or her needs being met immediately.
   ② The infant has not identified the difference between self and others.
   ③ Same as #2.
   ④ Same as #2.

19 TEST-TAKING TIP ● The word "highest" is a key word in the stem that sets a priority.
   ① Stress units for life events have been determined based on the readjustment required by an individual to adapt to a particular situation or event; the mean stress unit for retirement is 45 and is less than marriage, which is 50.
   ② The mean stress unit for a change in residence is 20 and is less than marriage, which is 50.
   ③ The mean stress unit for pregnancy is 40 and is less than marriage, which is 50.
 * ④ The mean stress unit for marriage is 50, which is higher than the other options presented.

20 TEST-TAKING TIP ● The word "cognitive" is a clue in the stem. Option 3 is unique because it is the only option that is concerned with "what is" rather than "how to." Options 1, 2, and 4 all relate to the performance of a skill.
   ① This statement focuses on the performance of a skill that relates to the psychomotor domain, not the cognitive domain, because it involves the performance of a skill.
   ② Same as #1.
 * ③ This is the cognitive domain because it deals with the comprehension of information.
   ④ Same as #1.

21 TEST-TAKING TIP ● The word "most" is the key word in the stem that sets a priority.

① Although this can be used for learning a skill (psychomotor domain), it is not as effective as demonstration and return demonstration; it is more appropriate for learning and comprehending information (cognitive domain).

② Same as #1.

③ Learning via discussion is appropriate for the cognitive (knowing) and affective (feeling) domains.

* ④ Demonstration uses a variety of senses such as sight, hearing, and touch. The opportunity to observe and manipulate the equipment promotes learning a skill.

22 TEST-TAKING TIP ● The word "priority" is the key word in the stem.

* ① Safety and security needs, second-level needs according to Maslow, are ranked after basic physiological needs and before the need for love and belonging; people need to feel physically and emotionally safe.

② Belonging needs, third-level needs according to Maslow, are ranked after safety and security needs and before self-esteem needs. A bond of affection is necessary for well-being.

③ Self-esteem needs, fourth-level needs according to Maslow, are ranked after love and belonging needs and before self-actualization needs. People need to feel competent and respected.

④ Self-actualization needs are ranked fifth, and this is the final level according to Maslow; maximizing abilities and feeling content within the self are necessary for self-satisfaction.

23 TEST-TAKING TIP ● The word "most" is a key word in the stem that sets a priority. The words "inadequacy and inferiority" in the stem provide a clue.

① Birth to 1 year of age is a time of concern with resolving the conflict of trust versus mistrust, not industry versus inferiority.

② During the ages of 4 to 8 years, the child is concerned with resolving the conflict of initiative versus guilt, not industry versus inferiority.

* ③ During the ages of 8 to 12 years, the child is concerned with resolving the conflict of industry versus inferiority; when a child is unable to develop physical, social, or cognitive skills well enough to perceive him- or herself as competent, the child feels inadequate; these feelings of inferiority can be carried throughout adulthood.

④ During the ages of 13 to 20 years, the child is concerned with resolving the conflict of identity versus role confusion, not industry versus inferiority.

24 ① Air pollution is a chemical stress, not a physical stress; physical stresses include temperature, sound, pressure, light, motion, gravity, and electricity.

* ② Burning wood releases toxic substances and gases into the air; these are considered chemical stresses. Acids, alkalies, drugs, and exogenous hormones are also considered chemical stresses.

③ Air pollution is a chemical stress, not a physiological stress; disturbances in structure or function of any tissue, organ, or system of the body are considered physiological stresses.

④ Air pollution is a chemical stress, not a microbiological stress; bacteria, viruses, molds, and parasites are considered microbiological stresses.

25 TEST-TAKING TIP ● The words "basic to most" provide the clue that the answer is a common component of most definitions of health. Option 3 is patient centered. Options 1 and 4 are equally plausible.

① Health fluctuates on a continuum that has extremes of wellness to illness; movement can occur up or down the continuum, not only in one direction.

② The World Health Organization's definition of health is "A state of complete physical, mental and social well being, and not merely the absence of disease or infirmity"; some people who have a chronic illness consider themselves healthy because they are able to function independently.

* ③ A definition of health is highly individualized; it is based on each person's own experiences, values, and perceptions. Health can mean different things to each individual; people tend to define health based on the presence or absence of symptoms, their perceptions of how they feel, and their capacity to function on a daily basis.

④ Although high-level wellness is one extreme of the wellness-illness continuum and severe illness the other, where one plots a position on the continuum is based on the individual's value system. An individual's perception of health is based on his or her physical, emotional, social, mental, and spiritual sense of wellness.

26 TEST-TAKING TIP ● The word "unexpected" causes this stem to have negative polarity. You need to identify the behavior that is not usually associated with the grieving process.

① Although talking about the illness occurs throughout the grieving response, it is most expected during the early stage of denial and disbelief ("No, not me").

② Anger is expected and occurs when there is a developing awareness of the impending loss ("Why me?").

* ③ Although some people who are terminally ill attempt suicide, it is not a normal expected response to loss.

④ Seeking alternative therapies occurs most often during the stage of bargaining ("Yes, me, but").

27 TEST-TAKING TIP ● An important word in the stem is "psychosocial." When examining the options, you see that one of them contains the word "society." "Society" is closely related to "psychosocial." Carefully consider this option. More often than not it will be the correct answer.

① Food is only one aspect of a society and its culture; the primary purpose of food is to meet physiological needs.

* ② A person's cultural environment, which includes the family and the community, has the greatest impact on psychosocial development.

③ Although alcohol meets some individuals' psychological needs and is served in social situations, it is not the factor that most influences psychosocial development.

④ Although genetics has been identified by some theorists as a factor related to personality and behavior, it is not the most influential factor in psychosocial development.

28 TEST-TAKING TIP ● The word "only" in option 1 and the word "always" in option 4 are specific determiners.

① Infants void very light yellow urine because they are unable to concentrate urine and reabsorb water efficiently, not because they ingest only fluids.

② Although it is true that infants have not developed neuromuscular control of urination, the inability to control micturition voluntarily has no impact on the color of the urine voided.

* ③ An infant's kidneys are unable to concentrate urine and reabsorb water efficiently. When the body is too immature to concentrate urine, urine is diluted and very light yellow in color.

④ Although this is a correct statement by itself, it is not related to the content in the stem. Infants' bladders are smaller than adults' bladders and they can only retain a small volume of urine. Also, infants cannot concentrate urine and reabsorb water efficiently; therefore, they void a larger percentage of urine per day compared to most adults. However, frequency is not related to the color of urine.

29* ① Trauma can be life threatening and interfere with basic physiological functioning.

    ② Although physiological changes are associated with the growth spurt and development of secondary sexual characteristics during puberty, self-identity and self-esteem often take priority at this time.

    ③ Restraints meet safety and security needs because they protect the patient from harm.

    ④ Although physiological changes are associated with menopause, love, self-esteem and self-actualization are often the priorities at this time.

30 TEST-TAKING TIP ● The word "Us" in Option 1 addresses both sides of an interpersonal relationship. It is a word that reflects a united front. "Me," "You," and "Them" reflect just one side of an interpersonal relationship.

  * ① During the conflict of initiative versus guilt, the child aged 4 to 8 strives to adjust to social spheres outside the home. The child begins to evolve as a social being seeking relationships with a small number of peers with a focus on "Us."

    ② During the conflict of autonomy versus shame and doubt, the child aged 2 to 4 strives to develop a sense of autonomy. Children this age view themselves as independent, separate beings focusing on "Me."

    ③ During the conflict of intimacy versus isolation, the young adult aged 20 to 30 strives to select a relationship partner. A relationship partner in one's life is the important "You."

    ④ During the conflict of industry versus inferiority, the school-age child 7 through 12 years strives to become a productive group member. The school-age child joins a "gang," becomes less self centered, and is more concerned with "Them."

31 ① High blood pressure in elderly people is generally caused by smoking, obesity, lack of exercise, and stress, not thicker blood.

    ② A decreased contractile strength of the myocardium results in a decreased cardiac output. The body compensates for this by increasing the heart rate, not the blood pressure.

    ③ This is a generalization that may or may not be true. The older adult has physical, cognitive, and social changes, and how the person perceives them and adapts to them determines if the individual's lifestyle is stressful and if it influences blood pressure.

  * ④ Vascular changes and the accumulation of sclerotic plaques along the walls of vessels make them more rigid.

32 TEST-TAKING TIP ● The words "eventually achieve" constitute a specific determiner that implies that everyone will obtain homeostasis. This specific determiner is more obscure than a word such as "always."

    ① The general adaptation syndrome is a common physiological response to stress that follows a uniform, not unique, pattern in everyone.

    ② An iatrogenic stress is a stimulus caused by a treatment or diagnostic procedure. It is a stress that can stimulate the general adaptation syndrome.

    ③ Not everyone achieves homeostasis. Some individuals reach the stage of exhaustion.

  * ④ Stressors precipitate the general adaptation syndrome, which is a neuroendocrine response and part of the autonomic nervous system.

33 TEST-TAKING TIP ● Options 3 and 4 are opposites, an individual versus a group, and can be eliminated from consideration.

* ① An explanation imparts information that is within the cognitive domain. An explanation defines, describes, and interprets information so that it is understood.
② A demonstration is most effective when dealing with skills, which are part of the psychomotor domain.
③ A group discussion is most effective when dealing with feelings, which are part of the affective domain.
④ Practice is most effective when dealing with skills, which are part of the psychomotor domain.

34 TEST-TAKING TIP ● The term "school-age child" is the clue in the stem. A school-age child would have homework

① A stuffed animal would be appropriate for an infant or toddler.
② Although this would be appropriate, it does not address the task of initiative versus guilt.
* ③ This is an appropriate activity for a school-age child. School-age children are interested in doing and producing.
④ Same as #2.

35 TEST-TAKING TIP ● The word *directly* is an important word in the stem. The correct option must have a direct, specific relationship to the likelihood that a person would adapt to a particular action; the other options may relate indirectly.

① According to the Health-Belief Model, this is an individual perception, not a factor that directly influences the likelihood of action.
* ② If the outcome or result of the intervention is viewed as positive and probable, the person will believe that the intervention will make a difference and is therefore worthwhile.
③ Same as #1.
④ Perceived self-efficacy is a cognitive-perceptual factor in the Health Promotion Model by Pender.

Communication and Meeting Patients' Emotional Needs

This section includes questions related to assessing and meeting patients' sociocultural, psychological, and spiritual needs. It also includes questions that focus on the principles of communication, communication skills, interventions that support emotional needs, and communicating with the confused or disoriented patient. Additional questions focus on patterns of behavior in response to illness, nursing interventions that assist patients to adapt to illness, caring for the dying patient's emotional needs, defense mechanisms, and responding to the crying patient.

Questions

1 To provide the most therapeutic communication with a patient, the nurse should:
① Use probing questions
② Teach about self-care
③ Ask direct questions
④ Listen attentively

TEST-TAKING TIP ● Identify the key word in the stem that sets a priority. Identify the unique option.

2 A patient's son has just died. The patient states, "I can't believe that I have lost my son. Can you believe it?" The nurse's BEST response is to:
① Say, "It is sad. I can't believe it either."
② Touch the patient's hand and say, "I am very sorry."
③ Encourage a family member to stay and provide support.
④ Leave the room and allow the patient to grieve privately.

TEST-TAKING TIP ● Identify the key word in the stem that sets a priority. Identify the patient-centered options. Identify the option that denies the patient's feelings.

3 Which nursing intervention would be least effective in meeting a patient's psychosocial needs?
① Addressing a patient by name
② Assisting a patient with meals
③ Identifying achievement of goals
④ Explaining care before it is to be given

TEST-TAKING TIP ● Identify the key word in the stem that indicates negative polarity. Identify the clue in the stem.

4 Which is an accurate statement about communication?
① Patients with expressive aphasia cannot communicate.
② Nurses' notes are a form of nonverbal communication.
③ Touch has various meanings to different people.
④ Words have the same meaning for all people.

TEST-TAKING TIP ● Identify specific determiners in options.

5 The nurse recognizes that a usually talkative patient is withdrawn. The nurse's best response would be:
① "You are very quiet today."
② "Tell me what you're upset about."

③ "Why are you so withdrawn today?"
④ "Something seems to be bothering you."

TEST-TAKING TIP ● Identify the key word in the stem that sets a priority. Identify equally plausible options.

6 A patient's spouse died 1 week ago. When reminiscing about their life together the patient begins to cry. The nurse's best response would be to:
① Leave the patient alone to provide privacy
② Say, "Things will get better as time passes."
③ Encourage the patient to get grief counseling
④ State, "This must be a very difficult time for you."

TEST-TAKING TIP ● Identify the key word in the stem that sets a priority. Identify the options that deny the patient's feelings. Identify options that are patient centered.

7 A patient has a history of verbally aggressive behavior. One afternoon the patient starts to shout at another patient in the lounge. The most appropriate statement by the nurse would be:
① "Stop what you are doing."
② "Let's go talk in your room."
③ "Please sit down and be calm."
④ "Do not raise your voice in a hospital."

TEST-TAKING TIP ● Identify the key words in the stem that set a priority. Identify the unique option.

8 A patient is being discharged to a nursing home. While preparing the discharge summary, the patient says, "I feel that nobody cares about me." The nurse's *best* response would be:
① "You feel as if nobody cares."
② "You sound angry at your family."
③ "We all care about you and are concerned."
④ "Your family doesn't have the skills to care for you."

TEST-TAKING TIP ● Identify the key word in the stem that sets a priority. Identify the clue in the stem that is a clang association in relation to an option. Identify the options that deny the patient's concerns.

9 A female patient talks about her children when they were young and states, "I was a very strict mother." A response by the nurse that reflects the technique of paraphrasing would be:
① "It must have been difficult to be a disciplinarian."
② "Sometimes we are sorry for our past behaviors."
③ "You believe you were a firm parent."
④ "You were a very strict mother."

TEST-TAKING TIP ● Identify the clue in the stem.

10 Which behavior would support the conclusion that a patient with a chronic illness is depressed?
① Wishing to attend a nephew's wedding
② Seeking multiple medical opinions
③ Evading activities of daily living
④ Being sarcastic to caregivers

TEST-TAKING TIP ● Identify the clue in the stem.

11 A patient who has been withdrawn says, "When I have the opportunity I am going to commit suicide." The *best* response by the nurse would be:
① "You have a lovely family. They need you."
② "Let's explore the reasons you have for living."
③ "You must feel overwhelmed to want to kill yourself."
④ "Suicide does not solve problems. Tell me what is wrong."

TEST-TAKING TIP ● Identify the key word in the stem that sets a priority. Identify the options that deny the patient's feelings. Identify the unique option.

12 A patient who is hard of hearing tells the nurse, "I cannot hear what people say to me." The nurse should:
① Provide pencil and paper for communication
② Ask questions that require a yes or no answer
③ Shout with a loud voice in the patient's better ear
④ Encourage the patient to use gestures when talking

13 A patient asks for advice regarding a personal problem. The <u>most</u> appropriate response by the nurse would be to:
① Encourage the patient to speak with a family member
② Explain that nurses are not permitted to give advice
③ Ask the patient what would be the best thing to do
④ Offer an opinion after listening to the patient

TEST-TAKING TIP ● Identify the key word in the stem that sets a priority. Identify the option that denies the patient's concerns. Identify opposites in options. Identify the patient-centered option.

14 A dying patient is withdrawn and depressed. The most therapeutic action by the nurse would be:
① Explaining that the patient still can accomplish goals
② Assisting the patient to focus on positive thoughts
③ Accepting the patient's behavioral adaptation
④ Offering the patient advice when appropriate

TEST-TAKING TIP ● Identify the key word in the stem that sets a priority. Identify the options that deny the patient's feelings. Identify the unique option.

15 The sense that is most important to a patient who appears to be in a coma is:
① Taste
② Smell
③ Touch
④ Hearing

TEST-TAKING TIP ● Identify the key word in the stem that sets a priority.

16 To best assist an agitated patient, the nurse should:
① Focus on something other than the patient's agitation
② Point out the agitated behavior to the patient
③ Encourage the patient to share feelings
④ Keep the patient as active as possible

TEST-TAKING TIP ● Identify the key word in the stem that sets a priority. Identify the clue in the stem. Identify opposites in options.

17 An elderly patient reminisces extensively and attempts to keep the nurse from leaving the room. The nurse's *most* therapeutic response would be:
① Encouraging the patient to focus on the present and future
② Limiting the amount of time the patient talks about the past
③ Setting aside time to listen to the stories about the patient's past
④ Suggesting that the patient reminisce with other patients the same age
TEST-TAKING TIP ● Identify the key word in the stem that sets a priority. Identify the options that deny the patient's needs. Identify opposites in options.

18 A patient who is incontinent becomes upset. When changing the gown and linens, the nurse's *best* intervention would be to say:
① "I am a nurse. This is part of my job."
② "This doesn't bother me. It often happens."
③ "This occurs all the time. Try not to feel bad."
④ "I am your nurse. I will change your gown and linens."
TEST-TAKING TIP ● Identify the key word in the stem that sets a priority. Identify the unique option.

19 A patient is friendly, has many visitors, and appears happy. However, when the patient's daughter visits, the patient cries and complains of pain. When the daughter becomes upset the nurse should:
① Encourage the patient to be more positive
② Continue to observe this situation from a distance
③ Explore the situation with the patient and daughter
④ Tell the daughter that the patient usually does not cry
TEST-TAKING TIP ● Identify the option that denies the patient's feelings. Identify the patient-centered option.

20 A patient has difficulty communicating verbally (aphasia) because of a stroke. To increase the patient's ability to communicate, the nurse should:
① Encourage the patient to elaborate with gestures
② Anticipate the patient's needs to reduce frustration
③ Talk to the patient, but not expect a verbal response
④ Ask the patient questions that require a yes or no response
TEST-TAKING TIP ● Identify the opposites in options.

21 Several times a day, every day, a patient asks when medication will be given. The patient receives medication at the same time every day. The most therapeutic intervention would be to:
① Inform the patient every time when it is time for medication
② Tell the patient to go to the nurse when it is time for medication
③ Encourage the patient to remember when it is time for medication
④ Make a sign for the patient's room indicating the times for medication
TEST-TAKING TIP ● Identify the key word in the stem that sets a priority. Identify equally plausible options. Identify the option that contains a specific determiner.

22 A patient is upset and rambles about an incident that occurred earlier in the week. The nurse should first:
① Ask the patient what is wrong
② Identify the concerns of the patient

③ Recognize that the patient is confused
④ Encourage the patient to focus on the present

TEST-TAKING TIP ● Identify the key word in the stem that sets a priority. Identify the patient-centered options. Identify the option that denies the patient's feelings.

23 Defense mechanisms can be classified as:
① Relief behaviors
② Conscious behaviors
③ Somatizing behaviors
④ Manipulative behaviors

24 A true statement about Kübler-Ross's theory on death and dying is that people:
① Ultimately reach the stage of acceptance
② Generally pass through the stages smoothly
③ Can move back and forth between the stages
④ Always move progressively forward through the stages

TEST-TAKING TIP ● Identify opposites in options. Identify the specific determiner in an option.

25 A dying patient says, "All my life I was fairly religious, but I am still worried about what happens after death." The nurse's best response would be:
① "The unknown is often very frightening."
② "If you were religious, you know God is forgiving."
③ "People with after-death experiences say it is peaceful."
④ "You must feel good about being religious all your life."

TEST-TAKING TIP ● Identify the key word in the stem that sets a priority. Identify equally plausible options. Identify the options that deny the patient's feelings.

26 A patient has metastatic lung cancer and the physician discusses the diagnosis and prognosis in detail with the patient. After a severe episode of coughing and shortness of breath later in the day, the patient says to the nurse, "This is just a cold. I'll be fine once I get over it." The nurse's best response would be:
① "Remember what the doctor told you this morning."
② "The doctor had some bad news for you today."
③ "Tell me more about your illness."
④ "It's not a cold, it's lung cancer."

TEST-TAKING TIP ● Identify the word in the stem that sets a priority.

27 A dying patient says to the nurse, "I was much more religious when I was young." The nurse's best response would be:
① "Do you still believe in God?"
② "Do you want us to pray for you?"
③ "Would you like me to call a chaplain?"
④ "Are you concerned about life after death?"

TEST-TAKING TIP ● Identify the word in the stem that sets a priority. Identify the unique option.

28 A female patient becomes upset whenever anyone mentions her upcoming birthday and does not want to talk about age. The nurse recognizes this behavior as:
① Denial
② Sorrow

③ Loneliness
④ Suppression

29 A patient who is usually verbal appears sad and withdrawn. The nurse should:
① Describe the behavior to the patient
② Continue to observe the patient's behavior
③ Ensure that the patient has time to be alone
④ Attempt to engage the patient in cheerful conversation
TEST-TAKING TIP ● Identify the unique option.

30 A terminally ill patient appears sad and withdrawn. The nurse should respond by being:
① Demonstrative
② Cheerful
③ Present
④ Aloof
TEST-TAKING TIP ● Identify the equally plausible options.

31 A patient is confused and disoriented. The route of communication used by the nurse that would be most effective would be:
① Touch
② Writing
③ Talking
④ Pictures
TEST-TAKING TIP ● Identify the unique option.

32 What is the best response by the nurse to the patient who is crying?
① "Sometimes it helps to talk about it."
② "I hope things will get better by tomorrow."
③ "Deep breathing may help you regain control."
④ "Crying helps because it gets it out of your system."
TEST-TAKING TIP ● Identify the unique option.

33 A patient receiving chemotherapy for cancer says to the nurse, "I just want to be well enough to enjoy the holidays." The nurse recognizes that, according to Kübler-Ross, the patient is in the stage of grieving known as:
① Denial
② Bargaining
③ Acceptance
④ Depression

34 A patient is admitted to the hospital, and when the family leaves, the patient begins to cry. The probably etiology of the crying is:
① Guilt
② Anger
③ Denial
④ Anxiety

35 Before entering a patient's room the nurse knocks on the door. This behavior incorporates the concept of:
① Perception
② Critical time
③ Territoriality
④ Confidentiality

194 Rationales

1 **TEST-TAKING TIP** ● The word "most" in the stem sets a priority. Option 4 is unique because it is a receptive, nonverbal action, whereas the other options are all active verbal interventions.

① Although this might be done later, listening comes first; open-ended questions are more therapeutic.

② Although teaching self-care might be done, listening comes first.

③ Same as #1.

* ④ Reception of a message must occur before the nurse can intervene; by listening, the nurse collects information that will influence future care.

2 **TEST-TAKING TIP** ● The word BEST in the stem is the key word that sets a priority. Options 1 and 2 are patient centered. Option 4 denies the patient's feelings.

① Although this statement identifies feelings, it supports denial.

* ② Touch denotes caring; this statement is direct and supportive while not reinforcing denial.

③ Although this may be done later, the patient needs immediate support.

④ Leaving the room is a form of abandonment.

3 **TEST-TAKING TIP** ● The word "least" in the stem indicates negative polarity. The word "psychosocial" in the stem is a clue.

① Calling a patient by name individualizes care and supports dignity and self-esteem.

* ② Usually eating is an independent activity of daily living; for an adult, assistance with meals may precipitate feelings of dependence and regression.

③ Identifying the achievement of goals is motivating and supports independence, self-esteem, and self-actualization.

④ Explaining care provides emotional support because it reduces fear of the unknown and involves the patient in care.

4 **TEST-TAKING TIP** ● In Option 1 the word "all" is understood; this option is really saying, "All patients with expressive aphasia cannot communicate." Option 4 contains the word "all," which is a specific determiner.

① Patients with expressive aphasia can often communicate using nonverbal behaviors, a picture board, or written messages.

② Words, whether they are spoken or written, are verbal communication.

* ③ Touch is a form of nonverbal communication that sends a variety of messages depending on the person's culture, sex, age, past experiences, and present situation; touch also invades a person's personal space.

④ People from different cultures and people in subgroups within the same culture place different values on words.

5 **TEST-TAKING TIP** ● The word best is a key word in the stem that sets a priority. Options 2 and 3 are equally plausible because they are both probing questions.

* ① This statement identifies the behavior and provides an opportunity for the patient to verbalize further.

② This statement is too direct; it may put the patient on the defensive and cut off communication.

③ Same as #2.

④ This statement is inappropriate because it comes to a conclusion that may be inaccurate.

6 TEST-TAKING TIP ● The word "best" is the key word in the stem that sets a priority. Options 1 and 2 deny the patient's feelings. Options 3 and 4 are patient centered.
   ① Leaving the room abandons the patient at a time when emotional support would be beneficial. Abandonment is an ultimate form of denial.
   ② This statement is false reassurance and denies the patient's feeling.
   ③ Encouraging grief counseling may eventually be done, but the patient needs immediate support.
 * ④ This statement identifies feelings, focuses on the patient, and provides an opportunity for the patient to share feelings.

7 TEST-TAKING TIP ● The words "most appropriate" in the stem set a priority. Option 2 is unique because it is the only option that removes the patient from the room.
   ① This statement is a command that may demean the patient; it challenges the patient and may precipitate more abusive behavior.
 * ② This statement interrupts the behavior and protects the other patient; walking to another room uses energy and talking promotes verbalization of feelings and concerns.
   ③ This statement is judgmental; this implies the patient is not calm. An agitated patient has too much energy to sit quietly.
   ④ This statement is inappropriate because it challenges the patient and puts the patient on the defensive.

8 TEST-TAKING TIP ● The word *best* is the key word in the stem that sets a priority. The words "nobody cares" appear in the stem and Option 1; this repetition is a clang association. Options 3 and 4 deny the patient's feelings.
 * ① Repeating the patient's statement allows the patient to focus on what was said, validates what was said, and encourages communication.
   ② This patient's statement reflects feelings of sadness and isolation, not anger.
   ③ This statement may or may not be true and does not encourage verbalization of feelings.
   ④ Same as #3.

9 TEST-TAKING TIP ● The word "paraphrasing" is the clue in stem.
   ① This response uses reflective technique, not paraphrasing, because it identifies a feeling.
   ② The patient's statement does not reflect feelings of sorrow or guilt.
 * ③ This response restates the message using different words; paraphrasing focuses on content rather than the feeling or underlying emotional theme.
   ④ This response is echolalia, not paraphrasing, because it uses the exact same words used by the patient.

10 TEST-TAKING TIP ● The word "depressed" is the clue in the stem.
   ① Wishing to attend a future event is future-oriented thinking and may be a form of bargaining for more time.
   ② Seeking multiple opinions is associated with denial and bargaining.
 * ③ When patients are depressed, they may feel a loss of control, alone, and withdrawn. In depression, there is little physical energy, a lack of concern about the activities of daily living, and a decreased interest in physical appearance.
   ④ Sarcasm generally reflects feelings of anger.

11 TEST-TAKING TIP ● The word *best* is the key word in the stem that sets a priority. Options 1, 2, and 4 deny the patient's feelings. Option 3 is unique because it is the only option that addresses feelings.
   ① This statement denies the patient's feelings. The patient is unable to cope, is select-

ing the ultimate escape, and is not capable of meeting the needs of others. This response may also precipitate feelings such as guilt.

(2) This statement denies the patient's feelings; the patient must focus on the negatives before exploring the positives.

* (3) Open-ended statements identify feelings and invite further communication.

(4) This response is judgmental, denies the patient's feelings, and may cut off communication. In addition, this response is too direct and the patient may not consciously know what is wrong.

12 * (1) Communication can be promoted in written rather than verbal form; this reduces social isolation and promotes communication.

(2) Communication is a two-way process; the patient is not having difficulty sending messages; the patient is having difficulty receiving messages. This intervention is more appropriate for a patient with expressive aphasia.

(3) Shouting is demeaning and unnecessary; enunciating words slowly and directly in front of the patient supports communication.

(4) The patient is having difficulty receiving messages, not sending messages.

13 **TEST-TAKING TIP** ● The word <u>most</u> is the key word in the stem that sets a priority. Option 2 denies the patient's concern. Options 2 and 3 are opposites. Option 3 is patient centered.

(1) Although this might eventually be done, the patient's concerns and perceived alternatives should be explored first; also the patient may never want to talk about a particular concern with family members.

(2) This approach puts the focus on the nurse and cuts off communication.

* (3) This response provides an opportunity for the patient to explore concerns and options without others influencing the decision making.

(4) Offering opinions is inappropriate; opinions involve judgments that are based on feelings and values that may be different from the patient's.

14 **TEST-TAKING TIP** ● The word "most" is the key word in the stem that sets a priority. Options 1 and 2 deny the patient's feelings. Option 3 is unique because it is the only option that uses the word "patient's," the possessive form of the word "patient."

(1) This denies the patient's feelings; the patient needs to focus on the future loss.

(2) Same as #1.

* (3) Depression is the fourth stage of dying according to Dr. Kübler-Ross; patients become withdrawn and noncommunicative when feeling a loss of control and recognizing future losses. The nurse should accept the behavior and be available if the patient wants to verbalize feelings.

(4) It is never appropriate to offer advice; people must explore their alternatives and come to their own conclusions.

15 **TEST-TAKING TIP** ● The word "most" is the key word in the stem that sets a priority.

(1) Although all the senses are important, hearing is the most important sense to an unconscious person. The nurse should assume that an unconscious patient is able to hear and make attempts to communicate verbally.

(2) This sense is not usually as significant as hearing to a patient who is in a coma.

(3) Same as #2.

* (4) Hearing is the most important sense to an unconscious patient because it is believed to be the last sense that is lost; the senses receive stimuli from the environment and hearing keeps one in contact with others.

16 TEST-TAKING TIP ● The word "best" is a key word in the stem that sets a priority. The word "agitated" is the clue in the stem. Options 1 and 2 are opposites.

① All behavior has meaning; therefore, the agitation cannot be ignored.

② This is confrontational and could precipitate a defensive response by the patient.

* ③ Agitation is a response to anxiety; the patient's feelings and concerns must be addressed to help relieve the anxiety and agitation.

④ This could increase the agitation, particularly if the cause of the agitation is ignored.

17 TEST-TAKING TIP ● The word *most* is the key word in the stem that sets a priority. Options 1 and 2 deny the patient's needs. Options 2 and 3 are opposites.

① Avoiding reminiscing is inappropriate; the developmental task of elderly people is to perform a life review.

② Same as #1.

* ③ The nurse is responsible for assisting the patient to explore the past and deal with the developmental conflict of integrity versus despair.

④ Patients should not be responsible for meeting each other's needs.

18 TEST-TAKING TIP ● The word *best* is the key word in the stem that sets a priority. Option 4 is unique because it is the only option that does not minimize the patient's feelings.

① This response cuts off communication and puts the focus on the nurse rather than the patient.

② This response generalizes rather than individualizes care. It minimizes the patient's concern and may cut off communication.

③ Same as #2.

* ④ This response meets the patient's right to know who is providing care and what will be done. This is a nonjudgmental, respectful response that reduces fears of the unknown. Although this response does not address the patient's feelings, it is the best response of the options offered.

19 TEST-TAKING TIP ● Option 1 denies the patient's feelings. Option 3 is patient centered.

① This approach denies the patient's feelings and cuts off communication.

② The nurse has a responsibility to intervene; the patient and the daughter both have needs that must be met.

* ③ This intervention provides an opportunity for both the patient and the daughter to explore their feelings; all behavior has meaning and talking about the situation may provide insight.

④ This information could further upset the daughter and may precipitate feelings such as guilt or anger.

20 TEST-TAKING TIP ● Options 3 and 4 are opposites.

* ① Communication can be both verbal and nonverbal. The use of gestures facilitates communication.

② Although anticipating needs may be done occasionally, it does not increase the patient's ability to communicate.

③ Communication is a two-way process and the patient should be involved. The patient should be encouraged to respond in some way.

④ Although this may be done occasionally, it does not increase the patient's ability to communicate; a yes or no response is too limited.

21 TEST-TAKING TIP ● The word "most" in the stem sets a priority. Options 2 and 3 are equally plausible. Option 1 contains the word "every," which is a specific determiner.

① Although reminding the patient every time might be done, it is not the most therapeutic intervention because it addresses only the next dose.

② The patient probably would not be capable of remembering. Too challenging a task can be frustrating.

③ Same as #2.

* ④ A sign promotes independence and does not demean the patient; the patient can refer to the schedule when necessary.

22 **TEST-TAKING TIP** ● The word "first" is a key word in the stem that sets a priority. Options 1 and 2 are patient centered. Option 4 denies the patient's feelings.

① This is too direct a statement; the patient may not be able to put into words what is wrong.

* ② Active listening is necessary for data collection; once data are collected, the patient's feelings and concerns can be identified.

③ When people are anxious, their conversation may ramble, but it does not necessarily mean they are confused.

④ This denies the patient's feelings; the patient will have to talk about the situation further to reduce anxiety.

23 * ① Defense mechanisms are used to lower anxiety, manage stress, maintain the ego, and shelter self-esteem; although they can be productive or eventually detrimental, they do provide relief by releasing physical and emotional energy.

② Most defense mechanisms are used on an unconscious level, except for suppression, which is used by the conscious mind.

③ A somatizing behavior is identified when a patient experiences a psychological conflict as a physical symptom; physical symptoms distract the patient from the actual emotional distress as the patient internally manages the anxiety physiologically.

④ Manipulative behaviors are not known as defense mechanisms but rather as purposeful behaviors used to meet personal needs; manipulative behaviors can be adaptive or maladaptive; they are maladaptive when they are the primary method used to meet needs, the needs of others are ignored, or others are dehumanized to meet the needs of the manipulator.

24 **TEST-TAKING TIP** ● Options 3 and 4 are opposites. In Option 4 the word "always" is a specific determiner.

① Some people never progress past denial, the first step in Kübler-Ross's theory of grieving.

② Although passing through the stages may be smooth for some people, it is not smooth for most individuals; the intensity and speed of progression depend on many factors such as extent of loss, level of growth and development, cultural and spiritual beliefs, sex roles, and relationships with significant others.

* ③ The stages are not concrete and the patient's behavior changes as different levels of awareness and/or coping occur. Kübler-Ross's theory of grieving is behaviorally oriented.

④ Progression is not always forward. Patients tend to move back and forth among stages or may remain in one stage.

25 **TEST-TAKING TIP** ● The word "best" is the key word in the stem that sets a priority. Options 2 and 3 are equally plausible. Options 2, 3, and 4 deny the patient's feelings.

* ① This statement uses reflective technique to identify the patient's feelings regarding fear of the unknown.

② This statement denies the patient's feelings and cuts off communication; also the patient's message did not indicate a need for forgiveness.

③ This statement focuses on other people's experiences rather than the patient's feelings or concerns.

④ This statement puts the emphasis on the wrong part of the message; it ignores the patient's concern about what happens after death.

26 **TEST-TAKING TIP** ● The word "best" sets a priority in the stem.
① This response would take away the patient's coping mechanism, is demeaning, and could cut off communication; the patient is using denial to cope with the diagnosis.
② Same as #1.
* ③ This provides an opportunity to discuss the illness; eventually a developing awareness will occur, and the patient will probably move on to other coping mechanisms.
④ Same as #1.

27 **TEST-TAKING TIP** ● The word *best* in the stem sets a priority. Option 3 is unique because it makes a referral to someone other than the nurse.
① This is inappropriate probing and would violate the patient's right to privacy or may put the patient on the defensive.
② This is an inappropriate question; not all the nurses on the team may want to assume this intervention.
* ③ This response recognizes that the patient is considering personal spiritual needs; it provides an opportunity that the patient can accept or reject.
④ Same as #1.

28 ① Denial is an unconscious defense mechanism; this patient consciously and voluntarily refuses to talk about the birthday.
② This is an assumption; there are not enough data to come to this conclusion.
③ Same as #2.
* ④ This is a conscious protective mechanism in which a person actively puts anxiety-producing feelings or concerns out of the mind.

29 **TEST-TAKING TIP** ● Option 1 is the only response that directly addresses the patient's behavior. The other options avoid the patient (Option 2), abandon the patient (Option 3), or deny the patient's feelings (Option 4).
* ① Pointing out the patient's behavior brings it to the attention of the patient and provides an opportunity to explore feelings.
② The patient's behavior needs to be addressed more fully than just by continued observation.
③ This would be abandonment; sad, withdrawn patients need to know that they are accepted and that the nurse is available for support.
④ This denies the patient's feelings.

30 **TEST-TAKING TIP** ● Options 1 and 2 are equally plausible and can be eliminated from consideration.
① This is inappropriate. The patient is in the fourth stage of grieving, depression; during this stage people become quiet and withdrawn. The nurse should be quiet and available, not demonstrative.
② This is inappropriate; cheerfulness denies the patient's feelings and cuts off communication.
* ③ The patient is developing a full awareness of the impact of dying and is expressing sorrow; this stage of coping should be supported by the quiet presence of the nurse.
④ This would be a form of abandonment; the nurse must be present and accessible.

31 **TEST-TAKING TIP** ● Option 1, touch, is the only intervention that involves the patient's personal space.
* ① Touch is a simple form of communication that is easily understood even by confused, disoriented, or mentally incapacitated individuals.
② This requires interpretation of symbols, which is a more complex form of communication than touch.
③ Same as #2.
④ Same as #2.

32 **TEST-TAKING TIP** ● Option 1 is unique. Options 2, 3, and 4 all imply that everything will get better; these are Pollyanna-like responses.
* ① This recognizes the patient's behavior and provides an opportunity to verbalize feelings and concerns.
② This is false reassurance.
③ This is inappropriate and implies that the patient is out of control. This interferes with the patient's coping mechanisms and may not help the patient regain control.
④ This is false reassurance; crying may or may not help this patient.

33 ① Denial is the first stage of disbelief, in which the person avoids reality, is noncompliant, and uses emotional energy to deny the truth.
* ② Bargaining is the third stage, in which the person is willing to do anything to change the prognosis, accepts new forms of therapies, and negotiates for more time.
③ Acceptance is the fifth and final stage, in which the person reminisces about the past, completes financial arrangements, and accepts death.
④ Depression is the fourth stage, in which the person recognizes the future loss, withdraws from relationships to avoid feelings, and has feelings of loneliness.

34 ① Guilt is usually expressed by statements of sorrow and regret and by behavior that attempts to make amends.
② Anger is usually expressed by acting-out, aggressive behavior.
③ Denial is a refusal to acknowledge facts that are consciously or unconsciously intolerable; a disregard for physical limitations or noncompliance with a medical regimen are examples of denial.
* ④ A change in a patient's emotional status, such as crying, usually reflects increased anxiety; crying releases physical and emotional tension and energy.

35 ① This is unrelated to personal space. Perception relates to having insight.
② Critical time refers to a specific span of time during which an individual is most vulnerable to certain stressors.
" ③ Territoriality refers to the concept of personal space. Nurses need to request permission to enter patients' personal space.
④ This is unrelated to personal space. Confidentiality refers to entrusting someone with private or secret information.

Physical Assessment of Patients

This section includes questions related to various aspects of physical and psychosocial assessment. Questions focus on temperature, pulse, respirations, blood pressure, level of consciousness, level of orientation, and principles related to specimens and the collection of specimens, such as wound cultures and stool specimens. Questions also address assessments common to infection, the general adaptation syndrome, and the inflammatory process. Additional questions focus on whether assessment data are subjective or objective in nature, whether sources are primary or secondary, the responsibilities of the nurse regarding data collected during assessment, the sources of data, and the use of common physical examination techniques.

Questions

1 A primary source for assessing how a patient slept is the:
① Nurse
② Patient
③ Physician
④ Roommate
TEST-TAKING TIP ● Identify the clue in the stem. Identify the unique option.

2 How long should the nurse wait to take an oral temperature after a patient has just had a cup of coffee?
① 5 minutes
② 7 minutes
③ 15 minutes
④ 30 minutes
TEST-TAKING TIP ● Identify the clue in the stem. Identify the options that are opposites.

3 Which signs and symptoms of respiratory distress should be reported to the physician?
① Respiratory rate of 16 with an irregular rhythm
② Respiratory rate of 26 with an irregular rhythm
③ Respiratory rate of 18 with a regular rhythm
④ Respiratory rate of 20 with a regular rhythm
TEST-TAKING TIP ● Identify the duplicate facts among the options.

4 When obtaining a radial pulse rate, the nurse understands that it reflects the function of the:
① Arteries
② Veins
③ Blood
④ Heart
TEST-TAKING TIP ● Identify the clue in the stem. Identify the options that are opposites.

5 An individual's body temperature would be at its lowest at:
① 6 AM
② 10 AM
③ 6 PM
④ 9 PM
TEST-TAKING TIP ● Identify the clue in the stem. Identify the options that are opposites.

6 When making rounds, the nurse finds a patient in bed with eyes closed. The nurse should:
① Suspect that the patient is feeling withdrawn
② Return in 30 minutes to check on the patient
③ Collect more information about the patient
④ Allow the patient to continue sleeping

TEST-TAKING TIP ● Identify the equally plausible options. Identify the options that are opposites.

7 Which is an example of objective data?
① Pain
② Fever
③ Nausea
④ Fatigue

TEST-TAKING TIP ● Identify the clue in the stem. Identify the unique option.

8 Immediately after removing a glass thermometer from a patient's mouth, the nurse should first:
① Wipe it with a tissue
② Rinse it with warm water
③ Soak it in antiseptic solution
④ Wash it with soap and cool water

TEST-TAKING TIP ● Identify the key word in the stem that sets a priority. Identify the clue in the stem. Identify the unique option.

9 The intervention that should be included in the assessment of a patient's orientation would be:
① Asking the patient to state the time of day
② Inquiring if the patient remembers the nurse's name
③ Ascertaining if the patient can follow simple directions
④ Determining if the patient follows movement with the eyes

TEST-TAKING TIP ● Identify the unique option.

10 When taking the resting pulse rate of an elderly patient, the nurse recognizes which of the following pulse ranges as normal?
① 50 to 60 beats per minute and irregular
② 80 to 90 beats per minute and regular
③ 105 to 115 beats per minute and irregular
④ 120 to 130 beats per minute and regular

TEST-TAKING TIP ● Identify the clue in the stem. Identify the duplicate facts among the options. Identify the options that are opposites.

11 Which rectal temperature is within the normal range?
① 96.4°F
② 97.6°F
③ 99.8°F
④ 101.2°F

TEST-TAKING TIP ● Identify the clue in the stem. Identify the options that are opposites.

12 A patient has a history of heart disease. After walking to the lounge, the patient sits in a chair, places a fist against the chest, and complains of a severe upset stomach. The nurse should first:
① Take the patient's vital signs
② Walk the patient back to bed
③ Administer an antacid to the patient
④ Listen to the complaints of the patient
TEST-TAKING TIP ● Identify the key word in the stem that sets a priority.

13 The general adaptation syndrome (GAS) is primarily controlled by the:
① Endocrine system
② Respiratory system
③ Integumentary system
④ Cardiovascular system
TEST-TAKING TIP ● Identify the key word in the stem that sets a priority.

14 An example of subjective data is that the patient:
① Appears jaundiced
② Has a headache
③ Looks tired
④ Is crying
TEST-TAKING TIP ● Identify the clue in the stem. Identify the unique option.

15 When assessing a patient for an emotional response to stress, monitor the patient for:
① Pain
② Headaches
③ Irritability
④ Hypertension
TEST-TAKING TIP ● Identify the clue in the stem. Identify the equally plausible options.

16 To ensure the most accurate results of a urine culture and sensitivity, the nurse should:
① Utilize a 24-hour urine collection
② Collect a midstream urine sample
③ Use only the first voiding of the day
④ Obtain a double-voided urine specimen
TEST-TAKING TIP ● Identify the key word in the stem that sets a priority. Identify the option that contains a specific determiner.

17 Which statement regarding blood pressure (BP) is true?
① A BP differs 5 to 10 mm Hg between arms.
② A BP remains consistent regardless of the patient's position.
③ The arm must be kept at the level of the clavicles to obtain a correct BP.
④ The arm must be kept below the apex of the heart to obtain an accurate BP.
TEST-TAKING TIP ● Identify the options that are opposites. Identify the option that is unique.

18 When assessing for a systemic adaptation to an inflammatory response, the nurse should monitor the patient for:
① Pain
② Fever

③ Edema
④ Erythema
TEST-TAKING TIP ● Identify the clue in the stem.

19 Which blood pressure reading would be considered the most hypertensive?
① 90/70
② 120/80
③ 160/90
④ 150/115
TEST-TAKING TIP ● Identify the key word in the stem that sets a priority.

20 A concern that is common to the collection of specimens, regardless of their source, for culture and sensitivity tests is that:
① The specimen should be collected in the morning
② Gloves, a gown, and a mask should be worn
③ Two specimens should always be obtained
④ Surgical asepsis should be maintained
TEST-TAKING TIP ● Identify the phrase in the stem that is a clue. Identify the option that contains a specific determiner.

21 When assessing the pulse of a patient, the nurse identifies a change in rate from 88 to 56. The nurse should first:
① Wait 15 minutes and retake the patient's pulse
② Ask the patient about recent activity
③ Assess the other vital signs
④ Alert the nurse in charge
TEST-TAKING TIP ● Identify the key word in the stem that sets a priority.

22 When obtaining a specimen from a wound for culture and sensitivity, the nurse should swab the wound at the:
① Top
② Edge
③ Bottom
④ Middle
TEST-TAKING TIP ● Identify the options that are opposites.

23 When assessing a patient for a response associated with the general adaptation syndrome (GAS), the nurse should monitor the patient for:
① Fluctuating blood pressure
② Wavering mental acuity
③ Rising respiratory rate
④ Decreasing heart rate

24 When collecting a stool specimen for parasites, a consideration that is unique from other stool specimens is the need to:
① Wear protective gloves
② Obtain three successive daily specimens
③ Send the specimen to the laboratory while it is still warm
④ Take feces from several areas of the bowel movement
TEST-TAKING TIP ● Identify the clue in the stem.

25 The nurse needs to recognize the patient's health beliefs before giving care. Therefore, the nurse must first:
① Identify the patient's level of wellness
② Individualize the patient's plan of care
③ Understand the patient's frame of reference
④ Teach the patient acceptable values related to health
TEST-TAKING TIP ● Identify the key word in the stem that sets a priority. Identify the option that denies the patient's feelings, concerns, or needs.

26 Who is the *best* source of information about a newly admitted alert patient with a fractured leg?
① Emergency Department nurse
② Patient's family
③ Physician
④ Patient
TEST-TAKING TIP ● Identify the word in the stem that sets a priority.

27 How long should the nurse wait to take an oral temperature if the patient has just had a cold drink?
① 3 minutes
② 5 minutes
③ 15 minutes
④ 30 minutes

28 To determine the presence of orthostatic hypotension, when is the most significant time for a patient's blood pressure to be assessed?
① After standing
② Between meals
③ During activity
④ Before standing
TEST-TAKING TIP ● Identify the options that are opposites.

29 A patient's urine specific gravity is 1.035, indicating a need for:
① Fluids
② Protein
③ Glucose
④ Antibiotics

30 Which physiological action is reflected by the diastolic blood pressure?
① Contraction of the ventricles
② Volume of cardiac output
③ Resting arterial pressure
④ Pulse pressure
TEST-TAKING TIP ● Identify the options with a clang association.

31 When obtaining a pedal pulse, the nurse is assessing the function of the patient's:
① Veins
② Heart
③ Blood
④ Arteries
TEST-TAKING TIP ● Identify the options that are opposites.

32 Which physical examination techniques would elicit the most significant information concerning a patient's respiratory status?
① Palpation
② Inspection
③ Percussion
④ Auscultation

33 When assessing cardiac function, the nurse should recognize which principle of blood pressure physiology?
① A trough pressure occurs during systole.
② The pulse pressure occurs during diastole.
③ The BP reaches a peak followed by a trough.
④ A peak pressure occurs when the ventricles relax.
TEST-TAKING TIP ● Identify the options that are opposites.

34 Which adaptation indicates that the an inflammatory response has entered the second phase?
① Pain
② A fever
③ Erythema
④ An exudate

35 What does the sensitivity part of a culture and sensitivity report indicate?
① All of the microorganisms present
② The virulence of the organisms in the culture
③ The antibiotics that would be effective treatment
④ The extent of the patient's response to the pathogens
TEST-TAKING TIP ● Identify the option that contains a specific determiner.

Rationales

1 **TEST-TAKING TIP** ● The word "primary" is a clue in the stem. Option 2 is unique. Options 1, 3, and 4 involve people other than the patient.
   ① The nurse is a secondary source of data. The nurse may not be totally aware of how well the patient slept.
 * ② Patients are primary sources and the only sources able to provide subjective data concerning how they slept.
   ③ The physician is a secondary source of information.
   ④ Patients should not be held responsible for other patients.

2 **TEST-TAKING TIP** ● The word "oral" is a clue in the stem. Options 1 and 4 are opposites on the continuum of times offered in the options.
   ① This is too short a period of time for the mouth to recover from the hot fluid; the dilated vessels in the mouth and the warmth of the tissues from the hot fluid would cause an inaccurate elevation in the temperature reading.
   ② Same as #1.
 * ③ It takes at least 15 minutes for the vessels in the mouth and the mucous membranes to recover from the hot fluid and for the mouth to return to the patient's core temperature.
   ④ Waiting 30 minutes is unnecessary; this is too long a time period.

3 **TEST-TAKING TIP** ● Options 1 and 2 contain the duplicate fact that the patient's respirations are irregular. Options 3 and 4 contain the duplicate fact that the patient's respirations are regular. If you know that respirations should be regular, then Options 3 and 4 are distractors.
   ① This is within the normal range of 12 to 20 breaths per minute. An irregular rhythm without other signs of distress would not necessitate notifying the physician.
 * ② Tachypnea, a respiratory rate above 24 breaths per minute, along with an irregular rhythm, indicates that the body is in respiratory distress.
   ③ Normal breathing is usually regular and within the range of 12 to 20 breaths per minute.
   ④ Same as #3.

4 **TEST-TAKING TIP** ● The word "radial" is a clue in the stem. Options 1 and 2 are opposites. Arteries carry blood away from the heart; veins carry blood to the heart. In this question these options are distractors.
   ① Elasticity and rigidity of the vessel walls and the quality and equality of pulses provide data about the status of the arteries.
   ② A pulse is palpated in an artery, not a vein.
   ③ Blood is assessed through laboratory tests performed on blood specimens.
 * ④ The heart is a pulsatile pump that ejects blood into the arterial system with each ventricular contraction; the pulse is the vibration transmitted with each contraction.

5 **TEST-TAKING TIP** ● The word "lowest" is a clue in the stem. Options 1 and 3 are opposites.
 * ① A person's body temperature is at its lowest in the early morning; core temperatures vary with a predictable pattern over 24 hours (diurnal or circadian temperature variations) because of hormonal variations.
   ② Body temperature is not at its lowest at 10 AM; body temperature steadily rises as the day progresses.

③ Body temperature peaks between 5 and 7 PM

④ Body temperature is not at its lowest at 9 PM; body temperature is still falling from its peak.

6 TEST-TAKING TIP ● Options 2 and 4 are equally plausible. Options 3 and 4 are opposites.

① This is an assumption based on insufficient data. A further assessment should be performed.

② Waiting 30 minutes is unsafe; more data need to be collected at this time.

* ③ More information must be collected to make a complete assessment and come to an accurate conclusion.

④ Same as #1.

7 TEST-TAKING TIP ● The word "objective" is a clue in the stem. Option 2 is unique because it is measurable. Options 1, 3, and 4 are similar because the adaptations can be described only by the patient.

① This is subjective; subjective data are a patient's perceptions, feelings, sensations, or ideas.

* ② This is objective because it can be measured with a thermometer.

③ Same as #1.

④ Same as #1.

8 TEST-TAKING TIP ● The word "first" is the key word in the stem that sets a priority. "Immediately after" are words in the stem that provide a clue. The words "rinse," "soak," and "wash" in Options 2, 3, and 4 are similar because they all use a solution to clean the thermometer. Option 1 is unique because wiping does not require a fluid.

* ① Wiping removes mucus that may distort the level of the mercury or the numbers on the thermometer, resulting in an inaccurate reading.

② Warm water would raise the mercury in the thermometer, producing an inaccurate reading; this also could damage the thermometer.

③ Soaking in an antiseptic solution is done after the reading is taken and the thermometer is washed in soap and water.

④ Washing the thermometer with soap and water is done after the reading is taken.

9 TEST-TAKING TIP ● Option 1 is unique. In Options 2, 3, and 4 the words "inquiring," "ascertaining," and "determining" are all followed by the phrase "if the patient."

* ① Questions related to time, place, and person (assessing orientation in three ways) are essential when assessing a patient's level of orientation.

② This assesses recent memory, not orientation.

③ This can be done by confused, disoriented patients.

④ Same as #3.

10 TEST-TAKING TIP ● The word "resting" is a clue in the stem. Options 1 and 3 relate to an irregular pulse rate. Options 2 and 4 relate to a regular pulse rate. If you know that a pulse rate should be regular, then Options 1 and 3 are distractors. Options 1 and 4 are opposites on the continuum of ranges offered in the options.

① A rate of 50 to 60 is below the normal range of a pulse rate in an elderly patient.

* ② The normal heart rate in an elderly adult is between 60 and 100 beats per minute.

③ A rate of 105 to 115 is too high for a heart rate taken at rest; in elderly people a decreased contractile strength of the myocardium may cause the heart rate to increase to this rate during exercise.

④ A rate of 120 to 130 is too high for a heart rate taken at rest.

11 TEST-TAKING TIP ● The word "rectal" is a clue in the stem. Options 1 and 4 are opposites.

① This is below the normal range for a rectal temperature.

② Same as #1.

* ③ A temperature of 99.8°F is within the normal range of 98.6 to 100.6°F for a rectal temperature.

④ A temperature of 101.2°F would indicate a fever.

12 TEST-TAKING TIP ● The word "first" is the key word in the stem that sets a priority.

* ① A further assessment is necessary; vital signs reflect the cardiopulmonary status of the patient.

② Activity at this time would be unsafe; if the problem is cardiac rather than gastric, walking will increase the demands on the heart.

③ The nurse needs more information before concluding that the problem is gastritis; antacids require a physician's order.

④ Although listening is important, it is more important at this point for the nurse to collect objective data about the patient's cardiopulmonary status.

13 TEST-TAKING TIP ● The word "primarily" is the key word in the stem that sets a priority.

* ① The general adaptation syndrome (GAS) primarily involves the endocrine system and autonomic nervous system; the antidiuretic hormone (ADH), adrenocorticotropic hormone (ACTH), cortisol, aldosterone, epinephrine, and norepinephrine are all involved with the fight-or-flight response.

② The respiratory system will be stimulated by the hormone epinephrine.

③ The autonomic nervous system affects the integumentary system.

④ The cardiovascular system will be stimulated by the hormones epinephrine and norepinephrine.

14 TEST-TAKING TIP ● The word "subjective" is a clue in the stem. Option 2 is unique because the patient is the only one who can describe the headache. Options 1, 3, and 4 are similar because they include assessments that can be observed by another person.

① Jaundice is objective; objective data require the use of a sense to collect the data. Jaundice is a human response that is measured using the sense of vision and the assessment technique of inspection.

* ② Subjective data are data that can be described or verified only by the patient; a patient's descriptions of pain, concerns, feelings, or sensations are additional examples of subjective data.

③ This is a conclusion based on observation.

④ Crying is objective data because it can be observed by another person.

15 TEST-TAKING TIP ● The word "emotional" is a clue in the stem. Options 1 and 2 are equally plausible.

① Pain is a physiological response to stress.

② Headaches are a physiological response to stress.

* ③ Irritability is a behavioral-emotional response; the body is using physical and emotional energy to reduce stress.

④ Hypertension is a physiological response to stress.

16 TEST-TAKING TIP ● The word "most" is the key word in the stem that sets a priority. The word "only" in Option 3 is a specific determiner.

① A 24-hour collection is unnecessary; 24 hours of urine are needed for special tests such as the measurement of levels of adrenocortical steroids, hormones, and creatinine clearance tests, not for a urine culture and sensitivity.

* ② A midstream urine sample contains a specimen that is relatively free of microorganisms from the urethra; after perineal care the patient begins to urinate, avoiding the initial stream and collecting a specimen during the midportion of the stream. Perineal care and the initial stream clear the urethra of microoganisms, providing a specimen with the least amount of contamination.

③ Specimens collected from the first voiding of the morning should be avoided; stagnant urine does not reflect urine that is recently filtered by the urinary system. A first voiding does not allow for the clearing of the urethra of growing microorganisms as in the midstream collection method.

④ A double-voided specimen is taken for the measurement of glucose and ketones in the urine; stagnant urine from the bladder does not reflect the current level of glucose and ketones found in the urine at the time of the voiding.

17 **TEST-TAKING TIP** ● Options 3 and 4 are opposites. Option 1 is unique because it is the only option that does not focus on the position of the arm when taking a BP.

* ① Because of variations in structure and distance, there might be 5 to 10 mm Hg difference between arms; the arm with the higher blood pressure should be used for subsequent assessments.

② This is untrue; the blood pressure is higher when the arm is below heart level and lower when the arm is above heart level. The patient's arm should be at the apex of the heart when taking a BP.

③ When the arm is above the apex of the heart, the resulting blood pressure would be abnormally low.

④ When the arm is below the apex of the heart, the resulting blood pressure would be abnormally high.

18 **TEST-TAKING TIP** ● The word "systemic" is the clue in the stem.

① Pain is a local adaptation to stimulation of nerve endings; it is a localized response of the central nervous system to the stimulus of pain.

* ② The inflammatory response is stimulated by trauma or infection, which increase the basal metabolic rate; with infection, fever results from the affect of pyrogens on the temperature-regulating center in the hypothalamus.

③ Edema is a local adaptation resulting from local vasodilatation and increased vessel permeability.

④ Erythema is a local adaptation resulting from increased circulation and local vasodilation in the involved area.

19 **TEST-TAKING TIP** ● The word "most" is the key word in the stem that sets a priority.

① A blood pressure reading of 90/70 is hypotensive.

② A blood pressure reading of 120/80 is within the normal range; the normal range for the systolic pressure is 100 to 140, and for the diastolic pressure it is 60 to 90.

③ Although a systolic reading of 160 is high and needs to be reported to the physician, a blood pressure with a higher diastolic is more dangerous.

* ④ A blood pressure with a higher diastolic pressure is more hypertensive than a blood pressure with a higher systolic pressure but lower diastolic pressure. The diastolic pressure is the pressure exerted against the arterial walls when the ventricles are at rest; the higher the diastolic pressure, the more dangerous the situation.

20 **TEST-TAKING TIP** ● The phrase "common to" is a clue in the stem. Option 3 contains the word "always," which is a specific determiner.

① The time of day is irrelevant for the collection of most specimens for culture and sensitivity.

② Gloves may be worn when collecting specimens to protect the nurse, not to maintain sterility of the specimen; gowns and masks are generally unnecessary unless splashing of body fluids is likely.

③ Generally, if a specimen is collected using proper technique, one specimen is sufficient for testing for culture and sensitivity. However, blood cultures for a disease such as endocarditis may require several specimens over a 24- to 48-hour period.

* ④ The results of a culture and sensitivity are faulty and erroneous if the collection container is not kept sterile; a contaminated specimen container introduces extraneous microorganisms that falsify and misrepresent results. Surgical asepsis (sterile technique) must be maintained.

21 **TEST-TAKING TIP** ● The word "first" is the key word in the stem that sets a priority.
① Waiting is unsafe; when there is an alteration in one vital sign, the other vital signs should immediately be taken.
② Activity would increase, not decrease, the heart rate.
* ③ Corroborative data should be obtained; the vital signs reflect cardiopulmonary functioning. When there is an alteration in one vital sign, there is usually a change in another.
④ Alerting the nurse in charge might be necessary after taking the other vital signs.

22 **TEST-TAKING TIP** ● Options 1 and 3 are opposites.
① Specimens collected from this area could be contaminated from microorganisms from the skin, misrepresenting results.
② Same as #1.
③ Same as #1.
* ④ Swabbing from the center of a wound provides a specimen that is least likely to be contaminated by microorganisms from the skin; it also provides for a specimen that generally contains the most representative properties of the exudate.

23 ① Because of the effects of the sympathetic nervous system, the blood pressure will rise, not fluctuate.
② Because of the sympathetic nervous system response, the individual's mental ability is alert and constant in preparation for fight or flight; the mental acuity does not waver.
* ③ The sympathetic nervous system response results in bronchial dilation and an increased respiratory rate; this increases the amount of oxygen available for the elevated basal metabolic rate associated with the general adaptation syndrome (GAS).
④ Because of the effects of the sympathetic nervous system, the heart rate increases; it does not decrease.

24 **TEST-TAKING TIP** ● The word "unique" is the clue in the stem.
① Gloves should always be worn when dealing with body secretions or excretions.
② Three separate samples from stool are collected on consecutive days to screen for occult blood, not for parasites.
* ③ Stool specimens for ova and parasites should be sent to the laboratory while still warm; stool that is allowed to cool can alter the accuracy of the laboratory results.
④ Taking feces from several areas of the bowel movement is unnecessary; a 1-inch portion of stool provides an adequate sample for testing for parasites.

25 **TEST-TAKING TIP** ● The word "first" is the key word in the stem that sets a priority. Option 4 denies the patient's feelings, concerns, and needs because it implies that the patient's values are unacceptable.

(1) This should be done after the nurse understands the variables influencing the patient's attitudes, beliefs, and practices.

(2) Same as #1.

* (3) Attitudes and beliefs influence health practices and how one perceives self-health; the nurse must always "begin care where the patient is at."

(4) Teaching patients "acceptable values" is judgmental; people perceive *their* values as acceptable. Eventually the nurse may teach patients healthy practices, but these practices must be viewed as important by patients before being incorporated into their beliefs and values.

26 **TEST-TAKING TIP** ● The word *best* in the stem sets a priority. All of these people supply information, but the patient is the most important source of information.

(1) This is a secondary source; when a patient is alert, the patient is the best source for current information.

(2) Same as #1.

(3) Same as #1.

* (4) The patient is the center of the health team and is the primary source for current objective and subjective data.

27 (1) This is too short a time period; the mucous membranes will be cool and the vessels in the mouth will be constricted, resulting in an inaccurate reduction in temperature.

(2) Same as #1.

* (3) It takes 15 minutes for the mucous membranes and vessels in the mouth to recover from the cold fluid and return to the patient's core temperature.

(4) This is unnecessary; this is too long a period of time.

28 **TEST-TAKING TIP** ● Options 1 and 4 are opposites. These options should be given careful consideration. In this question, one of these options is correct.

* (1) When a patient moves from a lying-down to a sitting or standing position, normally an automatic vasoconstriction occurs in the lower half of the body; this prevents the pooling of blood and effectively maintains the blood pressure. When this vasoconstriction response is inadequate, the patient will experience orthostatic hypotension after moving from a horizontal to a vertical position.

(2) This is untrue; this is unrelated to positional changes.

(3) This is done during a stress test.

(4) Although a patient's blood pressure is often taken before and after standing to assess for orthostatic hypotension, the result of the blood pressure taken after standing is more significant.

29 * (1) Specific gravity indicates the degree of concentration of dissolved substances in the urine. Normal specific gravity is 1.010 to 1.025. The higher the specific gravity, the more concentrated the urine. Concentrated urine indicates dehydration; fluids are indicated when a patient is dehydrated.

(2) A negative nitrogen balance indicates the need for increased protein intake. Specific gravity is not designed to test for nitrogen balance.

(3) Glucose in the urine is measured by a Clinitest tablet or reagent strip, not specific gravity.

(4) An increased white blood cell count or a positive culture and sensitivity, not specific gravity, indicates the presence of infection and the need for antibiotics.

30 TEST-TAKING TIP ● The word "pressure" appears in the stem and in Options 3 and 4. Options 3 and 4 should be examined carefully. Option 3 is the correct answer.
① This is reflected by the systolic pressure.
② The volume of cardiac output is computed by multiplying the stroke volume by the number of heart beats per minute.
* ③ Diastole is the period when the ventricles are relaxed and reflects the pressure in the arteries when the heart is at rest.
④ This is the difference between the systolic and diastolic pressures.

31 TEST-TAKING TIP ● Options 1 and 4 are opposites. Arteries carry blood away from the heart and veins carry blood to the heart. These opposites are more difficult to identify than most opposites.
① Veins do not have a pulse.
② Radial, carotid, or apical pulses, not pedal pulses, readily assess heart function.
③ Laboratory tests assess blood and its components.
* ④ The presence, absence, or quality of a pedal pulse reflects the patency of the dorsalis pedis artery; peripheral pulses should be present, equal, and symmetrical.

32 ① Although the chest wall is palpated for bulges, tenderness, and respiratory excursion, which provide valuable information, auscultation of breath sounds provides the most significant information concerning a patient's respiratory status.
② Although inspection assesses the pattern of respirations, condition of the skin, and shape and symmetry of the thorax, auscultation of breath sounds provides the most significant information concerning a patient's respiratory status.
③ Although percussion of the thorax determines whether underlying tissue is filled with air, liquid, or solid material and identifies the boundaries of the lung, auscultation of breath sounds provides the most significant information concerning a patient's respiratory status.
* ④ Auscultation of the chest includes assessment of breath sounds (normal, diminished, absent), adventitious breath sounds (crackles, rhonchi, wheeze, friction rub), and vocal resonance (bronchophony, whispered pectoriloquy, egophony); this is the most significant information for assessing the patient's respiratory status.

33 TEST-TAKING TIP ● Options 1 and 4 are opposites. Consider these seriously or eliminate both or them. In this question they are both distractors and can be eliminated.
① Peak pressures occur during systole.
② Pulse pressure is the difference between the systolic and diastolic pressures.
* ③ Peak pressures occur when the ventricles contract and trough pressures occur when the ventricles relax; these occur with each contraction and relaxation of the heart.
④ Peak pressures occur when the ventricles contract.

34 ① Pain occurs during the first phase in response to the release of histamine at the injury site. Histamine promotes vessel permeability, which increases edema, causing pressure on nerve endings.
② Fever is a systemic, not a localized, adaptation and is not indicative of phase two of the inflammatory response.
③ During the first phase, histamine is released, resulting in increased blood flow to the area. Dilation of capillaries causes the area to be flooded with blood, which makes the area appear red and warm to the touch.
* ④ Phase two is characterized by the formation of an exudate; it consists of a combination of cells and fluids produced at the localized site of injury.

35 TEST-TAKING TIP ● Option 1 contains the word "all," which is a specific determiner. This option can be eliminated from consideration.

① Examination of a specimen under a microscope, not the sensitivity part of a culture and sensitivity test, identifies the microorganisms present.

② The ability to produce disease (virulence) is not determined by the sensitivity portion of a culture and sensitivity test; virulence is determined by statistical data concerning morbidity and mortality associated with the microorganisms.

* ③ Areas of lack of growth of microorganisms surrounding an antibiotic on a culture medium indicate that the microorganism is sensitive to the antibiotic and the antibiotic is capable of destroying the microorganism.

④ The clinical manifestation of the disease process reflects the extent of the patient's response to the microorganism present.

Meeting Patients' Physical Safety and Mobility Needs

This section includes questions related to maintaining patients' physical safety and mobility needs. In relation to patients' safety needs, an emphasis is placed on the concepts of the use of restraints, issues associated with smoking and fire, prevention of injury, electrical safety, protection of a patient experiencing a seizure, and safety related to oxygen use. In relation to patients' mobility needs, this section includes questions that address the maintenance and restoration of musculoskeletal function and the prevention of musculoskeletal complications. These questions focus on knowledge, principles, and devices related to the prevention of pressure (decubitus) ulcers, contractures, and other hazards of immobility. Additional questions test principles associated with body alignment, transfer, range of motion (ROM), ambulation, positioning, and dressing.

Questions

1 What is the *main* reason for accidents in hospitals?
① People sneak cigarettes.
② Equipment breaks unexpectedly.
③ Patients do not recognize hazards.
④ Safety precautions always take extra time.
TEST-TAKING TIP ● Identify the key word in the stem that sets a priority. Identify the option that contains a specific determiner.

2 Restraints are mainly used to:
① Immobilize patients
② Reduce agitation
③ Limit movement
④ Prevent injury
TEST-TAKING TIP ● Identify the key word in the stem that sets a priority. Identify the equally plausible options.

3 A patient sitting in a wheelchair begins to have a tonic-clonic (grand mal) seizure. The patient should be:
① Secured in the wheelchair to prevent falling
② Returned to bed to provide a soft surface
③ Wheeled immediately to a private area
④ Moved to the floor to prevent injury
TEST-TAKING TIP ● Identify the options that are opposites.

4 Disoriented, confused patients who are restrained often struggle against restraints primarily because they are:
① Attempting to gain control
② Responding to the discomfort
③ Trying to manipulate the staff
④ Unable to understand what is occurring
TEST-TAKING TIP ● Identify the key word in the stem that sets a priority. Identify the option that is unique.

5 In institutions that are not "smoke free," the nurse can BEST prevent accidents associated with smoking by:
① Supervising patients when they smoke
② Taking away the cigarettes of patients who smoke
③ Encouraging patients to smoke in designated areas
④ Asking family members not to bring cigarettes for patients

TEST-TAKING TIP ● Identify the key word in the stem that sets a priority. Identify options that deny patient feelings, concerns, and needs.

6 As part of postmortem care, the nurse should:
① Slightly raise the head of the bed
② Carefully remove the dentures
③ Firmly tie the wrists together
④ Gently close the eyes

7 When transporting a fire extinguisher to a fire scene on a different level of the building than the one on which the nurse is working, the nurse should:
① Use the stairs
② Pull the safety pin
③ Keep it from touching the floor
④ Always run as quickly as possible

TEST-TAKING TIP ● Identify the option that contains a specific determiner.

8 The first thing the nurse should review with a newly admitted patient is the:
① Use of the call bell
② Daily routine on the unit
③ Potential date of discharge
④ Name of the nurse in charge

TEST-TAKING TIP ● Identify the key word in the stem that sets a priority.

9 To prevent disorientation at night in the minimally confused patient, the most effective intervention would be to:
① Check on the patient regularly
② Put a small light in the room
③ Place a call bell in the bed
④ Describe the environment

TEST-TAKING TIP ● Identify the key word in the stem that sets a priority. Identify the clues in the stem. Identify the unique option. Identify the equally plausible options.

10 While walking, a patient becomes weak and the patient's knees begin to buckle. What should the nurse do?
① Hold the patient up.
② Call for extra help quickly.
③ Walk the patient to the closest chair.
④ Lower the patient to the floor gently.

TEST-TAKING TIP ● Identify the options that are opposites.

11 What should the nurse do when the electrical cord on a patient's radio is frayed near the plug?
① Report it to the supervisor.
② Unplug it and put it in the patient's closet.
③ Wrap the frayed area with nonconductive tape.
④ Remove it and send it home with a family member.

12 An unacceptable practice related to the application of wrist restraints is:
① Using a double knot to secure the straps
② Securing the ties to the base of the bed
③ Allowing the fingers free movement
④ Padding the wrists with sheepskin

TEST-TAKING TIP ● Identify the key word in the stem that indicates negative polarity.

13 When planning nursing interventions to prevent falls in elderly patients, the nurse recognizes that the frequency of falls increases:
① At night
② After meals
③ After surgery
④ During visiting hours

14 To provide for safety when administering oxygen, it is most important that the nurse first recognize that oxygen:
① Must have its flow rate adjusted
② Is drying to the nasal mucosa
③ Should be humidified
④ Supports combustion

TEST-TAKING TIP ● Identify the key words in the stem that set a priority. Identify the equally plausible options.

15 Sheepskin contributes to pressure (decubitus) ulcer prevention primarily by:
① Absorbing urine
② Minimizing friction
③ Eliminating pressure
④ Keeping the skin warm

TEST-TAKING TIP ● Identify the key word in the stem that sets a priority.

16 To best prevent a pressure (decubitus) ulcer in an elderly person, the nurse should provide:
① An air mattress
② A daily bed bath
③ A high-protein diet
④ An indwelling urinary catheter

TEST-TAKING TIP ● Identify the word in the stem that sets a priority.

17 When providing range-of-motion (ROM) exercises, touching the thumb to the small fifth finger of the same hand is called:
① Extension
② Abduction
③ Adduction
④ Opposition

TEST-TAKING TIP ● Identify the options that are opposites.

18 What is the most therapeutic exercise that can be done by a patient on bed rest?
① Active range of motion
② Passive range of motion
③ Active-assistive exercises
④ Contracting and relaxing muscles

TEST-TAKING TIP ● Identify the key word in the stem that sets a priority. Identify the options that are opposites.

19 To safely transfer a patient with one-sided weakness (hemiparesis) to a chair, the nurse should:
① Pivot the patient on the unaffected leg
② Stand next to the patient's affected side
③ Stand next to the patient's strong side
④ Keep the patient's feet together

TEST-TAKING TIP ● Identify the clue in the stem. Identify the unique option. Identify the opposites in options.

20 What is the primary purpose of an egg-crate pad?
① Absorb moisture
② Limit perspiration
③ Support the body in alignment
④ Distribute pressure over a larger area

TEST-TAKING TIP ● Identify the key word in the stem that sets a priority. Identify the equally plausible options.

21 The nurse is transferring a patient from the bed to a chair using a mechanical lift. As the nurse begins to raise the lift off the bed, the patient begins to panic and scream. The nurse should:
① Lower the patient back onto the bed
② Quickly continue and say, "It's almost over."
③ Say, "Relax" and slowly continue with the transfer
④ Stop the lift from rising until the patient regains control

TEST-TAKING TIP ● Identify the options that are opposites. Identify the options that deny the patient's feelings, concerns, and needs.

22 Which position would contribute to the development of a pressure (decubitus) ulcer in the sacral area?
① Sims' position
② Prone position
③ Lateral position
④ High-Fowler's position

TEST-TAKING TIP ● Identify the clue in the stem.

23 What should the nurse do when assisting a blind patient to walk?
① Walk in front while the patient uses the corridor handrail.
② Stand behind the patient and provide verbal directions.
③ Walk on the side while holding the patient's elbow.
④ Instruct the patient to hold onto the nurse's arm.

TEST-TAKING TIP ● Identify the options that are opposites.

24 While a patient is lying in the dorsal recumbent position, the patient's leg externally rotates. What equipment should the nurse use to prevent external rotation?
① Footboard
② Bed cradle
③ Trochanter roll
④ Elastic stockings

TEST-TAKING TIP ● Identify the clue in the stem.

25 A patient with the highest risk of developing a pressure (decubitus) ulcer is the patient who:
① Uses a reclining wheelchair
② Utilizies crutches to ambulate
③ Is ambulatory but is confused
④ Is on bed rest but able to move

TEST-TAKING TIP ● Identify the key word in the stem that sets a priority. Identify the clue in the stem. Identify the unique option.

26 The action of moving an extremity toward the midline and beyond if possible during range-of-motion exercises is:
① Internal rotation
② Lateral flexion
③ Adduction
④ Inversion

TEST-TAKING TIP ● Identify the clue in the stem.

27 A patient is afraid of falling and gets anxious when it is time to get out of bed (OOB) to a chair. The *best* action by the nurse to reduce the patient's anxiety would be to:
① Use a mechanical lift to transfer the patient
② Allow the patient to decide when to get OOB
③ Explain to the patient that a fall will not occur
④ Allow the patient to set the pace of the transfer

TEST-TAKING TIP ● Identify the key word in the stem that sets a priority. Identify the option that denies the patient's feelings, concerns, and needs. Identify the patient-centered options.

28 Flotation pads or gel cushions are used to:
① Deliver heat
② Permit air to circulate
③ Distribute body weight
④ Prevent trapping moisture

TEST-TAKING TIP ● Identify the equally plausible options.

29 What should the nurse do to **best** prevent a patient from developing contractures?
① Support the patient's joints with pillows.
② Transfer the patient to a chair twice a day.
③ Turn and reposition the patient every 2 hours.
④ Teach the patient to perform active range-of-motion exercises.

TEST-TAKING TIP ● Identify the key word in the stem that sets a priority.

30 A patient who had a stroke 3 days ago has left-sided hemiparesis. When dressing the patient, the nurse should plan to:
① Put the patient's left sleeve on first
② Encourage the patient to dress independently
③ Instruct the patient to wear clothes with zippers
④ Tell the patient to get clothes with buttons in the front

TEST-TAKING TIP ● Identify the clue in the stem. Identify the equally plausible options. Identify the unique option. Identify the option that denies the needs of the patient.

31 When transferring a patient from the bed to a chair, the nurse sits the patient on the side of the bed for several minutes primarily to:
① Allow the patient to regain energy expended while sitting
② Enable the body to adapt to a drop in blood pressure
③ Provide time for the heart rate to return to normal
④ Permit the patient to take several deep breaths

TEST-TAKING TIP ● Identify the key word in the stem that sets a priority.

32 When positioning a patient, what is the *most* important principle of body mechanics?
① Elevating the arms on pillows
② Making the patient comfortable
③ Maintaining functional alignment
④ Keeping the head higher than the heart

TEST-TAKING TIP ● Identify the key word in the stem that sets a priority.

33 What is the main cause of pressure (decubitus) ulcers?
① Gravity
② Pressure
③ Skin breakdown
④ Cellular necrosis

TEST-TAKING TIP ● Identify the key word in the stem that sets a priority. Identify the equally plausible options.

34 The nurse is assisting a patient with range-of-motion exercises. The action of turning the palm of the hand up toward the ceiling is:
① Eversion
② Inversion
③ Supination
④ Circumduction

TEST-TAKING TIP ● Identify the options that are opposites.

35 When positioning a patient in a lateral position, which action by the nurse would MOST contribute to the patient's functional alignment?
① Using a footboard
② Utilizing a bed cradle
③ Positioning a pillow under the waist
④ Putting a pillow under the upper leg

TEST-TAKING TIP ● Identify the key word in the stem that sets a priority. Identify the equally plausible options.

Rationales

1 **TEST-TAKING TIP** ● The word *main* in the stem is a key word that sets a priority. The word "always" in Option 4 is a specific determiner.
   ① Statistics do not support cigarette smoking as the most common cause of hospital accidents. Most hospitals are smoke free.
   ② Equipment is usually monitored for preventive maintenance; equipment generally shows wear and tear before it breaks.
   * ③ Patients can be cognitively impaired, deny their physical impairments, or have limited perception which impedes their ability to recognize hazards.
   ④ It more often takes the same amount of time to do something correctly as it takes to do it incorrectly.

2 **TEST-TAKING TIP** ● The word "mainly" in the stem is a key word that sets a priority. Options 1 and 3 are equally plausible because they both focus on reducing movement.
   ① Restraints should be snug, yet loose enough for some movement; immobilization is not the purpose of restraints.
   ② Restraints can increase agitation; if used when a patient is severely agitated, they can cause injury.
   ③ The purpose of restraints is to prevent injury, not limit movement.
   * ④ The primary reason for the use of restraints is to prevent patient injury; restraints are used only as a last resort to protect the patient from self-injury or from hurting others.

3 **TEST-TAKING TIP** ● Options 1 and 3 are opposites.
   ① Securing a patient in a wheelchair during a tonic-clonic (grand mal) seizure could cause muscle strain, bone fractures, or other injury and is an unsafe action.
   ② Attempting to return a patient to bed during a tonic-clonic (grand mal) seizure could cause muscle strain, bone fractures, or other injury. Returning the patient to bed should be done once the seizure is over.
   ③ Physical safety is the priority, not the need for privacy. Transporting a patient in a wheelchair during a tonic-clonic (grand mal) seizure could cause muscle strain, bone fractures, or other injury and is an unsafe action.
   * ④ Moving the patient to the floor is the safest action; it provides free movement on a supported surface.

4 **TEST-TAKING TIP** ● The word "primarily" is the key word in the stem that sets a priority. Option 4 is unique because it is the only option that does not contain an action verb ending in "ing." The words "attempting," "responding," and "trying" in Options 1, 2, and 3 all end in "ing" and are therefore similar.
   ① Confused, disoriented patients who are restrained may become agitated and respond in a reflexlike way; attempts to gain control require problem solving, which confused, disoriented patients usually are unable to perform.
   ② A restraint should not cause discomfort if it is correctly applied and checked frequently.
   ③ A patient usually struggles against a restraint to get free, not to manipulate staff.
   * ④ Disoriented and confused patients do not have the cognitive ability to always understand what is happening to them and will often struggle against restraints.

5 **TEST-TAKING TIP** ● The word BEST is the key word in the stem that sets a priority. Options 2 and 4 deny patients feelings, concerns, and needs.
   * ① If a facility allows smoking, supervision provides for patient safety because the nurse can intervene if the condition becomes unsafe.

② Patients have a right to have cigarettes in their possession. Taking cigarettes away from patients who smoke is punitive and should be done only if attempts to teach safety precautions and policies fail to foster safe smoking behavior.

③ Although this would be done, this option does not take into consideration that patients who smoke should be supervised.

④ Asking family members not to bring in cigarettes for patients who smoke denies patients' feelings, concerns, and needs and is punitive.

6 ① A supine position is preferred; once rigor mortis sets in, it is difficult to reposition the body.

② Dentures should remain in the mouth to maintain facial structure and minimize facial distortion.

③ Firmly tying the patient's wrists together can cause permanent marks; wrists should be well padded and securely, yet loosely, tied so as not to cause permanent marks.

* ④ The patient's eyelids should be gently closed to avoid injury; once rigor mortis sets in, it is difficult to reposition the eyelids.

7 **TEST-TAKING TIP** ● The word "always" in Option 4 is a specific determiner.

* ① Using the stairs during a fire is safe practice; elevators must be avoided because they could break down and trap a person.

② The safety pin is pulled only when the extinguisher is going to be used, not when en route to a fire.

③ Often extinguishers are dragged along the floor en route to a fire because they are heavy; this is an acceptable practice.

④ Running should be avoided; it can cause injury and panic.

8 **TEST-TAKING TIP** ● The word "first" is the key word in the stem that sets a priority.

* ① Explaining the use of a call bell meets basic safety and security needs; the patient must know how to signal for help.

② Although this is important and should be done, safety needs come first.

③ Identifying the potential date of discharge is the physician's, not the nurse's, responsibility.

④ Same as #2.

9 **TEST-TAKING TIP** ● The word "most" is the key word in the stem that sets a priority. The words "night" and "minimally confused" are the clues in the stem. Option 2 is the only option that states an action that is unique to the nighttime. Options 1, 3, and 4 are equally plausible and are implemented regardless of the time of day or orientation of the patient.

① Although checking on the patient regularly is something the nurse should do to provide for patient safety, turning on a small light would be most effective in minimizing disorientation.

* ② A small light in the room would provide enough light for visual cues for a minimally confused patient, which would help prevent or limit disorientation when the patient awakens at night.

③ The patient has to be oriented enough to be aware of the presence of the call bell before it can be used; a small light would enable the patient to see the room and the call bell.

④ The patient may not remember the description of the environment on awakening and could become disoriented in the dark.

10 **TEST-TAKING TIP** ● Options 1 and 4 are opposites.

① Trying to hold the patient up could injure the nurse and cause both the nurse and the patient to fall.

② By the time help arrives, the patient may already be on the floor; calling out can scare the patient and others.

③ The patient is already falling; walking the patient to the closest chair is not an option.

* ④ Lowering the patient to the floor is the safest action; guiding the patient to the floor helps to break the patient's fall and minimize injury.

11 ① Reporting the frayed wire is ineffective in preventing the risk of injury; it should be removed from use.

② Putting the radio in the patient's closet does not preclude that it could be taken out and used again.

③ Attempting to repair an electrical cord is unsafe; it should be repaired by a trained person.

* ④ Removing the radio and sending it home with a family member is the safest option; this option removes it from use.

12 **TEST-TAKING TIP** ● The word "unacceptable" is the key word in the stem that indicates negative polarity.

* ① The use of a double knot prevents easy release in the event of an emergency and is an unsafe practice.

② Securing restraint ties to the base of the bed is safe practice. Restraint straps should be tied to an immovable underpart of the bed. This prevents injury when side rails are lowered, and also places the straps out of the patient's reach.

③ Allowing the patient's fingers free movement with the use of wrist restraints is acceptable practice; the wrists, not the fingers, are restrained.

④ Padding the patient's wrists with sheepskin when applying wrist restraints is safe practice; the wrist has several bony prominences and little muscle or adipose tissue to protect this area from pressure and skin breakdown.

13* ① Because of a dark, unfamiliar environment at night, elderly patients may become confused and disoriented, which contributes to the occurrence of falls.

② Mealtimes are generally unrelated to falls.

③ All patients, including postoperative patients, should be assisted when ambulating until they are able to ambulate safely on their own; therefore, these patients should not fall.

④ Visiting hours are generally unrelated to falls.

14 **TEST-TAKING TIP** ● The words "first" and "most" are the key words in the stem that set a priority. Options 1 and 3 are equally plausible options because they both address how to administer oxygen. Options 2 and 3 are equally plausible because they both address the drying effects of oxygen therapy.

① Although this is true, safety is the priority.

② Same as #1.

③ Same as #1.

* ④ Although oxygen by itself will not burn or explode, it facilitates combustion; the greater the concentration of oxygen, the more rapidly fires start and burn.

15 **TEST-TAKING TIP** ● The word "primarily" in the stem sets a priority.

① Sheepskin is not designed to absorb urine; wet sheepskin will contribute to skin breakdown.

* ② Soft tufts of sheepskin reduce friction and allow air to circulate under the patient.

③ Sheepskin will not eliminate pressure. Turning the patient off a body part is the most effective measure to relieve pressure.

④ Sheepskin helps to keep skin cool, not warm, by allowing air to circulate through the tufts of lamb's wool.

16 TEST-TAKING TIP ● The word "best" in the stem sets a priority.

* ① An air mattress is effective because it distributes body weight over a larger surface and reduces pressure over bony prominences.

② Although bathing removes secretions and promotes clean skin, it can also be very drying, which can compromise skin integrity.

③ Protein does not prevent pressure (decubitus) ulcers. Protein is the body's only source of nitrogen and is essential for building, repairing, or replacing body tissue.

④ An indwelling urinary catheter should never be used to prevent a pressure (decubitus) ulcer; however, a catheter may be used to prevent contamination of a pressure (decubitus) ulcer once it is present.

17 TEST-TAKING TIP ● Options 2 and 3 are opposites.

① Straightening the finger joints is extension.

② Spreading the fingers out in relation to one another is abduction.

③ Bringing the fingers in alignment next to one another is adduction.

* ④ Opposition is the correct term to describe touching the thumb to the tip of each finger of the hand.

18 TEST-TAKING TIP ● The word "most" is the key word in the stem that sets a priority. Options 1 and 2 are opposites.

* ① Active range-of-motion (ROM) exercise is preferable because it is an isotonic exercise that causes muscle contraction; active ROM exercise increases joint mobility, circulation, and muscle tone because the patient actively moves the joints through full range of motion.

② Passive range-of-motion (PROM) exercise is when a joint is moved by a source other than the muscles articulating to the joint; PROM exercise puts a joint through full range and prevents contractures, but does not increase muscle tone because the muscles are not contracted.

③ Active-assistive range-of-motion exercise is when the patient attempts active range of motion and receives some support and assistance from the nurse; active-assistive ROM exercise does not provide for as much isotonic exercise as active ROM exercise.

④ Isometric exercise involves contracting and relaxing a muscle without moving the joint; this improves muscle tone but does not put joints through the full range of motion.

19 TEST-TAKING TIP ● The words "one-sided weakness" are a clue in the stem. Option 1 is unique because it does not use the possessive form of the word patient (patient's). Options 2 and 3 are opposites.

* ① Pivoting the patient on the unaffected leg is a safe method to transfer this patient; this method avoids extra unnecessary movement by directly transferring the patient to the chair while supporting body weight on the unaffected leg.

② Standing next to the affected side when transferring this patient is unsafe; when transferring this patient, the nurse should stand in front of the patient.

③ Standing next to the strong side when transferring this patient is unsafe; when transferring this patient, the nurse should stand in front of the patient.

④ Keeping the patient's feet together narrows the base of support and decreases the patient's stability.

20 TEST-TAKING TIP ● The word "primary" is the key word in the stem that sets a priority. Options 1 and 2 are equally plausible.
  ① The purpose of an egg-crate pad is to distribute weight, not absorb moisture. A wet egg-crate pad should not be used because moisture against the skin can contribute to skin breakdown.
  ② The opposite may be true. Because egg-crate pads are made of synthetic materials, they often promote, rather than limit, perspiration.
  ③ Pillows and wedges, not an egg-crate pad, are used to keep the body in functional alignment.
 * ④ Intermittent raised areas on the egg-crate pad help to evenly distribute body weight over the entire body surface that is in contact with the pad.

21 TEST-TAKING TIP ● Options 1 and 2 are opposites. Options 2 and 3 deny the patient's feelings of fear.
 * ① Lowering the patient back onto the bed recognizes the cause of the anxiety and responds to the source.
  ② Continuing with the transfer denies the patient's fears and can intensify the anxiety.
  ③ Same as #2.
  ④ Not lowering the patient back onto the bed and leaving the patient up in the air can intensify the anxiety.

22 TEST-TAKING TIP ● The phrase "sacral area" is the significant clue in the stem.
  ① The Sims' position avoids pressure on the sacral area; weight is on the anterior ilium, the humerus, and clavicle.
  ② The prone position avoids pressure on the sacral area; prone is lying on the abdomen.
  ③ In the lateral position pressure is off the sacral area; the body is side-lying with weight on the dependent hip and shoulder.
 * ④ In the high-Fowler's position most of the weight is placed on the sacral area; this causes sacral pressure.

23 TEST-TAKING TIP ● Options 1 and 2 are opposites.
  ① Corridor rails are not continuous and standing in front does not position the nurse in a way that will protect the patient; this method does not inspire confidence and is not as safe as instructing the patient to hold onto the nurse's arm.
  ② Standing behind a blind patient and providing directions is unsafe; the patient cannot see and should not lead.
  ③ Walking on the side while holding the patient's elbow is one method used to assist a patient who has a mobility, not visual, deficit.
 * ④ Instructing the blind patient to hold onto the nurse's arm allows the nurse to guide and the patient to follow; it supports the patient's comfort and contributes to his or her confidence.

24 TEST-TAKING TIP ● The words "prevent external rotation" are the clue in the stem.
  ① A footboard prevents planter flexion, not external rotation.
  ② A bed cradle keeps linen off the feet and legs; it supports patient comfort and does not prevent external rotation.
 * ③ A trochanter roll prevents the hip and leg from externally rotating by positioning the leg in functional alignment.
  ④ Elastic stockings do not prevent external rotation; they are used to increase venous return in the lower legs.

25 TEST-TAKING TIP ● The word "highest" is the key word in the stem that sets a priority. The word "risk" is a clue in the stem. Option 1 is unique because it is the only option that does not mention that the patient is able to move independently.

    * ① A patient using a reclining wheelchair would have minimal lower- or upper-body control; the reclining features of the chair prevent a patient with decreased body control from falling forward. A reclining position places excessive pressure on the sacral area; a patient with decreased mobility positioned in a semi-Fowler's position would be at risk for skin breakdown because of pressure.

     ② As long as a person can move, positioning can be changed to relieve pressure.

     ③ Same as #2.

     ④ Same as #2.

26 TEST-TAKING TIP ● The word "toward" is a clue in the stem. One could say that the act of moving a body part "toward" another is like "adding" one to another. The first three letters of the word "adduction" in Option 3 are "add."

     ① Internal rotation is the act of rolling the leg and foot toward the midline, thereby internally rotating the hip joint, not moving an extremity toward the midline and beyond.

     ② Lateral flexion is when the head is tilted as far as possible to one shoulder and then the other shoulder, not moving an extremity toward the midline and beyond.

    * ③ The word "adduction" correctly represents the action of moving an extremity toward the midline and beyond.

     ④ Inversion is when the sole of the foot is turned medially, not moving an extremity toward the midline and beyond.

27 TEST-TAKING TIP ● The word *best* is the key word in the stem that sets a priority. Option 3 denies the patient's feelings. Options 2 and 4 are patient centered.

     ① Using a mechanical lift could contribute to feelings of dependence and loss of control. Also, a mechanical lift is used to safely transfer an immobile patient; the question identifies a fearful patient, not an immobile patient.

     ② Waiting and thinking about the transfer can increase anxiety, not reduce it; the patient may decide never to get out of bed.

     ③ Explaining that a fall will not occur is false reassurance and denies the patient's fears.

    * ④ Allowing the patient to set the pace of the transfer supports the need of the patient to be in control; the patient's anxiety is generally reduced in proportion to an increase in control.

28 TEST-TAKING TIP ● Options 2 and 4 are equally plausible.

     ① Flotation pads or gel cushions do not have a heat source; they are designed to distribute weight over the entire cushion.

     ② The body makes close contact with the cushion; air does not circulate between the patient and the cushion.

    * ③ When body weight is distributed across the cushion, pressure is reduced on the tissue over bony prominences.

     ④ Flotation pads and gel cushions are designed to spread body weight and reduce pressure, not limit moisture.

29 TEST-TAKING TIP ● The word **best** is the key word in the stem that sets a priority.

     ① Supporting joints contributes to maintaining functional alignment, which can help to prevent contractures. However, of the options offered, range-of-motion exercises best contribute to preventing contractures.

     ② Although movement of joints experienced during activity will contribute to preventing contractures, it will not move all joints through their full range; also, prolonged sitting can cause flexion contractures of the hips and knees.

③ Turning and positioning a patient every 2 hours will reduce pressure, not prevent contractures.

* ④ Range-of-motion exercises, which involve the flexing and extending of muscles, prevent shortening or lengthening of muscles that can result in contractures.

30 TEST-TAKING TIP ● The phrase "3 days ago" is a significant clue in the stem. Options 3 and 4 are equally plausible. Options 2, 3, and 4 are similar because they contain the verbs "encourage," "instruct," and "tell," which all require verbal interaction with the patient. Option 1 is unique because it is the only option in which the nurse is actually dressing the patient and that uses the possessive form of the word patient (patient's). Option 2 denies the patient's need for assistance during the acute phase of this illness.

* ① Affected joints should be dressed first to avoid unnecessary strain; the unaffected side generally has greater joint range.

② It is unreasonable to expect self-sufficiency during the acute phase.

③ Zippers are difficult to close with one hand. Velcro closures may be more appropriate.

④ Buttons are difficult to close with one hand. Velcro closures may be more appropriate.

31 TEST-TAKING TIP ● The word "primarily" in the stem sets a priority.

① This is not the primary reason for sitting on the side of the bed prior to transfer.

* ② Orthostatic hypotension is a condition that contributes to impaired stability. When moving to a sitting or standing position from lying or sitting, cerebral circulation is impaired, resulting in light-headedness and dizziness; sitting on the side of the bed allows the circulation time to adjust to a change in position.

③ Same as #1.

④ Although the patient might take several deep breaths, it is not the main reason for sitting on the side of the bed before transfer.

32 TEST-TAKING TIP ● The word *most* is the key word in the stem that sets a priority.

① The arms do not have to be elevated to be in functional alignment.

② A comfortable position for the patient may not provide the alignment necessary to prevent complications; although comfort is important, functional alignment takes priority.

* ③ Anatomical alignment maintains physical functioning, minimizes strain and stress on muscles and joints, and prevents contractures.

④ The head can be at the same level as the heart; it does not have to be higher.

33 TEST-TAKING TIP ● The word "main" is the key word in the stem that sets a priority. Options 3 and 4 are equally plausible.

① It is pressure that causes reduced oxygenation to local tissue, not gravity.

* ② Pressure causes ischemia to local tissue; when deprived of oxygen and nutrients, pathological changes begin within 1 to 2 hours. If pressure is not relieved, tissue breakdown and cellular death (necrosis) occur.

③ Skin breakdown is the adaptation to pressure, not the cause of a pressure ulcer; also, skin breakdown may be caused by stressors other than pressure.

④ Cellular necrosis is the death of tissues in response to prolonged pressure and oxygen deprivation; cellular necrosis is the adaptation to pressure, not the cause of a pressure ulcer.

34 TEST-TAKING TIP ● Options 1 and 2 are opposites.

① Eversion refers to when the sole of the foot is turned laterally.

② Inversion refers to when the sole of the foot is turned medially.

* ③ Supination is the word that describes the turning of the lower arm and hand so that the palm is up.

④ Circumduction refers to when an arm or a leg is moved in a circle.

35 TEST-TAKING TIP ● The word MOST is the key word in the stem that sets a priority. Options 1 and 2 are equally plausible.

① When a patient is in the lateral position, the feet are not against the footboard and the footboard only keeps the linen off the feet and legs.

② A bed cradle keeps linen off the feet and legs for comfort; it does not contribute to functional alignment.

③ A pillow under the waist is used when a patient is positioned in the supine position, not the lateral position.

* ④ Putting a pillow under the upper leg positions the upper leg and hip in functional alignment and reduces stress and strain on the hip joint.

Meeting Patients' Hygiene and Comfort Needs

This section includes questions related to meeting patients' hygiene and comfort needs. Questions focus on theories of pain, assessment of pain, pain relief measures, rest and sleep, the backrub, bedmaking, the use of heat and cold, principles associated with bed baths, principles associated with preventing skin breakdown, perineal care, and care of the hair, feet, and oral cavity.

Questions

1 A patient has a high temperature, is diaphoretic, and did not sleep well during the night. When planning for this patient's hygiene needs, the nurse should:
① Give a complete bath
② Do a partial bed bath
③ Delay the bath until later
④ Provide only perineal care

TEST-TAKING TIP ● Identify the options that are opposites. Identify the equally plausible options. Identify the option that contains a specific determiner.

2 When the nurse is giving a patient a bed bath, the water temperature should be:
① 80 to 90°F
② 95 to 105°F
③ 110 to 115°F
④ 120 to 130°F

TEST-TAKING TIP ● Identify options that are opposites.

3 When administering perineal care, the nurse can *best* provide emotional comfort by:
① Placing the patient in the supine position
② Pulling the curtain around the bed
③ Using warm water for washing
② Calling the patient by name

TEST-TAKING TIP ● Identify the word in the stem that sets a priority. Identify the clue in the stem.

4 When providing a partial bed bath, the nurse should:
① Help the patient to wash his or her face, hands, underarms, back, and perineal area
② Direct the patient to wash as much as possible and assist with the rest
③ Instruct the patient to wash his or her face, hands, and perineal area
④ Assist the patient to wash only one part of the body at a time

TEST-TAKING TIP ● Identify the clue in the stem. Identify the option that contains a specific determiner.

5 When the physician orders that a patient be kept NPO, the MOST important action by the nurse should be to:
① Allow the patient to sip clear fluids with medication
② Give the patient mouth care every 4 hours
③ Measure the patient's intake and output
④ Permit the patient to suck on ice chips

TEST-TAKING TIP ● Identify the key word in the stem that sets a priority. Identify the equally plausible options. Identify the clue in the stem.

6 When administering a bed bath, the nurse rinses the patient after applying soap and water mainly to:
① Increase circulation
② Promote rest and comfort
③ Minimize decubitus ulcers
④ Remove residue and debris

TEST-TAKING TIP ● Identify the key word in the stem that sets a priority.

7 When planning care for a patient with offensive mouth odor, the most effective intervention would be to encourage the patient to:
① Eat foods that do not generate odors
② Brush the teeth and tongue after meals
③ Rinse the mouth with mouthwash every shift
④ Flush the mouth with peroxide and baking soda

TEST-TAKING TIP ● Identify the key word in the stem that sets a priority. Identify the option that contains a specific determiner. Identify the equally plausible options.

8 Which action would be least effective in preventing hair from tangling and matting?
① Using conditioners after shampooing
② Washing the hair with soap
③ Placing the hair in braids
④ Brushing the hair daily

TEST-TAKING TIP ● Identify the key word in the stem that indicates negative polarity.

9 To prevent pressure (decubitus) ulcers, the bottom sheet should be:
① Covered by a draw sheet
② Made with a toe pleat
③ Kept free of wrinkles
④ Changed every day

TEST-TAKING TIP ● Identify the option that contains a specific determiner.

10 Before discharge an elderly patient complains of dry, itchy skin. To limit these problems, the nurse should teach the patient to apply a lubricating lotion and:
① Avoid the sun
② Bathe every day
③ Wear short-sleeved clothing
④ Rub the itchy areas with a soft towel

TEST-TAKING TIP ● Identify the option that contains a specific determiner.

11 The nurse makes the assessment that a patient's feet are dirty. When planning to clean this patient's feet, the <u>most</u> effective intervention would be to:
① Ask the patient to take a shower
② Lubricate them with lotion to soften the dirt
③ Soak each foot in a basin with soap and water
④ Use an antiseptic to prevent a fungal infection

TEST-TAKING TIP ● Identify the key word in the stem that sets a priority.

12 What is the most important action by the nurse when washing the perineal area of a male patient?
① Handling the genitalia always with a light touch
② Washing the scrotum before the shaft of the penis

③ Repositioning the foreskin after washing the penis
④ Cleansing down the length of the penis toward the glans
TEST-TAKING TIP ● Identify the key word in the stem that sets a priority. Identify the option that contains a specific determiner.

13 A patient is incontinent of urine and stool and is cognitively impaired. To BEST prevent skin breakdown in this patient, the nurse should:
① Frequently check the perineal area and wash if necessary
② Gently instruct the patient to call the nurse when soiled
③ Place sheepskin on the bed and apply a diaper
④ Turn and position the patient every 2 hours
TEST-TAKING TIP ● Identify the key word in the stem that sets a priority. Identify the option that contains a specific determiner.

14 A patient has a nasogastric tube inserted into the stomach. A daily intervention that would contribute to hygiene would include:
① Replacing the positioning tape on the nose
② Instilling 30 mL of water into the tube
③ Suctioning the oral pharynx
④ Lubricating the nares
TEST-TAKING TIP ● Identify the words that are clues in the stem.

15 A psychological reaction to chronic pain that the nurse should monitor for is:
① Dyspnea
② Depression
③ Self-splinting
④ Hypertension
TEST-TAKING TIP ● Identify the clues in the stem.

16 To promote sleep, the nurse should encourage the patient to:
① Exercise daily
② Drink a cup of tea
③ Eat only light meals
④ Review the day's events
TEST-TAKING TIP ● Identify the option that contains a specific determiner.

17 A behavioral response to moderate pain that the nurse should assess for is:
① Rapid, irregular breathing
② Increased muscle tension
③ Self-splinting
④ Fatigue
TEST-TAKING TIP ● Identify the words that are clues in the stem.

18 During a clinic visit an elderly patient complains about cold feet. The nurse should:
① Explain to the patient that this is normal in elderly people
② Teach the patient to place a heating pad over the feet
③ Instruct the patient in how to use a hot water bottle
④ Encourage the patient to wear warm socks
TEST-TAKING TIP ● Identify the clue in the stem. Identify the equally plausible options. Identify the option that denies the patient's concerns or needs.

19 In normal daily living, sleep is **most** often interfered with by:
① Environmental noise
② Emotional concerns
③ Room temperature
④ Body discomfort
TEST-TAKING TIP ● Identify the key word in the stem that sets a priority.

20 When planning care to relieve pain, the nurse could use an intervention that incorporates the gate-control theory of pain such as:
① Encouraging activity
② Administering a narcotic
③ Promoting rest and sleep
④ Applying a warm compress
TEST-TAKING TIP ● Identify the clue in the stem. Identify the options that are opposites.

21 Cold is effective in reducing the discomfort associated with a local inflammatory response because it:
① Anesthetizes nerve endings and causes vasoconstriction
② Stimulates nerve endings and causes vasoconstriction
③ Anesthetizes nerve endings and causes vasodilation
④ Stimulates nerve endings and causes vasodilation
TEST-TAKING TIP ● Identify the duplicate facts among the options.

22 To best promote rest and sleep in the hospital for all patients, the nurse should:
① Administer a sleeping medication
② Provide a backrub before sleep
③ Turn the lights off at night
④ Encourage usual routines
TEST-TAKING TIP ● Identify the key word in the stem that sets a priority. Identify the clue in the stem.

23 A backrub promotes comfort and rest because it:
① Causes vasodilation
② Stimulates circulation
③ Increases O_2 to tissues
④ Relieves muscular tension
TEST-TAKING TIP ● Identify the clue in the stem. Identify the unique option.

24 Heat effectively reduces discomfort at a local inflammatory site because it:
① Decreases local circulation and limits capillary permeability
② Decreases tissue metabolism and increases local circulation
③ Increases local circulation and promotes muscle relaxation
④ Provides local anesthesia and decreases local circulation
TEST-TAKING TIP ● Identify the duplicate facts among the options.

25 Which signs should the nurse expect when assessing the patient in acute pain?
① Decreased respiratory rate and pallor
② Flushed skin and increased respiratory rate
③ Increased blood pressure and dilated pupils
④ Constricted pupils and decreased blood pressure
TEST-TAKING TIP ● Identify the options that are opposites.

26 What should the nurse do to support dignity when providing oral hygiene for a patient with dentures?
　① Provide a denture cup for the patient.
　② Pull the curtain around the patient's bed.
　③ Support the patient in a high-Fowler's position.
　④ Resist looking at the patient while the dentures are out.
　TEST-TAKING TIP ● Identify the patient-centered option.

27 What should the nurse do when a patient has tangled, matted hair?
　① Braid the hair in sections
　② Use a comb instead of a brush
　③ Comb a small section at a time
　④ Brush from the roots toward the ends

28 When making an occupied bed, what is the most important action by the nurse?
　① Use new linen.
　② Raise both side rails.
　③ Keep the patient covered.
　④ Place a pad on the draw sheet.
　TEST-TAKING TIP ● Identify the word in the stem that sets a priority. Identify the patient-centered option.

29 Which is the most subjective characteristic of pain?
　① Intensity
　② Duration
　③ Location
　④ Quality
　TEST-TAKING TIP ● Identify the word in the stem that sets a priority. Identify the clue in the stem.

30 Which individuals require the least amount of sleep?
　① Adolescents
　② Older adults
　③ Young adults
　④ Middle-age adults
　TEST-TAKING TIP ● Identify the word in the stem that indicates negative polarity. Identify the options that are opposites.

31 A perioperative patient talks about being afraid of pain because of a previous experience with painful surgery. What should the nurse do *first* to help the patient deal with this fear?
　① Encourage the patient not to be afraid.
　② Teach the patient relaxation techniques.
　③ Listen to the patient's concerns about pain.
　④ Inform the patient that medication is available.
　TEST-TAKING TIP ● Identify the word in the stem that sets a priority. Identify the unique option. Identify the option that denies the patient's feelings, concerns, or needs.

32 A female patient who has cancer that has metastasized to the bone experiences pain when moving. What should the nurse do when the patient refuses to move?
　① Reassure her that she will not be hurt.
　② Complete nursing care as quickly as possible.

③ Let her perform her own activities of daily living.

④ Touch her gently when assisting with required care.

TEST-TAKING TIP ● Identify the option that denies the patient's feelings, concerns, or needs.

33 Pain perception is MOST influenced by the:

① Duration of the stimulus

② Characteristics of the pain

③ Activity of the cerebral cortex

④ Level of endorphins in the blood

TEST-TAKING TIP ● Identify the word in the stem that sets a priority.

34 Which description would indicate that a patient had sordes?

① Accumulation of debris on the teeth and gums

② Deposits of hard plaque at the gumline

③ Inflammation of the oral mucosa

④ Lesions on the tongue and gums

35 What should the nurse do when providing perineal care for a female patient?

① Use a new area of the washcloth for each stroke

② Wash from the rectum toward the pubis

③ Clean the dirtiest area first

④ Use only warm tap water

TEST-TAKING TIP ● Identify the option that contains a specific determiner.

Rationales

1   **TEST-TAKING TIP** ● Options 1 and 3 are opposites. Options 2 and 4 are equally plausible. Option 4 contains the word "only," which is a specific determiner.
 * ① Diaphoresis is a profuse secretion of sweat associated with an elevated body temperature, physical exertion, or emotional stress. The secretions must be removed from the entire body to limit the growth of microorganisms and promote comfort; evaporation during the bed bath may help lower the patient's temperature.
   ② A partial bed bath is inadequate; a complete bed bath is necessary.
   ③ Delaying the bed bath is unsafe; the patient needs immediate physical hygiene.
   ④ Same as #2.

2   **TEST-TAKING TIP** ● Options 1 and 4 are opposites in the ranges offered in the item.
   ① This temperature range is too cool; this would promote chilling.
   ② Same as #1.
 * ③ The temperature of bath water should be between 110 and 115°F to promote comfort, dilate blood vessels, and prevent chilling.
   ④ This temperature range is too hot; this would be uncomfortable and could injure tissue.

3   **TEST-TAKING TIP** ● The word *best* is the key word in the stem that sets a priority. The word "emotional" is a clue in the stem.
   ① Correct positioning provides for physical, not emotional, comfort.
 * ② Perineal care is a private activity, and measures should be taken to provide for privacy.
   ③ Warm water provides physical comfort.
   ④ Although calling the patient by name is a respectful, individualized approach, it does not address the patient's right to privacy during a procedure that exposes the genitalia.

4   **TEST-TAKING TIP** ● The word "partial" in the stem is a clue. Option 4 contains the word "only," which is a specific determiner.
 * ① These areas should be washed daily because they harbor the most microorganisms.
   ② This intervention would be considered a complete bed bath with assistance.
   ③ The axillary areas and the back must also be washed in a partial bed bath.
   ④ Same as #2.

5   **TEST-TAKING TIP** ● The word MOST is a key word in the stem that sets a priority. Options 1 and 4 are equally plausible. "NPO" is the clue in the stem.
   ① Fluids of any kind are contraindicated; *non per os* (NPO) means nothing by mouth.
 * ② When people are NPO, they tend to have dry mucous membranes and thick secretions on the tongue and gums; mouth care cleans the oral cavity.
   ③ Although monitoring the patient's intake and output (I&O) may be done, the priority is direct physical care of the patient.
   ④ Same as #1.

6   **TEST-TAKING TIP** ● The word "mainly" is the key word in the stem that sets a priority.
   ① Friction from firm, long strokes used during rinsing increases circulation; however, it is not the reason for rinsing.
   ② A backrub and positioning in functional alignment, not rinsing, promote rest and comfort.
   ③ Local massage and repositioning every 2 hours, not rinsing, prevent decubitus ulcers.
 * ④ Rinsing flushes the skin with clean water, which removes debris and soap residue.

7 **TEST-TAKING TIP** ● The word "most" is a key word in the stem that sets a priority. Option 3 contains the word "every," which is a specific determiner. Options 3 and 4 are equally plausible.

① Although some foods can cause halitosis, it is more often caused by inadequate oral hygiene, a local infection, or a systemic disease; brushing uses friction, which most often effectively cleans the oral cavity.

* ② Halitosis is often caused by decaying food particles and gingivitis; brushing the teeth and tongue cleans the oral cavity and promotes healthy teeth and gums.

③ Rinsing or flushing the mouth is done after brushing the teeth and tongue; rinsing or flushing alone will not remove debris caught between the teeth.

④ Same as #3.

8 **TEST-TAKING TIP** ● The word "least" in the stem indicates negative polarity.

① Conditioners moisturize the hair, which makes the strands more supple, preventing tangles.

* ② Soap is drying because it removes natural secretions, which keep the hair supple.

③ Braids organize the strands of hair, which limits movement of hair into mats and tangles because of friction and pressure.

④ Brushing distributes oils along hair shafts, keeping them supple and preventing tangles and matting.

9 **TEST-TAKING TIP** ● Option 4 contains the word "every," which is a specific determiner.

① A draw sheet is an additional sheet that could add to the number of wrinkles; the purpose of a draw sheet is to keep the bottom sheet clean.

② A toe pleat should be placed in the top sheet and spread, not the bottom sheet. A toe pleat prevents footdrop.

* ③ Wrinkles exert pressure and friction against the skin, promoting the formation of pressure (decubitus) ulcers.

④ The bottom sheet does not have to be changed every day unless the sheet is wet or dirty.

10 **TEST-TAKING TIP** ● The word "every" in Option 2 is a specific determiner.

* ① The sun promotes loss of fluid from the skin, and the ultraviolet rays could cause a burn.

② Elderly patients often avoid daily baths because they dry the skin. Soap and water irritate and dry the skin because they remove natural secretions that lubricate the skin.

③ Exposure of the skin to the environment promotes drying.

④ Itchy areas should be patted, not rubbed, to prevent damage to tissues.

11 **TEST-TAKING TIP** ● The word <u>most</u> is the key word in the stem that sets a priority.

① Showering is not as effective as submerging the feet in soapy water.

② A lubricant would be applied after the feet are clean.

* ③ Soaking in soap and water softens the debris on the skin, between the toes, and under the toenails, facilitating cleaning.

④ The application of an antiseptic requires a physician's order.

12 **TEST-TAKING TIP** ● The word "most" is a key word in the stem that sets a priority. Option 1 contains the word "always," which is a specific determiner.

① A light touch would be stimulating and could precipitate a penile erection; a firm but gentle touch should be used.

② This action violates the principle of working from clean to dirty. The tip of the penis at the urethral meatus is washed first; bathing should then progress down the shaft of the penis toward the perineum and then the scrotum.

   * ③ Repositioning the foreskin protects the head of the penis and prevents drying and irritation; if it is allowed to remain retracted, the tightening of the foreskin around the shaft of the penis could cause local edema and discomfort.

    ④ Cleaning should occur in the opposite direction, starting at the urinary meatus and then progressing down the shaft of the penis away from the urinary meatus.

13 TEST-TAKING TIP ● The word BEST in the stem a sets a priority. Option 4 contains the word "every," which is a specific determiner.

   * ① When patients are incontinent they should be cleaned immediately; feces contain digestive enzymes and urine contains ammonia and other irritating substances that cause skin breakdown.

    ② This is an unrealistic instruction for this patient; a cognitively impaired patient would have difficulty with this task.

    ③ Sheepskin and an incontinence pad (the word diaper should be avoided) hold moisture next to the skin and their use should be avoided.

    ④ Turning may be necessary more frequently than every 2 hours in a patient at risk.

14 TEST-TAKING TIP ● The words "daily" and "contribute to hygiene" in the stem are significant clues.

    ① It is not necessary to replace the tape daily; the tape should be reapplied if the nares become irritated or the tape becomes soiled.

    ② After placement is established, instillation of solution may be done to promote patency, not hygiene.

    ③ Suctioning is not necessary; cleaning the oral cavity when necessary with a tooth brush, dental floss, and mouthwash, and applying a lubricant to the lips are sufficient.

   * ④ Lubricating the nares keeps the skin supple and prevents drying, which limits the development of encrustations.

15 TEST-TAKING TIP ● The words "psychological" and "chronic" in the stem are clues.

    ① This is a physiological adaptation to a stress, not a psychological adaptation.

   * ② Patients with chronic pain commonly experience depression; this is a psychological adaptation to lack of control over relentless pain.

    ③ Self-splinting is a physical attempt to minimize pain.

    ④ Same as #1.

16 TEST-TAKING TIP ● Option 3 contains the word "only," which is a specific determiner.

   * ① Exercise contributes to physical and mental relaxation, which reduces tension and promotes sleep.

    ② Tea contains caffeine, which contributes to wakefulness.

    ③ The opposite is true. Moderate to heavy meals promote sleep; the body's energy is engaged in the process of digestion.

    ④ Reviewing the day's events can cause an increase in tension that can prevent a person from falling asleep.

17 TEST-TAKING TIP ● The words "behavioral" and "moderate" are clues in the stem.

    ① Rapid, irregular breathing is a physiological response to pain; pain generally activates the flight-or-fight mechanism of the general adaptation syndrome (GAS). The GAS stimulates the sympathetic branch of the autonomic nervous system, which results in these symptoms; this response provides greater oxygen transport.

    ② The GAS stimulates the sympathetic branch of the autonomic nervous system, which results in increased muscle tension; it is a physiological response that prepares muscles for action.

     * ③ Self-splinting is a behavioral attempt to protect the area in pain and minimize stress and strain to the area, for example, supporting the area or leaning in the direction of the pain.

     ④ Fatigue is a physiological response to pain; physical and emotional responses to pain can use a great deal of physical and emotional energy and leave a person fatigued.

18 **TEST-TAKING TIP** ● The word "cold" in the stem is a clue. Options 2 and 3 are equally plausible. Option 1 denies the patient's comfort needs.

     ① This response ignores the patient's comfort needs.

     ② The application of heat is not as safe as socks; externally produced heat can burn the feet in elderly people, who have reduced peripheral sensation.

     ③ Same as #2.

     * ④ Wearing socks is the safest way to keep the feet warm; socks contain the heat generated by the body.

19 **TEST-TAKING TIP** ● The word **most** in the stem sets a priority.

     ① Although this can interfere with sleep, emotional concerns have been proved most often to interfere with sleep.

     * ② Research studies suggest that emotional concerns impede sleep because they interfere with the patient's ability to relax the mind and body and fall asleep.

     ③ Same as #1.

     ④ Same as #1.

20 **TEST-TAKING TIP** ● The term "gate-control theory" is the clue in the stem. Options 1 and 3 are opposites.

     ① Activity uses distraction, not the gate-control theory, to focus attention on stimuli other than the pain. When in pain, patients often do not have the physical or emotional energy to concentrate on activities.

     ② Narcotics do not work through the gate-control theory; they act on the higher centers of the brain to modify the perception of pain.

     ③ Rest, sleep, and relaxation associated with pain relief are not based on the gate-control theory.

     * ④ The gate-control theory assumes that pain fibers that originate in the peripheral areas of the body synapse in the gray matter of the dorsal horns of the spinal cord. Large nerve fibers stimulated by heat, cold, and touch transmit impulses through the same synapses as those that transmit pain. When larger fibers are stimulated, they close the gate to painful stimuli, and the perception of pain is reduced.

21 **TEST-TAKING TIP** ● There are four hypotheses being tested in this option: cold anesthetizes nerve endings, causes vasocontriction, stimulates nerve endings, and causes vasodilation. If you know that one of these hypotheses is wrong, then you can eliminate two distractors.

     * ① Cold is a form of cutaneous stimulation that slows the nervous conduction of impulses, thereby anesthetizing nerve endings, which relaxes muscle tension and relieves pain. Vasoconstriction decreases the flow of blood to the affected area; this limits the development of edema, which puts pressure on nerve endings, resulting in pain.

     ② Cold anesthetizes rather than stimulates nerve endings; it does cause vasoconstriction.

     ③ Although cold does anesthetize nerve endings, it causes vasoconstriction, not vasodilation.

     ④ Cold anesthetizes, rather than stimulates, nerve endings and causes vasoconstriction.

22 TEST-TAKING TIP ● The word "best" in the stem sets a priority. The words "all patients" in the stem are a clue.

① Sleeping medication should not be administered until all nondrug approaches fail to achieve sleep.

② A backrub invades personal space and should be administered according to a patient's need and preference; a backrub may be contraindicated in certain clinical situations such as myocardial infarction or back surgery.

③ In an unfamiliar environment, turning the lights off can precipitate confusion or disorientation; a small light provides visual cues if a person should awaken at night.

* ④ Usual routines meet self-identified needs and reduce anxiety because they provide a familiar pattern.

23 TEST-TAKING TIP ● The words "comfort and rest" are the clue in the stem. Option 4 is unique because it addresses muscles. Options 1, 2, and 3 all refer to the circulatory system.

① The friction of a backrub causes heat, which in turn causes vasodilation. Vasodilation improves circulation by bringing oxygen and nutrients to the area; these physiological effects help prevent pressure (decubitus) ulcers.

② Same as #1.

③ Same as #1.

* ④ Effleurage, applying long, smooth strokes while moving the hands up and down the back without losing contact with the skin, has a relaxing and sedative effect. Its effect may be related to the gate-control theory of pain relief; rubbing the back stimulates large muscle fiber groups, which close the synaptic gates to pain or uncomfortable stimuli, permitting a perception of relaxation.

24 TEST-TAKING TIP ● The words "increases local circulation" in Options 2 and 3 and "decreases local circulation" in Options 1 and 4 are examples of duplicate facts.

① Heat increases, rather than decreases, local circulation, capillary vasodilation, and permeability.

② Although heat increases local circulation, it increases, rather than decreases, tissue metabolism. Heat causes vasodilatation, facilitating the exchange of nutrients and waste products and increasing cellular metabolism.

* ③ Heat increases circulation because of its vasodilating effect. Heat is known to relax muscle spasms and the discomfort associated with muscle spasm; this mechanism is unknown.

④ Cold, not heat, provides local anesthesia and decreases local circulation.

25 TEST-TAKING TIP ● Options 1 and 2 are opposites and options 3 and 4 are opposites.

① Although the patient with acute pain exhibits pallor, there will be an increased, not decreased, respiratory rate.

② Although the respiratory rate will increase in response to the fight-or-flight mechanism, pallor rather than flushing is expected. Peripheral vasoconstriction occurs in an effort to shift the blood supply from the periphery to the skeletal muscles, viscera, and brain.

* ③ Sympathetic stimulation in response to the fight-or-flight mechanism increases vasomotor tone and peripheral vascular resistance, increasing the blood pressure. Also, the pupils will be dilated to increase visual acuity.

④ In the general adaptation syndrome the pupils dilate rather than constrict, and the blood pressure increases rather than decreases.

26 **TEST-TAKING TIP** ● Option 2 is patient centered. It addresses the patient's needs in the affective (emotional) domain.

   ① This would be used to store the dentures when the patient is sleeping.

* ② This provides privacy while the dentures are out of the mouth and supports the patient's dignity and self-esteem.

   ③ This supports the patient's physical needs.

   ④ This is unsafe; the nurse must look at the patient to inspect the oral cavity.

27 ① This should be done after the hair is combed and untangled.

   ② Either a comb or brush can be used.

* ③ Separating the hair into small sections promotes ease in combing and limits discomfort.

   ④ When removing tangles the hair should be grasped at the scalp and the loose ends combed; each stroke should start progressively higher than the preceding stroke up the shafts of hair strands.

28 **TEST-TAKING TIP** ● The word "most" in the stem sets a priority. The actions in Options 1, 2, and 4 could be done, but they are less important than the action in Option 3. Option 3 is the patient-centered option because it focuses on the patient rather than on the steps in a procedure.

   ① This is unnecessary unless the linens are wet or dirty.

   ② This does not support correct body mechanics when working and puts excessive stress on the nurse; the side rail may be lowered on the side where the nurse is working.

* ③ This supports privacy and dignity and prevents chilling.

   ④ This promotes the formation of pressure ulcers; it should be used only during perineal care or for patients who are incontinent.

29 **TEST-TAKING TIP** ● The word "most" in the stem sets a priority. The clue in the stem is the word "subjective," which modifies the word "characteristic." Options 2 and 3 are objective characteristics and can be eliminated from consideration.

* ① Intensity is the most subjective characteristic of pain; a patient's perception of pain influences the descriptive report of the severity of pain.

   ② This description is based on determining onset, periodicity, frequency, and duration; it is based on time frames, which can be objectively measured.

   ③ This description is based on anatomical landmarks in the patient's attempt to localize the pain.

   ④ Although subjective, quality is less subjective than intensity because there is more consistency in the language used to describe types of pain. For example, surgical pain is generally described as sharp and pain related to a myocardial infarction (heart attack) is described as crushing.

30 **TEST-TAKING TIP** ● The word "least" in the stem indicates negative polarity. Options 2 and 3 are opposites and must carefully be considered. In this question, Option 2 is the correct answer.

   ① Adolescents go through a growth spurt and need more sleep than older adults.

* ② Studies demonstrate that the older adult requires less sleep than people on any other developmental level.

   ③ Young adults may still be growing and are active, and need more sleep than older adults.

   ④ These adults are usually involved with activities related to growing children and developing a career; this age requires more sleep than the older adult.

31 TEST-TAKING TIP ● The word "first" in the stem sets a priority. Option 3 is unique because it receives information from the patient. Options 1, 2, and 4 all send messages to the patient. Option 1 denies the patient's fears about pain.
  ① This denies the patient's fears.
  ② Although this may eventually be done, it does not allow the patient to discuss fears.
  * ③ This supports the patient's need to verbalize the fears.
  ④ This is false reassurance and cuts off communication; it does not recognize the patient's need to verbalize fears.

32 TEST-TAKING TIP ● Option 2 ignores the patient's fear of moving.
  ① This is false reassurance; this is something the nurse cannot promise.
  ② This can intensity pain; also it can tire the patient, which may intensify pain.
  ③ The patient refuses to move now and will probably avoid any self-care that requires movement.
  * ④ This conveys that the nurse recognizes the patient's need to move slowly, gently, and carefully; a gentle touch with slow movements will contribute to the patient's comfort.

33 TEST-TAKING TIP ● The word MOST in the stem sets a priority. All of the options address factors that influence pain, but Option 3 is the MOST significant.
  ① Duration is one component of a description of pain once it is perceived.
  ② The characteristics of pain are the components of the description of pain once it is perceived.
  * ③ This controls the higher levels of the perceptual aspects of pain.
  ④ Although endorphin levels influence pain perception, it is the activity of the cerebral cortex that controls the higher levels of the perceptual aspects of pain.

34 * ① Sordes are crusts of food, epithelial cells, and/or microorganisms that collect on surfaces of the mouth when a patient is febrile, or NPO, or in response to inadequate mouth care.
  ② Plaque is a thin film of mucin and colloidal material on the teeth, particularly around the base of the crown at the gum margins.
  ③ Inflammation of the oral mucosa is a protective response to irritation or injury and is indicated by redness, heat, swelling, and discomfort, not the formation of crusts.
  ④ Lesions refer to any wound, injury, or pathologic change in body tissue causing a sore, not crusts of food, epithelial cells, and/or microorganisms.

35 TEST-TAKING TIP ● The word "only" in Option 4 is a specific determiner and can be eliminated from consideration.
  * ① This is a basic principle of medical asepsis. This would be done so that contaminated material would not be carried by the washcloth to another area of the perineum.
  ② The opposite is true. Cleaning from the pubis toward the rectum prevents contaminating the urinary meatus and vagina with fecal material.
  ③ The area closest to the urinary meatus and vagina is cleaned first because it is considered the cleanest area of the perineum.
  ④ Soap can be used on the perineal area.

242 Meeting Patients' Fluid and Nutritional Needs

This section includes questions related to basic fluid balance and nutrition. Specific questions focus on principles associated with therapeutic diets, enteral feedings, fluid and electrolyte balance, intake and output, dehydration, feeding patients, vitamins, total parenteral nutrition, intralipids, and medications associated with meeting patients' nutritional needs.

Questions

1 When planning for the nutritional needs of a patient who is receiving chemotherapy and is nauseated, the nurse should:
① Provide meals and supplements as previously planned
② Serve the ordered diet in small quantities frequently
③ Withhold food by mouth until the nausea subsides
④ Obtain an order for a full liquid diet

TEST-TAKING TIP ● Identify the options that are opposites.

2 What should the nurse do FIRST when caring for a patient on intake and output?
① Remove the pitcher of water from the bedside.
② Measure the fluid that the patient drinks and voids.
③ Post an intake and output sign over the patient's bed.
④ Explain the meaning of intake and output to the patient.

TEST-TAKING TIP ● Identify the key word in the stem that sets a priority.

3 To prevent burns during mealtime in patients with mental and physical impairments, the nurse should:
① Assist patients with warm drinks
② Use plastic instead of metal utensils
③ Serve unsteady patients just cold drinks
④ Wait until the food is cool before serving

TEST-TAKING TIP ● Identify the options that deny the patient's feelings, concerns, and needs. Identify the option that contains a specific determiner. Identify the patient-centered option.

4 When a patient drinks 9 oz of milk, which calculation should the nurse enter on the intake and output record?
① 30 mL
② 90 mL
③ 240 mL
④ 270 mL

TEST-TAKING TIP ● Identify the options that are opposites.

5 Which action is LEAST therapeutic when caring for an obese patient who is on a 1000-calorie diet?
① Teaching the patient to avoid starches on the meal tray
② Identifying low-calorie snacks that the patient can eat
③ Encouraging the patient to chew and eat slowly
④ Recognizing when the patient has lost weight

TEST-TAKING TIP ● Identify the key word in the stem that indicates negative polarity.

6 What is the **most** accurate way to measure the amount of urine in a drainage collection bag?
① With a urometer
② With a marked graduate
③ By the markings on the bag
④ By emptying it in a bedpan

TEST-TAKING TIP ● Identify the key word in the stem that sets a priority.

7 When the amount of calories ingested is not sufficient for the patient's basal metabolic rate, the patient will:
① Become dehydrated
② Develop edema
③ Lose weight
④ Sleep more

TEST-TAKING TIP ● Identify the options that are opposites.

8 To avoid trauma to the oral mucous membranes from hot food being served to a cognitively impaired patient, the nurse should:
① Request a menu that includes many cold foods
② Always touch the food to test its temperature
③ Mix the hot food with appropriate cold food
④ Wait for the hot food to cool slightly

TEST-TAKING TIP ● Identify the option that contains a specific determiner. Identify the options that deny the patient's feelings, concerns, and needs.

9 To meet the nutritional needs of an easily confused patient, the most appropriate nursing intervention would be:
① Assisting the patient to eat
② Feeding the patient each meal
③ Explaining to the patient where everything is on the tray
④ Encouraging family members to take turns feeding the patient

TEST-TAKING TIP ● Identify the key word in the stem that sets a priority.

10 How much fluid should the nurse give a patient during 24 hours to maintain *normal* fluid balance?
① 500 mL
② 1000 mL
③ 2000 mL
④ 3000 mL

TEST-TAKING TIP ● Identify the clue in the stem. Identify the options that are opposites.

11 A patient who had a heart attack because of atherosclerotic plaques should obtain protein by primarily ingesting:
① White meats
② Legumes
③ Shrimp
④ Milk

TEST-TAKING TIP ● Identify the word in the stem that sets a priority.

12 A patient with a deficiency in vitamin K should be assessed for:
① Muscle cramps
② Signs of infection
③ Cardiac dysrhythmias
④ Bleeding irregularities
TEST-TAKING TIP ● Identify the clue in the stem.

13 When caring for a patient with a draining pressure (decubitus) ulcer, the nurse recognizes which loss as being most significant?
① Fluid
② Weight
③ Protein
④ Leukocytes
TEST-TAKING TIP ● Identify the clue in the stem. Identify the key word in the stem that sets a priority.

14 As a result of being on a low-calorie diet, all patients will:
① Break down adipose tissue for energy
② Have a decreased body metabolism
③ Have decreased energy levels
④ Require vitamin supplements
TEST-TAKING TIP ● Identify the equally plausible options.

15 An age group that has the highest energy requirements is:
① Birth to 1 year old
② 3 to 5 years old
③ 13 to 19 years old
④ Over 65 years old
TEST-TAKING TIP ● Identify the options that contain opposites.

16 When assessing a patient, which symptoms would support the nursing diagnosis of fluid volume deficit?
① Thready radial pulse and straw-colored urine
② Straw-colored urine and decreased skin turgor
③ Urine specific gravity of 1.015 and thready radial pulse
④ Decreased skin turgor and a urine specific gravity of 1.035
TEST-TAKING TIP ● Identify the duplicate facts among the options.

17 The nurse should encourage a patient on a low-sodium diet to ingest:
① Milk
② Fruit
③ Bread
④ Vegetables

18 Which breakfast foods would contribute the most to the healing of a patient's pressure (decubitus) ulcer?
① French toast and oatmeal
② Oatmeal and orange juice
③ French toast and poached eggs
④ Poached eggs and orange juice
TEST-TAKING TIP ● Identify the key word in the stem that sets a priority. Identify the duplicate facts among the options.

19 An essential vitamin for a patient with anemia would be:
① Ascorbic acid
② Riboflavin
③ Folic acid
④ Thiamine
TEST-TAKING TIP ● Identify the clue in the stem.

20 When a patient is receiving total parenteral nutrition (TPN) and intralipids, the nurse MUST administer the intralipids:
① Via an infusion pump
② Through a separate line
③ Piggybacked into the proximal port of the TPN catheter
④ After the total parenteral nutrition infusion is completed
TEST-TAKING TIP ● Identify the key word in the stem that sets a priority.

21 Increasing the flow rate of total parenteral nutrition (TPN) above the prescribed rate is dangerous because it can result in:
① Osmotic diuresis and hypoglycemia
② Hypoglycemia and dumping syndrome
③ Electrolyte imbalance and osmotic diuresis
④ Dumping syndrome and electrolyte imbalance
TEST-TAKING TIP ● Identify the duplicate facts among the options.

22 After a gastrostomy tube feeding is completed, the nurse should:
① Insert 30 mL of air into the tube
② Gently instill 30 mL of water
③ Check the dressing site
④ Encourage activity
TEST-TAKING TIP ● Identify the clue in the stem.

23 Supplemental iron is most needed by:
① Menstruating women
② Active adolescents
③ Growing children
④ Elderly men
TEST-TAKING TIP ● Identify the key word in the stem that sets a priority.

24 To maintain life, the most important nutrients are:
① Carbohydrates
② Vitamins
③ Proteins
④ Fluids
TEST-TAKING TIP ● Identify the key word in the stem that sets a priority.

25 The group of individuals with the GREATEST need for calcium is:
① Postmenopausal women
② School-age children
③ Pregnant women
④ Working men
TEST-TAKING TIP ● Identify the key word in the stem that sets a priority.

26 A patient who has a fluid intake of 500 cc over 24 hours will:
① Produce urine with a specific gravity of 1.020
② Urinate small amounts at each voiding
③ Develop an atonic bladder
④ Have dark amber urine

27 What intervention by the nurse is most important when feeding a patient with hemi-paresis?
① Ensure that food is pureed.
② Provide foods that require chewing.
③ Offer fluids with each mouthful of food.
④ Allow time to empty the mouth between spoonfuls.
TEST-TAKING TIP ● Identify the options that contain opposites.

28 When urine output is less than fluid intake, the nurse can expect the patient to:
① Gain weight
② Void frequently
③ Become jaundiced
④ Experience nausea

29 What should the nurse do if a patient's pulse is full and bounding?
① Measure the patient's urine specific gravity.
② Monitor the patient's serum glucose.
③ Lower the head of the patient's bed
④ Check the flow rate of the IV fluids.
TEST-TAKING TIP ● Identify the unique option.

30 Which vitamin facilitates the absorption of iron?
① D
② C
③ A
④ K

31 Which foods should be removed from a tray for a patient on a full liquid diet?
① Ice cream
② Prune juice
③ Cream of Wheat
④ Raspberry gelatin
TEST-TAKING TIP ● Identify the words in the stem that suggest negative polarity.

32 Which factor related to normal aging influences the nutritional status of elderly people?
① Additional need for milk products
② Greater production of gastric acid
③ Deterioration in taste perception
④ Increased need for kilocalories
TEST-TAKING TIP ● Identify the unique option.

33 A patient is experiencing diarrhea and needs to replace potassium. The nurse recognizes that additional teaching is necessary when the patient says that he should increase his intake of:
① Orange juice
② Warm tea

③ Bananas
④ Raisins

TEST-TAKING TIP ● Identify the phrase in the stem that suggests negative polarity. Identify the option that is unique.

34 Patients with cancer are at risk for altered nutrition, less than body requirements, because:
① Anabolism exceeds catabolism
② Of an inability to use nutrients
③ Cancer increases metabolic demands
④ Cell division causes an altered nitrogen balance

TEST-TAKING TIP ● Identify the clang association in the stem.

35 Which patient statement would indicate the need for further teaching about vitamins?
① "Vitamins can be taken without the fear of toxic effects."
② "I don't need vitamins because I eat a balanced diet."
③ "Some vitamins can be manufactured by the body."
④ "My need for vitamins will change as I get older."

TEST-TAKING TIP ● Identify the phrase in the stem that suggests negative polarity.

Rationales

1 **TEST-TAKING TIP** ● Options 1 and 3 are opposites.
   ① Meals served with regular-size portions can be overwhelming for the patient experiencing nausea.
 * ② Small quantities of food frequently offered establish small realistic goals for the patient without being overwhelming.
   ③ The patient could be nauseated for a long period of time; adequate food and fluid must be ingested to meet physiological needs
   ④ A full liquid diet will not reduce the nausea.

2 **TEST-TAKING TIP** ● The word FIRST is the key word in the stem that sets a priority.
   ① Removing the water pitcher from the bedside could upset the patient if the reason were not explained first.
   ② Measuring intake and output (I&O) would be done after I&O is explained to the patient.
   ③ Posting signs violates a patient's right to privacy; signs directing the staff should not be posted at the bedside where they can be seen and violate patient confidentiality.
 * ④ Before any procedure is implemented, the patient has the right to know what is being done and why; knowledge increases compliance.

3 **TEST-TAKING TIP** ● Options 3 and 4 deny the patient's right to have food and drinks served at warm temperatures. Option 3 contains the word "just," which is a specific determiner. Option 1 is patient centered.
 * ① Patients with mental and physical deficits need assistance with warm drinks; this prevents burns.
   ② The use of plastic utensils will not prevent spilling hot liquids; plastic utensils need to be used only when utensils need to be discarded to prevent the transmission of microorganisms.
   ③ Patients have a right to have a variety of foods presented at different temperatures; serving only cold drinks would violate a patient's rights.
   ④ Hot foods should be served hot and cold foods should be served cold.

4 **TEST-TAKING TIP** ● Options 1 and 4 are opposites in relation to the values presented in the offered options.
   ① 30 mL is only 1 ounce
   ② 90 mL is only 3 ounces
   ③ 240 mL is only 8 ounces
 * ④ 270 mL is equal to 9 ounces; 1 oz is equal to 30 mL

5 **TEST-TAKING TIP** ● The word LEAST is the key word in the stem that indicates a negative polarity.
 * ① The patient is receiving a special diet that has been carefully calculated, and all food on the tray should be eaten.
   ② Identifying low-calorie snacks is supportive; it helps reduce caloric intake.
   ③ Encouraging thorough chewing and slow eating makes a meal take longer and allows more time for the body to feel full.
   ④ Recognizing weight loss is supportive; progress should be identified to provide motivation.

6 TEST-TAKING TIP ● The word **most** is the key word in the stem that sets a priority.
① A urometer is used to measure the specific gravity of urine, not the volume of urine.
* ② A graduate is a special container with volume markings on the side for measuring fluid; of all the options offered, it is the most accurate way to measure urine.
③ Using the markings on a urine collection bag is not as accurate as using a marked graduate because the plastic that the bag is made of often stretches, making the markings inaccurate.
④ Bedpans are designed to collect excreta when a person cannot use a toilet or commode, not to measure urine volume.

7 TEST-TAKING TIP ● Options 1 and 2 are opposites.
① Dehydration occurs when fluid intake is insufficient, not when calories are insufficient.
② Edema can occur if the patient experiences an inadequate intake of protein, not just in response to a reduction in caloric intake.
* ③ When calories are insufficient to meet metabolic needs, the body catabolizes fat, resulting in weight loss.
④ Sleeping is not directly related to a decreased caloric intake; however, a patient who is anemic may easily tire from an inadequate intake of iron or folic acid.

8 TEST-TAKING TIP ● The word "always" in Option 2 is a specific determiner. Options 1 and 3 deny the right of the patient to ingest foods of different temperatures.
① Patients have a right to a variety of foods, textures, and temperatures within the ordered diet.
② This would contaminate the food.
③ Foods should not be mixed; they should be served separately so that they retain their own flavor and texture.
* ④ Waiting for hot foods to cool slightly is the safest and most practical action; once hot food loses some of its heat, it will be safe to eat.

9 TEST-TAKING TIP ● The word "most" is the key word in the stem that sets a priority.
* ① Providing assistance will best keep the patient focused on the task of eating.
② Feeding the patient when only assistance is necessary would contribute to feelings of dependence.
③ Although this is something the nurse may do to orient the patient, the patient may forget or not understand the explanation; explaining where everything is on the tray will not keep the patient focused on eating during the meal.
④ Although family members can be helpful, it is the responsibility of the staff to care for the patient, not the family members. This request may precipitate guilt feelings in family members who are unable to help.

10 TEST-TAKING TIP ● The word *normal* is the clue in the stem. Options 1 and 4 are opposites among the volumes presented in the options.
① This is an inadequate intake to maintain life.
② Same as #1.
* ③ 2000 mL is an average daily intake necessary to maintain normal fluid balance.
④ 3000 mL is more fluid intake than the body needs for normal fluid balance.

11 TEST-TAKING TIP ● The word "primarily" is the key word in the stem that sets a priority.
① White meat contains less fat than red meat; however, white meat contains more fat than legumes.
* ② Legumes, such as beans, peas, and lentils, contain the least amount of cholesterol and

fat of the options presented and are high in protein, which is necessary for tissue regeneration.

③ Although shrimp is a protein source, it is high in cholesterol, which should be avoided because it contributes to plaque formation.

④ Milk contains fat, which contributes to plaque formation in atherosclerosis.

12 TEST-TAKING TIP ● The word "deficiency" is a significant clue in the stem.

① Calcium contributes to neuromuscular excitability, and therefore lowered calcium levels, not a deficiency in vitamin K, can result in muscle cramps and tetany.

② A deficiency in vitamin K does not contribute to the occurrence of infection. Vitamins A and C help build resistance to infection.

③ A deficiency of vitamin B_1 (thiamine), not vitamin K, can result in tachycardia and cardiac enlargement; deficiencies in calcium, magnesium, and potassium can also contribute to cardiac problems.

* ④ Vitamin K is essential for promthrombin formation and blood clotting; if a patient is deficient in vitamin K, the patient will experience a prolonged clotting time and be prone to bleeding.

13 TEST-TAKING TIP ● The word "loss" is a significant clue in the stem. The word "most" is the word in the stem that sets a priority.

① Although fluid is lost from a draining pressure ulcer, it is the loss of protein in that fluid that has the most serious implication.

② Weight loss is related to inadequate caloric intake, not the presence of a draining pressure ulcer.

* ③ Protein loss is a serious concern when a patient has a draining pressure ulcer. A patient can lose as much as 50 grams of protein daily from a draining pressure ulcer; this is a large percentage of the normal daily requirement of 60 grams of protein for women and 70 grams of protein for men. Patients with draining pressure ulcers should ingest 2 to 4 times the normal daily requirements of protein to rebuild epidermal tissue.

④ Leukocyte counts increase in response to the threat of infection. If a pressure ulcer is infected, the leukocyte count will increase, not decrease. Decreased white blood cell levels are a response to bone marrow depression caused by a stress other than a pressure ulcer.

14 TEST-TAKING TIP ● Options 2 and 3 are equally plausible because decreased energy levels are often associated with a decrease in the metabolic rate.

* ① When the number of calories ingested does not meet the body's energy requirements, the patient will catabolize body fat for energy and lose weight.

② Metabolism relates to the biochemical reactions that take place within the body to meet energy needs; metabolism will increase and decrease in response to the energy demands placed on the body, not as a result of a low-calorie diet.

③ Not all people experience a decrease in energy in response to a low-caloric diet; however, all individuals break down adipose tissue for energy if caloric intake is insufficient to meet metabolic needs. Age, body size, body and environmental temperatures, growth, sex, nutritional state, and emotional state affect energy levels.

④ A well-balanced low-calorie diet should contain adequate vitamins, requiring no supplementation.

15 TEST-TAKING TIP ● Options 1 and 4 are opposites in relation to the age groups in the options offered.

* ① During the first year of life the infant grows at a faster pace than at any other devel-

opmental stage; infants double their birth weight by 6 months and triple their birth weight during the first year.

② The preschool (3- to 5-year-old) child's growth rate is slower than during the first year of life; the preschool child gains only another 7 to 12 pounds in addition to the four times the birth weight gained during the first three years.

③ Although the adolescent goes through a dramatic physical growth spurt that reflects significant changes in height, weight, dentition, and skeletal and sexual development, it is not as spectacular as three times the growth rate seen in the first year of life.

④ No physical growth occurs when a person is over 65 years of age; different parts of the body begin to degenerate, and functions slow.

16 TEST-TAKING TIP ● Five adaptations are offered as symptoms of dehydration: the presence of straw-colored urine, a thready radial pulse, decreased skin turgor, and two different urine specific gravity measurements. If you are able to identify that straw-colored urine is unrelated to dehydration, you will be able to eliminate Options 1 and 2. If you are able to identify that decreased skin turgor is reflective of dehydration, you will be able to narrow the correct answer to Options 2 and 3. The specific gravity measurements in Options 3 and 4 are not helpful when trying to eliminate distractors using the duplicate fact strategy. However, recognize that they are opposites.

① Although a thready pulse would indicate a decrease in circulating blood volume and is a symptom of dehydration, a straw-colored urine indicates that the patient is probably in fluid balance.

② Skin turgor refers to normal skin fullness or the ability of the skin and underlying tissue to return to their regular position after being pinched and lifted; when there is decreased skin turgor due to dehydration, the skin remains pinched or "tented" for a longer period of time than well-hydrated skin after it is released. However, straw-colored urine is what is expected, and it indicates that the patient is probably in fluid balance.

③ A thready pulse would indicate a decrease in circulating blood volume and is a symptom of dehydration. However, a specific gravity of 1.015 is within the normal range of 1.010 to 1.030 and would indicate that the patient is in normal fluid balance.

* ④ Skin turgor refers to normal skin fullness or the ability of the skin and underlying tissue to return to their regular position after being pinched and lifted. When there is decreased skin turgor because of dehydration, the skin remains pinched or "tented" for a longer period of time than well-hydrated skin after it is released. A urine specific gravity of 1.035 would indicate that the patient has a fluid volume deficit.

17 ① Whole milk, depending on the brand, has approximately 6 to 130 mg of sodium per 8 oz.

* ② Fresh fruits contain the least amount of sodium per serving of the options presented; most fresh fruits such as apples, pears, bananas, peaches, and cantaloupe contain under 10 mg of sodium per serving.

③ White bread, depending on the brand, has approximately 55 to 225 mg of sodium per slice.

④ Fresh vegetables such as peas, beans, carrots, broccoli, cauliflower, corn, and celery contain approximately 40 mg of sodium per serving.

18 TEST-TAKING TIP ● The word "most" is the key word in the stem that sets a priority. Five different foods are offered as foods that contribute to healing. If you are able to identify the one food that would most contribute to healing, you have narrowed the correct answer to two options. If you are able to identify the one food that is the least beneficial to the healing process, then you have narrowed the correct answer to two options.

① Although French toast contains some egg coating, which is protein, it does not contain the amount of protein in two poached eggs. Oatmeal does not contain protein or vitamin C.

② Although orange juice contains vitamin C, which contributes to wound healing, oatmeal does not contain protein or vitamin C, which are essential for building cells and therefore for wound healing.

③ Each poached egg contains 6 to 8 g of protein; protein contains the amino acids necessary for building cells and therefore for wound healing. Although French toast contains some egg coating, which is protein, it does not contain vitamin C.

* ④ This is the best combination of foods in the options offered. Each egg contains 6 to 8 g of protein; protein contains the amino acids necessary for building cells and therefore for wound healing. Orange juice contains vitamin C, which contributes to wound healing. Vitamin C promotes collagen formation, enhances iron absorption, and maintains capillary wall integrity.

19 TEST-TAKING TIP ● The word "essential" is the significant clue in the stem.

① Ascorbic acid (vitamin C) promotes collagen formation, enhances iron absorption, and maintains capillary wall integrity.

② Riboflavin (vitamin B_2) functions as a coenzyme in the metabolism of carbohydrates, fats, amino acids, and alcohol.

* ③ Folic acid (vitamin B_9), or folacin, promotes the maturation of red blood cells. When red blood cells fall below the normal range of 4.2 million/mm^3 for women and 4.7 million/mm^3 for men, a person is considered anemic.

④ Thiamine (vitamin B_1) performs as a coenzyme in the metabolism of carbohydrates, fats, amino acids, and alcohol.

20 TEST-TAKING TIP ● The word MUST is the word in the stem that sets a priority.

① Because an intralipid solution is a concentrated source of nonprotein kilocalories, it would be desirable for an infusion pump to be used; however, an infusion pump does not have to be used because the solution can flow by gravity.

* ② This action ensures that the intralipid solution is NOT mixed with a dextrose–amino acid solution. If they are mixed, the fat emulsion will break down.

③ If an intralipid solution is mixed with a dextrose–amino acid solution, the fat emulsion will break down; the solutions must not be administered through the same line.

④ The solutions can be run at the same time but through different lines.

21 TEST-TAKING TIP ● Four adaptations are offered as undesirable results associated with an increase in the flow rate of TPN above the prescribed rate: osmotic diuresis, hypoglycemia, dumping syndrome, and electrolyte imbalance. If you are able to identify one adaptation that is unrelated to an increased TPN rate, you will be able to eliminate two distractors. If you are able to identify the two adaptations that are unrelated to an increased TPN rate, you will arrive at the correct answer. If you are able to identify one adaptation that is related to an increase in a TPN rate above the prescribed rate, you have narrowed the correct answer to two options.

① The hypertonic TPN solution pulls intracellular and interstitial fluid into the intravascular compartment; the increased blood volume increases circulation to the kidneys, raising urinary output (osmotic diuresis). Because of the high glucose load of total parenteral nutrition (TPN), hyperglycemia, not hypoglycemia, could result.

② Because of the high glucose load of TPN, hyperglycemia, not hypoglycemia, could result. Dumping syndrome, the sensation caused by rapid entry of food from the stomach into the jejunum, could occur with a tube feeding, not TPN.

* ③ The hypertonic TPN solution pulls intracellular and interstitial fluid into the intravascular compartment; the increased blood volume increases circulation to the kidneys, raising urinary output (osmotic diuresis). Potassium and sodium imbalances are common among clients receiving TPN. Therefore, TPN rates must be carefully controlled.

④ Potassium and sodium imbalances are common among clients receiving TPN. However, dumping syndrome occurs with a tube feeding, not TPN.

22 TEST-TAKING TIP ● The word "after" is the clue in the stem.

① Inserting 30 mL of air into the tube is part of the procedure that is done to determine if the tube is in the stomach before a tube feeding is initiated.

* ② Instilling 30 mL of water flushes the tube, preventing future blockage from a buildup of formula along the sides of the lumen of the tube.

③ Checking the gastrostomy site is not necessarily part of the procedure for administering a gastrostomy tube feeding. Checking the dressing site should be done routinely, such as every 4 hours or every shift. Also, the insertion site should be inspected routinely.

④ After a gastrostomy tube feeding, the patient should remain in a sitting or slightly elevated right lateral position for 30 minutes to limit the risk of aspiration.

23 TEST-TAKING TIP ● The word "most" is the key word in the stem that sets a priority.

* ① Iron is essential to the formation of hemoglobin, a component of red blood cells, which is lost in menstrual blood.

② Supplemental iron is unnecessary for active adolescents.

③ Supplemental iron is unnecessary in growing children (1 to 13 years). However, infants (birth to 1 year) who are breast fed need some iron supplementation from 4 to 12 months of age, and formula-fed infants need iron supplementation throughout the first year of life.

④ Supplemental iron is unnecessary for healthy elderly men.

24 TEST-TAKING TIP ● The word "most" is the key word in the stem that sets a priority.

① Although this is important, the body can survive longer without this nutrient than it can without water.

② Same as #1.

③ Same as #1.

* ④ The most basic nutrient needed is water; 60 percent of the body weight of an average healthy male is water. Women have a smaller percentage of water than men because they have proportionately more fat; all body processes require an adequate fluid balance in the body.

25 TEST-TAKING TIP ● The word GREATEST is the key word in the stem that sets a priority.

① Although postmenopausal women can benefit from calcium supplementation to prevent osteoporosis, the need is not as high as in pregnant women.

② This group of individuals does not have an increased need for calcium; an adequate intake of milk and dairy products will meet minimum daily requirements for calcium.

* ③ Calcium should be increased 50 percent to an intake of 1.2 grams per day to provide calcium for fetal tooth and bone development; this is essential during the third trimester when fetal bones are mineralized.

④ Same as #2.

26 ① Reduced fluid intake will produce a concentrated urine with a specific gravity higher than 1.025.

② This is not true; the bladder will still fill to the patient's normal capacity before there is a perceived need to void.

③ This is caused by a neurological problem; it is a loss of the sensation of fullness that leads to distention from overfilling.

* ④ This is the color of urine when fluid intake is below 1500 to 2000 mL per day; the urine is concentrated.

27 **TEST-TAKING TIP** ● Options 1 and 2 are opposites. Both can be eliminated or one of them is the correct answer. In this question, both can be eliminated from consideration.

① This may not be necessary; the patient may only need more time to thoroughly manage the food.

② This could be unsafe and possibly unreasonable because the patient has a reduced ability to move the muscles on one side of the face necessary for chewing.

③ This would increase the risk of aspiration; fluid is more difficult to control than pureed food when swallowing.

* ④ This minimizes food buildup in the mouth; also it does not rush the patient.

28* ① Fluid has mass; when fluid is retained the patient will gain weight; a patient can gain 6 to 8 pounds before edema can be identified through inspection.

② The opposite is true.

③ This is related to impaired liver function, not fluid volume excess.

④ This is not a common sign of fluid volume excess.

29 **TEST-TAKING TIP** ● Option 4 is unique. It is the only option that does not specifically refer to the patient.

① This reflects the concentrating ability of the kidneys, not the cardiovascular system.

② A full, bounding pulse is not related to hyperglycemia or hypoglycemia; a weak, thready pulse is a late sign of diabetic ketoacidosis.

③ A full, bounding pulse may indicate hypervolemia; in this compromised patient, lowering the head of the bed could impede respiration and is therefore contraindicated.

* ④ IV solutions are administered directly into the intravascular compartment; if the IV flow rate is excessive, it could cause a full, bounding pulse.

30 ① Vitamin D is essential for adequate absorption and utilization of calcium in bone and tooth growth; it does not facilitate the absorption of iron.

* ② Ascorbic acid (vitamin C) helps to change dietary iron to a form that can be absorbed by the body.

③ Vitamin A is essential for the growth and maintenance of epithelial tissue, maintenance of night vision, and promotion of resistance to infection, not the absorption of iron.

④ Vitamin K is essential for the formation of prothrombin, which prevents bleeding, not the absorption of iron.

31 **TEST-TAKING TIP** ● This question is really asking, what food is NOT permitted on a full liquid diet? Therefore, this stem has negative polarity.

① This food changes its state from a solid to a liquid at room temperature.

② This is a fluid and is permitted on a full liquid diet.

* ③ This is considered solid food and is not permitted on a full liquid diet.

④ Same as #1.

32 TEST-TAKING TIP ● Options 1, 2, and 4 have positive words (greater, additional, and increased). Options 3 includes the word "deterioration," which has a negative connotation.

① The need for food from all levels of the Food Guide Pyramid remains the same regardless of age; an increase in milk products is needed only by elderly people who are at risk for osteoporosis.

② Gastric secretions decrease, not increase, with aging.

* ③ Taste perception decreases because of atrophy of the taste buds and a reduced sense of smell; sweet and salty tastes are lost first.

④ The need for kilocalories decreases because of the lower metabolic rate and the reduction in physical activity associated with elderly people.

33 TEST-TAKING TIP ● In the stem, the phrase "additional teaching is necessary" suggests a negative polarity. Of the options provided, this question is asking, what food or drink contains the LEAST amount of potassium? Option 2 is unique because Options 1, 3, and 4 relate to fruit and tea is not a fruit.

① One cup of orange juice contains approximately 475 mg of potassium.

* ② One cup of tea contains approximately 35 mg of potassium.

③ One banana contains approximately 450 mg of potassium.

④ One ounce (⅛ of a cup) of raisins contains approximately 200 mg of potassium.

34 TEST-TAKING TIP ● The word "cancer" in both the stem and Option 3 is a clang association.

① The opposite is true. With cancer, catabolism exceeds anabolism.

② The ability to utilize nutrients is not impaired. Cancerous tumors use excessive amounts of the body's available nutrients.

* ③ The energy required to support the rapid growth of cancerous cells increases the metabolic demands one-and-a-half to two times the resting energy expenditure.

④ The byproducts of cell breakdown cause a negative nitrogen balance.

35 TEST-TAKING TIP ● The phrase "the need for further teaching" indicates negative polarity. This question is asking, which option contains inaccurate information?

* ① This is an inaccurate statement; therefore, this option is the correct answer to this question. Megadoses of vitamins can cause hypervitaminosis and result in toxicity.

② Ordinarily healthy persons who eat a variety of foods that reflect a balanced diet should not need vitamin supplements.

③ Vitamin D can be synthesized by the body. In addition to dietary intake, vitamin D is manufactured in the skin.

④ The National Academy of Sciences, National Academy Press, Washington, DC publishes the Recommended Dietary Allowances (RDA) of vitamins. The list reflects age, gender, and physical status differences.

256 Meeting Patients' Elimination Needs

This section includes questions related to bowel and bladder needs. Topics associated with intestinal elimination include incontinence, constipation, diarrhea, enemas, bowel retraining, and medications. Questions also focus on needs associated with urinary elimination and include topics such as incontinence, bladder retraining, toileting, and external and indwelling urinary catheters.

Questions

1   To help maintain continence in a patient who has urge incontinence, the nurse should:
   ① Toilet the patient every 4 hours
   ② Toilet the patient immediately on request
   ③ Encourage the patient to stay near the bathroom
   ④ Ask the patient to limit fluid intake in the evening

   TEST-TAKING TIP ● Identify the word in the stem that is a clue. Identify the patient-centered option. Identify the option that contains a specific determiner.

2   When a patient has an indwelling urinary catheter (Foley catheter), the collection bag should be:
   ① Carried at waist level when walking
   ② Kept below the level of the pelvis
   ③ Changed at least once a week
   ④ Clamped when out of bed

   TEST-TAKING TIP ● Identify the options that are opposites.

3   Which action would be included in <u>all</u> bladder-retraining programs?
   ① Providing 3000 mL of fluids a day
   ② Toileting the patient before sleep
   ③ Toileting the patient every 2 hours
   ④ Using adult incontinence underwear

   TEST-TAKING TIP ● Identify the clue in the stem. Identify the option that contains a specific determiner.

4   When changing a condom catheter (external catheter) for an uncircumcised patient, the nurse must:
   ① Replace the foreskin over the glans
   ② Lubricate the distal penis and glans
   ③ Secure the condom directly behind the glans
   ④ Retract the foreskin behind the head of the glans

   TEST-TAKING TIP ● Identify the clue in the stem. Identify the options that are opposites.

5   When a patient complains about being constipated, the nurse should encourage ingestion of:
   ① Fresh fruit and whole wheat bread
   ② Baked chicken and plain yogurt
   ③ Whole wheat bread and chicken
   ④ Plain yogurt and fresh fruit

   TEST-TAKING TIP ● Identify the clue in the stem. Identify the duplicate facts among the options.

6 Women have a higher incidence of urinary tract infections than men because:
① Urine flows toward the rectum via gravity when women void
② Women use bedpans, which harbor microorganisms
③ Women must sit rather than stand when toileting
④ The rectum is closer to the urinary meatus

TEST-TAKING TIP ● Identify the equally plausible options.

7 Which action comes <u>first</u> in a bladder-retraining program?
① Offer to toilet the patient every 2 hours.
② Design an individual schedule for toileting.
③ Provide adequate fluids during the retraining period.
④ Assess the patient's ability to cooperate with the program.

TEST-TAKING TIP ● Identify the key word in the stem that sets a priority. Identify the option that contains a specific determiner.

8 When administering a tap water enema, the nurse recognizes that its primary purpose is to:
① Minimize intestinal gas
② Cleanse the bowel of stool
③ Reduce abdominal distention
④ Decrease the loss of electrolytes

TEST-TAKING TIP ● Identify the clue in the stem. Identify the key word in the stem that sets a priority.

9 A confused patient asks to use the bathroom even though the patient was toileted only 30 minutes ago. The nurse should:
① Request a physician's order for an indwelling urinary catheter
② Persuade the patient to try to hold it for at least 1 hour
③ Take the patient to the bathroom and assist the patient
④ Remind the patient of the recent trip to the bathroom

TEST-TAKING TIP ● Identify the options that deny the patient's feelings, concerns, and needs. Identify the option that is patient centered.

10 The physician orders a 750-mL tap water enema. To best promote acceptance of the volume ordered, the nurse should:
① Administer the fluid slowly and have the patient take shallow breaths
② Place the patient in the left lateral position and administer the fluid slowly
③ Have the patient take shallow breaths and keep the fluid at body temperature
④ Keep the fluid at body temperature and place the patient in the left lateral position

TEST-TAKING TIP ● Identify the key word in the stem that sets a priority. Identify the duplicate facts among the options.

11 The patient at the highest risk for developing diarrhea would be a patient who:
① Is physically active
② Drinks a lot of fluid
③ Eats whole-grain cereal
④ Is experiencing emotional problems

TEST-TAKING TIP ● Identify the key word in the stem that sets a priority. Identify the clue in the stem.

12 Foods likely to cause constipation are:
① Cheese and broccoli
② Yogurt and cheese
③ Broccoli and peas
④ Peas and yogurt
TEST-TAKING TIP ● Identify the duplicate facts among the options.

13 Which solution would be most effective for a patient who is unable to tolerate a large amount of enema fluid?
① Hypertonic fluid
② Normal saline
③ Soapy water
④ Tap water
TEST-TAKING TIP ● Identify the key word in the stem that sets a priority.

14 Which patient is at greatest risk for developing constipation?
① Toddler
② Adolescent
③ Pregnant woman
④ Middle-aged man
TEST-TAKING TIP ● Identify the key word in the stem that sets a priority.

15 To best facilitate the expelling of urine from the bladder, the patient should be taught:
① Pelvic floor contractions
② The Valsalva maneuver
③ The Kegel exercises
④ The Credé method
TEST-TAKING TIP ● Identify the key word in the stem that sets a priority.

16 What normal physiological function of the body helps prevent infection?
① Elevated temperature
② High pH of gastric secretions
③ Flushing action of urine flow
④ Rapid peristalsis in the large intestine
TEST-TAKING TIP ● Identify the clues in the stem.

17 When preparing a soapsuds enema for an adult, how much fluid should the nurse use?
① 250 mL
② 500 mL
③ 750 mL
④ 900 mL
TEST-TAKING TIP ● Identify the options that are opposites.

18 The nurse understands that diarrhea causes skin irritation mainly because it consists of:
① Bile
② Fiber
③ Fluid
④ Enzymes
TEST-TAKING TIP ● Identify the key word in the stem that sets a priority.

19 When administering an enema, the nurse should position the patient in the:
① Dorsal recumbent position
② Right lateral position
③ Back-lying position
④ Left Sims' position

TEST-TAKING TIP ● Identify the equally plausible options. Identify the options that are opposites.

20 When planning for the elimination needs of a patient, the nurse recognizes which statement as being accurate?
① Peristalsis increases after ingesting food.
② Emotional stress initially decreases peristalsis.
③ Straining during defecation reduces intrathoracic pressure.
④ Enema solutions should be administered at room temperature.

TEST-TAKING TIP ● Identify the options that are opposites.

21 While sitting on a toilet, a person leans forward when attempting to defecate. Leaning forward specifically promotes fecal elimination because it:
① Raises intra-abdominal pressure
② Uses gravity to facilitate elimination
③ Elongates the curves of the sigmoid colon
④ Relaxes the internal and external rectal sphincters

TEST-TAKING TIP ● Identify the clues in the stem.

22 When voiding, the male patient on bed rest should be positioned in the:
① Supine position
② Lateral position
③ Contour position
④ Standing position

TEST-TAKING TIP ● Identify the option that denies the patient's needs.

23 In the morning a patient has a loose watery stool. To determine if the patient has diarrhea, the nurse should ask:
① "What did you have for dinner last night?"
② "Have you been drinking a lot of fluid lately?"
③ "When was the last time you had a similar stool?"
④ "Are you experiencing any abdominal cramping?"

24 When administering a soapsuds enema, the nurse understands the primary action of the soapsuds is to:
① Increase pressure in the bowel
② Distend the lumen of the bowel
③ Irritate the bowel mucosa
④ Exert an osmotic effect

TEST-TAKING TIP ● Identify the key word in the stem that sets a priority. Identify the equally plausible options.

25 Which is the safest form of a laxative?
① Softening agent
② Osmotic cathartic
③ Bulk-forming agent
④ Stimulant cathartic

TEST-TAKING TIP ● Identify the key word in the stem that sets a priority.

26 A patient has a full body cast and is experiencing diarrhea. This patient is at risk for developing:
① Pressure ulcers
② A wound infection
③ Urinary incontinence
④ A hip flexion contracture

27 Which is the most important nursing intervention to promote a successful bladder retraining program?
① Offering the patient a full liquid diet
② Following the scheduled program exactly
③ Maintaining a strict intake and output record
④ Washing the patient's perineal area every shift

TEST-TAKING TIP ● Identify the word in the stem that sets a priority.

28 When does stress incontinence occur?
① With a urinary tract infection
② In response to emotional strain
③ As a result of increased intra-abdominal pressure
④ When a specific volume of urine is in the bladder

29 A patient on a bladder retraining program is incontinent at 1:00 AM every morning. What should the nurse do to promote continence?
① Toilet the patient at 1:30 AM.
② Toilet the patient at 12:30 AM.
③ Limit the patient's intake of fluid after dinner.
④ Position the call bell within easy reach of the patient.

TEST-TAKING TIP ● Identify the options that are opposites.

30 What is the purpose of a rectal tube?
① Administer an enema
② Dilate the anal sphincters
③ Relieve abdominal distention
④ Visualize the intestinal mucosa

31 Which nursing diagnosis is associated with a physiological need of a patient with a colostomy?
① Knowledge deficit
② Body Image disturbance
③ Ineffective Individual coping
④ Risk for Impaired Skin Integrity

TEST-TAKING TIP ● Identify the clue in the stem.

32 Which statement about a tap water enema is accurate?
① The volume of instilled water stimulates peristalsis.
② The water can cause excessive interstitial fluid loss.
③ The surface tension of water is reduced by soapsuds.
④ The hypertonic nature of the water irritates the intestinal mucosa.

TEST-TAKING TIP ● Identify the clue in the stem.

33 What should the nurse assess for when establishing the patency of a urinary retention catheter (Foley)?
① Color
② Clarity

③ Volume
④ Constituents

34 What should the nurse do first when applying a condom catheter (Texas catheter) to an uncircumcised patient?
① Trim excessive pubic hair.
② Wash the genitals with soap and water.
③ Apply the adhesive band with a spiral motion.
④ Ensure that the foreskin is over the head of the glans.
TEST-TAKING TIP ● Identify the word in the stem that sets a priority.

35 Which is the most common psychological concern of patients who have a colostomy?
① Maintenance of skin integrity
② Frequency of defecation
③ Ability to control odor
④ Consistency of feces
TEST-TAKING TIP ● Identify the clue in the stem.

1 **TEST-TAKING TIP** ● The word "urge" is the significant clue in the stem. Option 2 is patient centered. The word "every" in Option 1 is a specific determiner.

① Toileting the patient every 2 hours is more appropriate; only when the patient feels the need to void does the patient need to be immediately toileted.

* ② Toileting the patient immediately on request supports continence because the person with urge incontinence must immediately void or lose control.

③ Encouraging the patient to stay near a bathroom promotes isolation and should be avoided.

④ Limiting fluid intake during the early evening and night may be part of a toileting program to provide uninterrupted sleep; however, it does not address the patient's need to urinate immediately when feeling the urge to void.

2 **TEST-TAKING TIP** ● Options 1 and 2 are opposites. The phrase "waist level" in Option 1 is opposite to "below the level of the pelvis" in Option 2. Waist level is above the pelvis.

① Carrying an indwelling urinary catheter collection bag at waist level is too high; it allows urine to flow back into the bladder, which can contribute to a urinary tract infection.

* ② Positioning an indwelling urinary catheter collection bag below the level of the pelvis prevents urine from flowing back into the bladder; urine flows away from the bladder by gravity.

③ Collection bags are attached to an indwelling urinary catheter and should not be disconnected; an indwelling urinary catheter and bag should be changed only every 4 to 6 weeks unless crusting or sediment collects on the inside of the tubing.

④ It is unnecessary to clamp an indwelling urinary catheter when a patient is out of bed; this is unsafe for some patients.

3 **TEST-TAKING TIP** ● The word <u>all</u> is a clue in the stem. The word "every" in Option 3 is a specific determiner.

① The volume of scheduled fluid intake is based on the individual needs of the patient.

* ② All patients on bladder-retraining programs are toileted before sleep; this contributes to less urine volume in the bladder during the night.

③ Toileting is not automatically implemented every 2 hours but is based on the individual needs of the patient.

④ Incontinence pads are generally not encouraged when implementing a bladder-retraining program; however, devices used depend on the individual needs and preferences of the patient.

4 **TEST-TAKING TIP** ● The word "uncircumcised" is the significant clue in the stem. Options 1 and 4 are opposites.

* ① Perineal care should be provided when changing a condom catheter; in the uncircumcised male, if the foreskin is not replaced to the normal position, it can tighten around the shaft of the penis, causing local edema and pain.

② The distal end of the penis should not be lubricated; this could prevent the condom device from securely staying in place.

③ A condom catheter (external catheter) should be secured further up the shaft of the penis, not immediately behind the glans.

④ The foreskin must be returned to its natural position over the head of the glans; if the foreskin is not returned to the normal position, it can tighten around the shaft of the penis, causing local edema and pain.

5 TEST-TAKING TIP ● The word "constipated" is a clue in the stem. Four different foods are offered as foods that will help a patient who is constipated. If you are able to identify one food that would contribute to increasing peristalsis and the relief of constipation, you can narrow the correct answer to two options. If you are able to identify one food that is not beneficial for the relief of constipation, you can delete two options.

* ① Fresh fruit and whole wheat bread contain roughage, which adds bulk to stool, increasing peristalsis.

② Chicken does not contain roughage and plain yogurt contains yeast, not roughage.

③ Although whole wheat bread contains roughage, chicken does not contain much roughage.

④ Although fresh fruit contains roughage, plain yogurt contains yeast, not roughage.

6 TEST-TAKING TIP ● Options 2 and 3 are equally plausible because both options indicate a fact related to the unique toileting needs of women.

① Urine that flows toward the rectum rarely causes infection; however, bacteria from the rectal area can cause urinary tract infections.

② If properly cleaned after use, bedpans are not a source of infection.

③ The act of sitting when toileting should not increase the prevalence of infection.

* ④ Stool wiped toward the urinary meatus can cause urinary tract infections; *Escherichia coli*, a common bacteria in stool, causes urinary tract infections.

7 TEST-TAKING TIP ● The word <u>first</u> is the key word in the stem that sets a priority. The word "every" in Option 1 is a specific determiner.

① Toileting times are not automatically every 2 hours; they are individually designed based on the patient's voiding pattern and fluid intake.

② Designing an individual toileting schedule would be the second step once it is determined that the patient is motivated and able to participate and cooperate with the program.

③ Although providing fluids would be done eventually, the nurse first must assess the patient's ability to participate and cooperate with the program.

* ④ Assessment is the initial step in a bladder-retraining program. The patient must be an active participant in a bowel- or bladder-retraining program and therefore a patient's cooperation is an essential component of a successful program.

8 TEST-TAKING TIP ● The words "tap water" are a significant clue in the stem. The word "primary" is the key word in the stem that sets a priority.

① A Harris drip (Harris flush), not a tap water enema, helps evacuate intestinal gas.

* ② A tap water enema introduces a hypotonic fluid into the intestinal tract; distention and pressure against the intestinal mucosa increase peristalsis and evacuation of stool.

③ The primary purpose of a tap water enema is to distend the bowel to stimulate the evacuation of stool; however, a secondary gain is that it can reduce abdominal distention because flatus and stool are evacuated along with the enema solution.

④ A tap water enema would increase, not decrease, the loss of electrolytes because it is a hypotonic solution.

9 TEST-TAKING TIP ● Options 2 and 4 deny the patient's feelings, concerns, and needs. Option 3 is the patient-centered option.

① Indwelling urinary catheters should not be used to avoid incontinence or the inconvenience of frequently toileting a patient.

② The patient has a need to void now; an hour is too long to postpone urination.

* ③ Immediate toileting meets the patient's need to void and promotes continence. Whether the patient is confused or not, the patient should be taken to the bathroom.

④ Reminding the patient that voiding occurred 30 minutes ago denies the patient's need to void now.

10 TEST-TAKING TIP ● The word "best" is the word in the stem that sets a priority. Four different interventions are offered as actions that will help a patient retain a 750-mL tap water enema. If you are able to identify one action that is based on a scientific principle associated with tap water enema administration, you can narrow the correct answer to two options. If you are able to identify one action that is not based on a scientific principle associated with tap water enema administration, you can delete two options from consideration.

① Although the slow administration of enema fluid minimizes the probability of intestinal spasm and premature evacuation of the enema fluid before a therapeutic effect is achieved, encouraging shallow breaths, versus deep breaths, may contribute to an increase in intra-abdominal pressure, which can interfere with the retention of enema fluid.

* ② Both of these actions contribute to retention of enema fluid. In the left lateral position the sigmoid colon is below the rectum, facilitating the instillation of fluid. The slow administration of enema fluid minimizes the probability of intestinal spasm and premature evacuation of the enema fluid before a therapeutic effect is achieved.

③ Encouraging shallow breaths and using a 98.6°F enema fluid interfere with the instillation and retention of enema fluid. Encouraging deep breaths, not shallow breaths, helps to prevent patients from holding their breath, which increases intra-abdominal pressure; increased intra-abdominal pressure can interfere with the instillation and retention of enema fluid. A water temperature of 98.6°F is too cool and can contribute to intestinal muscle spasm and discomfort.

④ Although placing the patient on the left side positions the sigmoid colon below the rectum, facilitating the instillation of fluid, a water temperature of 98.6°F is too cool and can contribute to intestinal muscle spasm and discomfort. Enema water temperature should be between 105 and 110°F because warm fluid promotes muscle relaxation and comfort.

11 TEST-TAKING TIP ● The word "highest" is the key word in the stem that sets a priority. The word "risk" in the stem is a significant clue.

① Physical activity, fluid, and fiber help to prevent constipation, not precipitate diarrhea.

② Same as #1.

③ Same as #1.

* ④ Psychological stress initially increases intestinal motility and mucus secretion, promoting diarrhea.

12 TEST-TAKING TIP ● Four foods are offered as likely to cause constipation: peas, yogurt, broccoli, and cheese. If you can identify one food that helps prevent constipation, you will be able to eliminate two distractors. If you are able to identify two foods that help prevent constipation or contribute to constipation, you will arrive at the correct answer. If you can identify one food that is constipating, then you can narrow the correct answer to two options.

① Although cheese can contribute to constipation, broccoli facilitates defecation.

* ② Dairy products are low in roughage and lack bulk; they produce too little waste to stimulate the defecation reflex. Low-residue foods move more slowly through the intestinal tract, permitting increased fluid uptake from stool, resulting in hard-formed stools and constipation.

③ Both broccoli and peas provide bulk that increases peristalsis, which facilitates defecation, not constipation.

④ Although yogurt contributes to constipation, peas provide bulk (undigested residue), which facilitates fecal elimination, not constipation.

13 TEST-TAKING TIP ● The word "most" in the stem sets a priority.

*   ① A hypertonic enema solution uses only 120 to 180 mL of solution. Hypertonic solutions expend osmotic pressure that draws fluid out of the interstitial spaces; fluid pulled into the colon and rectum distend the bowel, causing an increase in peristalsis resulting in bowel evacuation.

② A normal saline enema is isotonic and requires a volume of 500 mL to 750 mL to be effective; the volume of fluid, not its saline content, causes an evacuation of the bowel.

③ A soapsuds enema requires a volume of 750 to 1000 mL of fluid to result in an effective evacuation of the bowel.

④ A tap water enema usually requires a minimum of 750 mL of water, which is a large volume of fluid.

14 TEST-TAKING TIP ● The word "greatest" is the key word in the stem that sets a priority.

① A toddler usually drinks adequate fluids, eats a regular diet, and is very active; these activities contribute to bowel elimination, not the development of constipation.

② The adolescent usually eats more food than at earlier stages and may complain of indigestion, not constipation; indigestion is a response to increased gastric acidity that occurs during adolescence.

*   ③ The growing size of the fetus exerts pressure on the rectum and bowel, which impinges on intestinal functioning, contributing to constipation; the decreased motility causes increased absorption of water, promoting constipation.

④ As people advance through middle adulthood, they are at risk for gaining weight, not developing constipation.

15 TEST-TAKING TIP ● The word "best" is the key word in the stem that sets a priority.

① Pelvic floor exercises help to enable the person to start and stop a stream of urine. These exercises include trying to stop and start the stream of urine while urinating; they also include the contraction and relaxation of the anterior and posterior muscles of the pelvic floor while in a sitting or standing position. Pelvic floor exercises are done to improve one's ability to retain urine, not pass urine.

② Although some people use the Valsalva maneuver to expel urine, the majority of people use this maneuver to expel stool. The Valsalva maneuver is accomplished when people hold their breath during a forced expiration and contract the abdominal muscles; the levator ani muscle relaxes and permits feces to be expelled.

③ Kegel exercises are isometric exercises of the pubococcygeal muscle, which is the muscle associated with the urinary sphincter; this improves one's ability to retain urine, not pass urine.

*   ④ The Credé method stimulates micturition and relaxation of the urethral sphincter via external manual compression of the bladder.

16 TEST-TAKING TIP ● The words "normal" and "prevent" are important clues in the stem.

① An elevated temperature results from released toxins in the presence of infection; it may help to limit an already existing infection, but it will not prevent an infection.

② Gastric secretions are acidic and have a low pH.

* ③ Microorganisms congregate at the urinary meatus because it is warm, moist, and dark; when urine flows down the urethra and out the urinary meatus, the force of the urine carries microorganisms away, which minimizes ascending infections.

④ Rapid peristalsis results in diarrhea; this is not a normal physiological function.

17 TEST-TAKING TIP ● Options 1 and 4 are opposites.

① 250 mL is too little fluid to stimulate effective evacuation of the bowel when administering a soapsuds enema to an adult. This is the recommended amount the nurse might administer to a toddler.

② 500 mL is too little fluid to stimulate effective evacuation of the bowel when administering a soapsuds enema to an adult. This is the recommended amount of solution the nurse might administer to a large school-age child or small adolescent.

③ 750 mL is too little fluid to stimulate effective evacuation of the bowel when administering a soapsuds enema to an adult. This is the recommended amount of solution the nurse might administer to an average-sized adolescent. This is also the amount of volume suggested for saline and tap water enemas.

* ④ 900 mL is the average suggested volume of soapsuds solution administered to an adult to stimulate effective evacuation of the bowel. It provides enough fluid to fill the bowel and apply pressure to the intestinal mucosa, along with the irritating action of soap on the mucosa, to stimulate defecation.

18 TEST-TAKING TIP ● The word "mainly" sets a priority in the stem.

① Although irritating, bile is not as caustic as digestive enzymes. The components of bile include bilirubin, bile salts, cholesterol, lecithin, fatty acids, electrolytes, and water. Bile salts are the components that are metabolically active; bile salts increase fat solubility, which enables fat to pass through the intestinal wall.

② Fiber is bulk that distends the lumen of the bowel and, by itself, does not irritate the skin.

③ Although fluid on the skin contributes to tissue irritation, it is the enzymes in feces that erode the skin.

* ④ Enzymes are biological catalysts that speed up chemical reactions; digestive enzymes break down nutrient cells by hydrolysis and therefore are also extremely caustic to the skin.

19 TEST-TAKING TIP ● Options 1 and 3 are equally plausible. Options 2 and 4 are opposites.

① This position would not use the natural curve of the rectum and sigmoid colon to facilitate instillation of the enema solution.

② Same as #1.

② Same as #1.

* ④ The left Sims' position permits the solution to flow downward by gravity along the natural curve of the rectum and sigmoid colon, promoting instillation and retention of the solution.

20 TEST-TAKING TIP ● Options 1 and 2 are opposites.

* ① Food or fluid that enters and fills the stomach or the duodenum stimulates peristalsis; this is called the "gastrocolic reflex" or "duodenocolic reflex."

② Emotional stress initially increases peristalsis because the bowel will evacuate its contents to prepare for the "fight." As the sympathetic nervous system increases its control, in its response to stress, the action of the parasympathetic nervous system decreases. The parasympathetic nervous system stimulates peristalsis, and as its action decreases, peristalsis will also decrease.

③ Straining at defecation will increase, not decrease, intrathoracic pressure. Forcible exhalation against the closed glottis (the Valsalva maneuver) raises the intrathoracic pressure, which impedes venous return. When the breath is released, blood is propelled through the heart, causing tachycardia and an increased blood pressure; a reflex bradycardia immediately follows. With an increase in intrathoracic pressure, immediate tachycardia and bradycardia occur in succession; patients with heart problems can experience a cardiac arrest.

④ Enema solutions should be administered slightly above body temperature (105 to 110°F).

21 TEST-TAKING TIP ● The words "leaning forward" and "fecal elimination" are the clues in the stem.

* ① When a person leans forward while in the sitting position, intra-abdominal pressure increases, facilitating fecal elimination.

② The sitting position, not leaning forward, uses gravity to facilitate defecation.

③ When sitting and leaning forward, the curves of the sigmoid colon remain unchanged.

④ Relaxation of the internal and external rectal sphincters may result in response to this position; however, this relaxation of sphincters is in response to increased intra-abdominal pressure.

22 TEST-TAKING TIP ● Option 4 denies the patient's needs because standing is contraindicated. The stem informs you that the patient is on "bed rest."

① The supine position would not promote passage of urine through the urinary tract via gravity.

* ② The lateral position is the closest to the normal standing position used by men to void; the hips and knees are almost extended and the hands can be used for self-care.

③ In the contour position the hips and knees are flexed and the perineal area is dependent in relation to the knees; placing and using a urinal in this position without spilling would be difficult.

④ Standing is contraindicated because the patient is not allowed out of bed.

23 ① Although this answer may help determine if food influenced the patient's intestinal elimination, it will not further assess the presence of diarrhea.

② Excessive fluid intake is excreted through the kidneys, not the intestinal tract.

* ③ Diarrhea is the defecation of liquid feces and increased frequency of defecation; there should be more than one episode to be considered diarrhea.

④ Cramping is not specific to diarrhea; it can also be associated with constipation and intestinal obstruction.

24 TEST-TAKING TIP ● The word "primary" is the key word in the stem that sets a priority. Options 1 and 2 are equally plausible because they are both related to the effects of the volume of the enema solution, not the action of soapsuds, on the intestinal mucosa.

① This is the rationale for using a particular volume of fluid, not soapsuds.

② Same as #1.

* ③ Soap is an irritant that stimulates the intestinal mucosa, precipitating peristalsis and the eventual evacuation of stool.

④ Exerting an osmotic effect is the rationale for using a hypertonic solution, not soapsuds.

25 TEST-TAKING TIP ● The word "safest" is the key word in the stem that sets a priority.

① Softening (surfactant) laxatives reduce the surface tension of feces through detergent action; softening agents allow feces to absorb water and fat, causing stool to become large, soft, and easy to defecate. They inhibit fluid absorption and stimulate secretion of fluid and electrolytes into the intestinal lumen. These laxatives can contribute to fluid and electrolyte imbalances.

② Osmotic (saline) laxatives are the most rapid-acting and powerful laxatives. They draw water into the fecal mass via osmotic action; the body attempts to dilute the salt preparation in the cathartic by pulling water, causing lubrication and increased bulk of stool. Osmotic cathartics can contribute to electrolyte imbalances.

* ③ Bulk-forming laxatives absorb water and increase intestinal bulk. Bulk stretches the intestinal walls, stimulating peristalsis; bulk-forming agents are the least irritating and therefore the safest cathartic.

④ Stimulant (contact) laxatives cause local irritation to the intestinal mucosa; they also minimize absorption of water in the large intestines. Stimulant cathartics are more caustic than bulk-forming agents in stimulating peristalsis.

26 * ① In addition to being warm and moist, feces contain enzymes that promote tissue breakdown.

② There is no wound present to become infected; fecal material could cause a vaginal or urinary tract infection, not a wound infection.

③ Immobility may precipitate urinary retention rather than incontinence; diarrhea would not promote urinary incontinence.

④ With a full body cast the hips are usually in extension.

27 TEST-TAKING TIP ● The word "most" in the stem sets a priority.

① This is unnecessary; a balanced diet plus adequate fluid is all that is necessary.

* ② Toileting times are purposely scheduled in response to times of fluid intake and the patient's normal elimination pattern; to increase success, the schedule must be followed exactly.

③ Intake and output is unnecessary; it is not the volume of fluids/urine that is of interest but the pattern of voiding relative to fluid intake.

④ Although important, this will not contribute to a patient's ability to regain continence.

28 ① Urinary tract infections often cause frequency as a result of irritation of the mucosal wall of the bladder, not stress incontinence

② Emotional strain may cause frequency, not stress incontinence.

* ③ This is correct. When intra-abdominal pressure increases, the person with stress incontinence will experience urinary dribbling, or an approximate loss of 50 cc of urine or less.

④ This occurs in reflex incontinence, not stress incontinence.

29 TEST-TAKING TIP ● Options 1 and 2 are opposites. Consider these options carefully; either they are both distractors or one of them is the correct answer. In this item, one of them is the correct answer.

① This would be too late.

* ② This provides the patient with the opportunity to void before becoming incontinent; if effective, it will contribute to self-esteem and personal hygiene.

③ This will decrease the volume of urine voided; it will not prevent incontinence.

④ The patient may not have time to communicate the need to void or may be unaware of the need to void before being incontinent.

30 ① An enema tube is used to administer an enema; a rectal tube is different and is used to provide temporary relief from flatulence.

② This is not the purpose of a rectal tube.

    * ③ A rectal tube is inserted past the anal sphincters (6 inches in an adult and 2 to 4 inches in a child) and left in place for 30-minute intervals every 2 to 3 hours; rectal tubes are used to promote the passage of flatus, reducing abdominal distention.

    ④ A rectal tube is not designed to visualize the intestinal mucosa; a proctoscope is an instrument designed to visualize the rectum, a sigmoidscope is an instrument designed to visualize the sigmoid colon and the rectum, and a colonscope is an instrument designed to visualize the entire large intestine

31 TEST-TAKING TIP ● The word "physiological" is the clue in the stem; it modifies the word "need." The word "skin" in Option 4 is the only word in any of the options that relates to anatomy or physiology.

    ① A knowledge deficit is a psychosocial problem, not a physiological problem.

    ② Concern about body image is a psychological problem, not a physiological problem.

    ③ An inability to cope with a colostomy is a problem in the affective domain and is not considered a physiological problem.

    * ④ This is correct. Risk for Impaired Skin Integrity is a common physiological problem of a patient with a colostomy.

32 TEST-TAKING TIP ● The words "tap water" modify the word "enema." This is the clue in the stem.

    * ① The large volume of instilled tap water distends the colon, which in turn stimulates peristalsis; it also softens feces.

    ② Tap water is hypotonic, which can cause water intoxication and fluid and electrolyte imbalance, not excessive interstitial fluid loss.

    ③ Soap is not added to a tap water enema. Soapsuds enemas work by irritating the mucosa and distending the colon, which in turn stimulates peristalsis.

    ④ A tap water enema is hypotonic, not hypertonic.

33 ① The color of urine would reflect urine concentration or a reaction to specific drugs or foods, not whether or not the catheter was patent.

    ② The clarity of urine would indicate the presence of such products as red or white blood cells, bacteria, prostatic fluid, or sperm. Clarity would not indicate whether or not a catheter was patent.

    * ③ If urine volume was minimal or nonexistent it would indicate that the catheter was obstructed or the patient was not excreting urine.

    ④ The constituents of urine such as pus, mucus, or blood would indicate possible pathology, not whether or not the catheter was patent.

34 TEST-TAKING TIP ● The word "first" in the stem sets a priority because it is asking what is the most important thing to do for this patient.

    ① This is unnecessary. An external drainage condom catheter can be applied without having to trim pubic hair.

    * ② This is an essential first step in applying an external drainage condom catheter. Perineal care minimizes the risk of skin irritation and excoriation after the condom is applied.

    ③ Applying and securing the external drainage condom catheter in place occurs only after perineal care is provided and the foreskin is returned to normal position if the patient is uncircumcised. There are various types of external drainage condom catheters, and each has its own design to secure the condom in place. A spiral adhesive band is just one type.

    ④ During perineal care the foreskin is retracted back from the tip of the penis so that the area under the foreskin can be washed. Once washing is completed, the foreskin is returned to its normal position down and over the glans.

35 TEST-TAKING TIP ● The word "psychological" is the clue in the stem. It modifies the word "concern."

  ① The maintenance of skin integrity and frequency of defecation are physiological concerns, not a psychological concern.

  ② Same as #1.

* ③ This is a major psychological concern of people with a colostomy because the odor can be offensive.

  ④ The consistency of feces varies according to the location of the stoma along the intestinal tract. Stool that is less firm generally has more odor. It is the odor that is of more concern than the consistency.

Meeting Patients' Oxygen Needs

This section includes questions related to assessments and interventions associated with normal and abnormal respiratory and circulatory function. Questions focus on topics such as preventing aspiration, providing emergency care for aspiration, techniques and devices that assess or increase respiratory or circulatory function, and assessments and interventions associated with the administration of oxygen.

Questions

1 To prevent aspiration while administering physical hygiene to a patient receiving a nasogastric tube feeding, the nurse should:

① Lower the height of the bag
② Seek additional assistance
③ Slow the rate of flow
④ Shut the feeding off

TEST-TAKING TIP ● Identify the equally plausible options.

2 A patient walking in the hall complains of sudden chest pain. The initial intervention by the nurse should be to:

① Take the patient's vital signs
② Perform a detailed pain assessment
③ Walk the patient back to bed slowly
④ Get a chair so the patient can sit and rest

TEST-TAKING TIP ● Identify the key word in the stem that sets a priority. Identify the options that are opposites.

3 When oxygen therapy via nasal cannula is ordered for a patient, the <u>first</u> action by the nurse is to:

① Post an "oxygen in use" sign on the door to the room
② Adjust the oxygen level before applying the cannula
③ Explain the rules of fire safety and oxygen use
④ Lubricate the nares with water-soluble jelly

TEST-TAKING TIP ● Identify the key word in the stem that sets a priority. Identify the equally plausible options.

4 To prevent aspiration after meals by a patient who has difficulty swallowing, the nurse should *first:*

① Position the patient in the low-Fowler's position
② Provide a pitcher of water at the bedside
③ Encourage mouth care when necessary
④ Inspect the mouth for pocketed food

TEST-TAKING TIP ● Identify the key word in the stem that sets a priority. Identify the clue in the stem.

5 What should the nurse do first when a patient chokes on food and is unable to speak?

① Initiate the abdominal thrust maneuver.
② Clap between the scapulae several times.
③ Instruct the patient to swallow forcefully.
④ Wait to see if the patient can cough up the obstruction.

TEST-TAKING TIP ● Identify the key word in the stem that sets a priority.

6 A patient with a history of chronic respiratory disease begins to have difficulty breathing. The adaptations that are the most serious would be:
① Orthostatic hypotension when rising and the need to sit in the orthopneic position
② The need to sit in the orthopneic position and wheezing sounds on inspiration
③ Wheezing sounds on inspiration and mucus tinged with frank red streaks
④ Mucus tinged with frank red streaks and chest pain

TEST-TAKING TIP ● Identify the key word in the stem that sets a priority. Identify the duplicate facts among the options.

7 What is the MOST important intervention by the nurse to increase both circulation and respiration in a patient?
① Encourage the use of a spirometer
② Reposition the patient every 2 hours
③ Massage bony prominences with lotion
④ Teach the patient to cough and breathe deeply

TEST-TAKING TIP ● Identify the key word in the stem that sets a priority. Identify the clue in the stem.

8 To prevent skin breakdown around the nares of a patient receiving oxygen through a nasal cannula, the nurse should:
① Remove the tubing for 15 minutes every 2 hours
② Turn and position the patient every 2 hours
③ Provide oral hygiene whenever necessary
④ Adjust the cannula so it is comfortable

TEST-TAKING TIP ● Identify the clue in the stem. Identify the specific determiners in the options.

9 While eating, a patient clutches the upper chest with the hands, appears unable to breathe, and has a frightened facial expression. The most appropriate initial intervention by the nurse is to:
① Perform the abdominal thrust maneuver
② Slap the patient three times on the back
③ Ask the patient to attempt to speak
④ Start artificial respirations

TEST-TAKING TIP ● Identify the key word in the stem that sets a priority. Identify the unique option.

10 The following adaptations are observed by the nurse when giving mouth care to an unconscious patient. Which assessment requires immediate intervention?
① A gurgling sound the patient makes when breathing
② Saliva drooling out of the patient's mouth
③ Sordes found on the patient's hard palate
④ Lesions on the patient's gingival tissue

TEST-TAKING TIP ● Identify the key word in the stem that sets a priority. Identify the equally plausible options.

11 Which are the most appropriate sites of the patient's body to assess for the presence of cyanosis?
① Lower legs and around the mouth
② Fingernail beds and around the mouth

③ Conjunctiva of the eyes and lower legs

④ Fingernail beds and conjunctiva of the eyes

TEST-TAKING TIP ● Identify the key word in the stem that sets a priority. Identify the duplicate facts among the options.

12 To reduce anxiety related to the use of oxygen via a nasal cannula, the nurse should say to the patient:

① "Keep calm and everything will be OK."

② "This is oxygen; it will help your breathing."

③ "This is a treatment that was ordered by your doctor."

④ "The oxygen will be discontinued as soon as possible."

TEST-TAKING TIP ● Identify the clue in the stem. Identify the option that denies the patient's feelings, concerns, and needs.

13 When a patient complains of being short of breath, the nurse's initial action should be to:

① Obtain the vital signs

② Raise the head of the bed

③ Administer emergency oxygen

④ Encourage pursed-lip breathing

TEST-TAKING TIP ● Identify the key word in the stem that sets a priority.

14 When a patient has moderate chronic impaired peripheral arterial circulation, the nurse should assess for:

① Yellow toenails and cool extremities

② Cyanosis of the feet and yellow toenails

③ Cool extremities and continuous leg discomfort

④ Continuous leg discomfort and cyanosis of the feet

TEST-TAKING TIP ● Identify the clues in the stem. Identify the duplicate facts among the options.

15 What is the primary purpose of implementing chest physiotherapy?

① Alter the tracheobronchial mucosa

② Change the consistency of sputum

③ Mobilize secretions

④ Induce coughing

TEST-TAKING TIP ● Identify the key word in the stem that sets a priority.

16 When monitoring a patient's status through pulse oximetry, the nurse is assessing the patient's:

① Heart rate

② Vital signs

③ Blood pressure

④ Oxygen saturation

TEST-TAKING TIP ● Identify the clue in the stem.

17 Which individual would most likely have life-threatening complications when experiencing a respiratory infection?

① Infant

② Adolescent

③ Elderly person

④ School-age child

TEST-TAKING TIP ● Identify the key word in the stem that sets a priority.

18 A patient receiving oxygen by nasal cannula exhibits an elevation of the clavicles on inspiration. When you are assisting the patient with activities of daily living, which intervention should take priority?
① Monitoring the respiratory rate every hour
② Increasing the O_2 flow rate
③ Promoting bed rest
④ Pacing care

TEST-TAKING TIP ● Identify the key word in the stem that sets a priority. Identify the clue in the stem.

19 Which individual would have the most dramatic increase in the need for oxygen?
① Pregnant woman
② Man with a fever
③ Person exercising
④ Patient receiving general anesthesia

TEST-TAKING TIP ● Identify the key word in the stem that sets a priority. Identify the clue in the stem.

20 To BEST evaluate peripheral circulation in the lower extremities, the nurse should assess the:
① Pedal pulses and presence of hair on the toes
② Capillary refill in the toenails and pedal pulses
③ Presence of hair on the toes and blood pressure
④ Blood pressure and capillary refill in the toenails

TEST-TAKING TIP ● Identify the key word in the stem that sets a priority. Identify the duplicate facts among the options.

21 Which is most effective for maintaining a patent airway?
① Active coughing
② Incentive spirometry
③ Nebulizer treatments
④ Abdominal breathing

TEST-TAKING TIP ● Identify the key word in the stem that sets a priority.

22 A common local adaptation to pressure is specifically referred to as:
① Edema
② Ischemia
③ Orthopnea
④ Hypovolemia

TEST-TAKING TIP ● Identify the clues in the stem.

23 When inserting an oral airway, the initial action of the nurse is to:
① Insert it with the tip end toward the tongue
② Sweep the oral cavity with a gloved finger
③ Ensure that the airway is the correct size
④ Lightly lubricate the lips with Vaseline

TEST-TAKING TIP ● Identify the key word in the stem that sets a priority. Identify the clue in the stem.

24 The adequacy of tissue oxygenation is most accurately measured by:
① Hematocrit values
② Hemoglobin levels

③ Arterial blood gases
④ Pulmonary function tests

TEST-TAKING TIP ● Identify the key word in the stem that sets a priority. Identify the clue in the stem.

25 The nurse recognizes that a patient's fever can result in tachypnea because of the:
① Increase in the metabolic rate
② Need to retain carbon dioxide
③ Decrease in carbon dioxide levels
④ Attempt to compensate for respiratory alkalosis

TEST-TAKING TIP ● Identify the equally plausible options.

26 During meals, what should the nurse do to help prevent aspiration when a patient has difficulty swallowing?
① Allow enough time between spoonfuls for chewing.
② Cut up the meat and mix it with the soft food.
③ Encourage fluids before swallowing food.
④ Promote conversation during meals.

27 When do wheezing breath sounds occur?
① When fluid is in the lung
② When sitting in the orthopneic position
③ When air moves through a narrowed airway
④ When the pleural sack rubs against the lung surface

TEST-TAKING TIP ● Identify the unique option.

28 Kussmaul respirations are:
① Rapid and deep
② Slow and regular
③ Slow and shallow
④ Rapid and irregular

TEST-TAKING TIP ● Identify the duplicates in the options. Identify the options that are opposites.

29 The nurse assesses that the patient understands diaphragmatic breathing when the patient says, "I should:
① Feel my abdomen flatten on inspiration."
② Raise my shoulders and chest when I inhale."
③ Hold my breath for 3 seconds at the height of inspiration."
④ Use my hands to put pressure against the abdomen when I inhale."

TEST-TAKING TIP ● Identify the equally plausible options.

30 Anemia is related to the body's inability to:
① Transport oxygen
② Exchange oxygen
③ Perfuse oxygen
④ Diffuse oxygen

TEST-TAKING TIP ● Identify the unique option.

31 What should the nurse do when applying a pulse oximetry sensor to the patient's finger?
① Send the patient's rings home with a family member.
② Remove frosted nail polish from the patient's nails.

③ Keep the hand continuously elevated on a pillow.
④ Shave any hair on the finger.

32 When teaching the use of an incentive spirometer, the nurse knows that the patient understands its correct use when the patient:
① Snaps the ball to the top of the chamber and exhales rapidly
② Seals the lips around the tube and inhales rapidly
③ Inhales slowly and keeps the ball floating
④ Gets the ball to rise and lower smoothly

TEST-TAKING TIP ● Identify the equally plausible options. Identify the options that are opposites.

33 A productive cough means that the cough:
① Causes pain
② Results in sputum
③ Interferes with breathing
④ Gets progressively worse

34 What should the nurse do when implementing nasotracheal suctioning in an adult?
① Apply intermittent suction during removal of the catheter.
② Use wall suction with a pressure setting below 90 mm Hg.
③ Suction the nasotracheal area after the oropharyngeal area.
④ Employ continuous negative pressure during insertion of the catheter.

TEST-TAKING TIP ● Identify the options that are opposites.

35 Which principle is associated with the exchange of respiratory gases?
① Osmosis
② Invasion
③ Diffusion
④ Decompression

Rationales

1 TEST-TAKING TIP ● Options 1 and 3 are equally plausible.

① Lowering the height of the feeding bag will only slow the rate of the feeding, not halt its flow. Continuing the feeding adds a volume of fluid that could be aspirated.

② Seeking additional assistance will not reduce the risk of aspiration; the feeding should be temporarily halted.

③ The feeding needs to be shut off, not just slowed. The administration of an additional volume of feeding could promote aspiration.

* ④ Shutting off the feeding reduces the risk of aspiration by temporarily halting the administration of an additional volume of feeding.

2 TEST-TAKING TIP ● The word "initial" is the key word in the stem that sets a priority. Options 3 and 4 are opposites.

① Taking the vital signs at this time will delay meeting the heart's need to rest; vital signs can be taken once the patient is sitting.

② Performing a detailed assessment at this time will delay meeting the heart's need to rest. A detailed assessment can be done after the patient is sitting.

③ Walking should be avoided; activity increases the demand on the heart and will increase the pain.

* ④ Reducing activity decreases the oxygen demand on the heart; this will in turn reduce the pain. After the activity is interrupted, the nurse should obtain the vital signs and conduct a thorough pain assessment.

3 TEST-TAKING TIP ● The word <u>first</u> is the key word in the stem that sets a priority. Options 2 and 4 are equally plausible because both are distractors associated with possible "hands-on" intervention.

① Posting an "oxygen in use" sign on the door to the room is done after explaining the procedure to the patient.

② Adjusting the oxygen level before applying the cannula is done after explaining the procedure to the patient.

* ③ Safety is a priority; patients must understand the rules related to oxygen use and that oxygen supports combustion.

④ Lubricating the nares with water-soluble jelly is unnecessary; the nares should be cleaned only with soap and water daily and whenever necessary.

4 TEST-TAKING TIP ● The word *first* is the key word in the stem that sets a priority. The word "after" is the clue in the stem.

① A high-Fowler's, not a low-Fowler's, position facilitates food retention by gravity.

② Fluids can be easily aspirated by a patient who has difficulty swallowing; fluid intake should be supervised.

③ Frequent mouth care will provide comfort, but it will not reduce the risk of aspiration.

* ④ Inspecting the mouth for pocketed food is an important action; patients who have difficulty swallowing do not recognize that food can become trapped in the buccal cavity and eventually be aspirated.

5 TEST-TAKING TIP ● The word "first" is the key word in the stem that sets a priority.

* ① The abdominal thrust maneuver pushes trapped air out of the lungs, forcing out the obstructing food.

② Clapping between the scapulae could cause aspirated food to lodge deeper in the respiratory passages.

③ Swallowing forcefully will not clear the airway. Attempting to swallow could cause the food to move further down the respiratory passages.

④ Once it has been assessed that the patient cannot speak, the abdominal thrust maneuver should immediately be done. Waiting would be unsafe because an inability to speak indicates that the person is experiencing a total obstruction. Letting the patient cough would be appropriate if there were a partial obstruction.

6 TEST-TAKING TIP ● The word "most" is the key word in the stem that sets a priority. Five adaptations are offered in different combinations for you to choose from as being the most serious in this situation. If you are able to identify one adaptation that appears in two options and that is most serious, you can narrow the correct answer to two options. If you can identify one adaptation that appears in two options and is least significant, you can eliminate two distractors from consideration.

① Orthostatic hypotension when rising and the need to sit in the orthopneic position are common responses by individuals with chronic respiratory disease. Encouraging the patient to rise slowly from a lying to a sitting position and from a sitting to a standing position permits the circulation to adjust to the change in position, thereby minimizing orthostatic hypotension. Elevating the head helps breathing by lowering the abdominal organs by gravity, which allows the diaphragm to contract more efficiently on inspiration.

② The need to sit in the orthopneic position and wheezing on inspiration are common adaptations to respiratory disease. Raising the head of the bed helps breathing by lowering the abdominal organs by gravity, which allows the diaphragm to contract more efficiently on inspiration. Wheezing on inspiration is a response to an increase in airway resistance.

③ Although mucus tinged with frank red streaks is an uncommon adaptation to respiratory disease, wheezing is a common response.

* ④ Mucus tinged with frank red streaks and chest pain are not common responses to chronic respiratory disease and should be reported immediately.

7 TEST-TAKING TIP ● The word MOST is the key word in the stem that sets a priority. The word "both" in the stem is a clue. The intervention chosen must increase both circulation and respiration.

① The use of a spirometer helps only to prevent respiratory complications.

* ② Repositioning the patient every 2 hours prevents fluid from collecting in lung fields, which can contribute to infection, thereby promoting respirations; it also relieves pressure and increases activity, thereby promoting circulation.

③ Massaging bony prominences with lotion only increases local circulation.

④ Coughing and deep breathing only help to prevent respiratory complications.

8 TEST-TAKING TIP ● The word "prevent" is the clue in the stem. The word "every" in Options 1 and 2 is a specific determiner.

① Fifteen minutes is too long to remove oxygen from a patient who needs oxygen.

② Turning and positioning the patient every 2 hours will prevent pressure ulcers of dependent areas of the body, but will not prevent skin breakdown around the nares.

③ Although adequate oral hygiene is important, it is mainly pressure that causes skin breakdown; oral hygiene alone does not prevent skin breakdown.

* ④ If the cannula comfortably rests in the nares, it will avoid pressure on the nares that can cause skin breakdown.

9 TEST-TAKING TIP ● The word "initial" is the key word in the stem that sets a priority. Option 3 is unique because it is the only option that is an assessment. Options 1, 2, and 3 are all actions.

① The abdominal thrust maneuver is done once it is determined that the patient cannot speak.

② Slapping the patient on the back could cause the aspirated object to lodge deeper in the respiratory passages.

* ③ If the patient can speak, the airway is partially obstructed. If the patient cannot speak, the airway is totally obstructed. Assessment is the priority because each of the situations requires a different intervention.

④ The patient is not in respiratory arrest; food is lodged in the respiratory passages.

10 TEST-TAKING TIP ● The word "immediate" is the key word in the stem that sets a priority. Options 3 and 4 are equally plausible.

* ① A gurgling sound when breathing indicates fluid or mucus in the airway; it may be necessary to suction this material out of the airway of an unconscious patient if the patient does not cough.

② Saliva drooling out of the mouth is expected; saliva is exiting from the mouth and away from the airway and therefore is not a threat.

③ Although this indicates a need for more frequent mouth care, it is not an emergency.

④ Same as #3.

11 TEST-TAKING TIP ● The word "most" is the key word in the stem that sets a priority. Four different sites are presented as preferred sites to assess for the presence of cyanosis. If you are able to identify one site that is the least desirable to use for the assessment of cyanosis, you can dismiss two distractors and narrow the correct answer to two options. If you are able to identify one site that is desirable to use for the assessment of cyanosis, you can narrow the correct answer to two options.

① Although the lips and mucous membranes of the mouth are a primary site to assess for early signs of oxygen deprivation, the lower legs are not the first sites to assess for systemic oxygen deprivation.

* ② Nail beds, lips, and mucous membranes of the mouth are the primary sites to assess for early signs of oxygen deprivation.

③ Pallor of the conjunctiva of the eyes, not cyanosis, reflects reduced oxyhemoglobin. The lower legs are not the first sites to assess for systemic oxygen deprivation.

④ Although the nail beds are a primary site to assess for early signs of oxygen deprivation, pallor of the conjunctiva of the eyes, not cyanosis, reflects reduced oxyhemoglobin.

12 TEST-TAKING TIP ● The word "reduce" is a clue in the stem. Option 1 denies the patient's feelings because it is false reassurance.

① This statement is false reassurance and minimizes the patient's concerns.

* ② This statement provides information and an explanation; this generally reduces fear and increases understanding and compliance. Oxygen therapy generally helps patients breathe more easily, and therefore the statement is not false reassurance.

③ This statement does not address the fact that patients have a right to know what is being done and why.

④ This statement could intensify fear if the oxygen is not discontinued; also, it does not provide an explanation.

13 TEST-TAKING TIP ● The word "initial" is the key word in the stem that sets a priority.

  ① Obtaining vital signs does not facilitate breathing.

* ② Raising the head of the bed immediately facilitates breathing. Gravity aids the expansion of the thoracic cavity during inspiration; it also reduces the resistance of body weight on the chest during inspiration.

  ③ Administering oxygen can further compromise respiratory compensatory mechanisms if the cause of the shortness of breath is related to chronic obstructive pulmonary disease (COPD); oxygen can precipitate CO_2 narcosis in patients with COPD.

  ④ Pursed-lip breathing helps patients with emphysema to exhale; diaphragmatic breathing is most effective for patients who are short of breath.

14 TEST-TAKING TIP ● The words "moderate chronic" and "peripheral arterial" are the clues in the stem. Four different adaptations are offered as common responses to prolonged impaired peripheral arterial circulation. If you are able to identify one adaptation that is common to this situation, you can narrow the correct answer to two options. If you are able to identify one response that is unrelated to prolonged impaired peripheral arterial circulation, you can eliminate two distractors and narrow the correct answer to two options.

* ① Yellow toenails and cool extremities both indicate impaired arterial circulation; there is a decrease in oxygen and nutrients to the area.

  ② Although yellow toenails indicate prolonged tissue hypoxia of the extremity, it is ascending pallor from the toes and descending rubor from the knees, not cyanosis, that reflects impaired peripheral arterial perfusion.

  ③ Although cool extremities reflect inadequate peripheral arterial perfusion, intermittent claudication (leg pain on activity), not continuous leg discomfort, is a clinical manifestation of chronic peripheral arterial disease.

  ④ Leg discomfort related to decreased peripheral arterial perfusion is usually intermittent and associated with activity (intermittent claudication). Pallor ascending from the toes and rubor descending from the knees, not cyanosis, reflect moderate chronic impaired peripheral arterial perfusion.

15 TEST-TAKING TIP ● The word "primary" is the key word in the stem that sets a priority.

  ① Chest physiotherapy will not alter the tracheobronchial mucosa; it mobilizes secretions within the respiratory tract.

  ② Chest physiotherapy does not change the consistency of sputum; it mobilizes sputum. An increased fluid intake will promote a less tenacious sputum.

* ③ Chest percussion (cupping, clapping) and vibration mechanically dislodge tenacious secretions from the walls of the respiratory passages, while postural drainage drains secretions from various lung segments via gravity. Collectively these actions are called "chest physiotherapy."

  ④ The mobilization of secretions may eventually induce coughing. Coughing without the mobilization of secretions is less effective and may even be futile.

16 TEST-TAKING TIP ● The "ox" in "oximetry" is the clue in the stem because it is similar to the word "oxygen" in Option 4. Both words begin with the letters "ox."

  ① When palpating a peripheral pulse or auscultating the apical rate, the nurse obtains the heart rate.

  ② The vital signs include temperature, pulse, respirations, and blood pressure, not oxygen saturation.

  ③ Blood pressure is one of the vital signs, and it reflects the pressure exerted by the blood as it pulsates through the arteries.

* ④ Oxygen saturation via pulse oximetry measures the degree to which hemoglobin is saturated with oxygen; it provides some indication of the efficiency of lung ventilation.

17 TEST-TAKING TIP ● The word "most" is the key word in the stem that sets a priority.

* ① Because of the small lumens of their respiratory passages, infants and toddlers are at serious risk for airway obstruction, which can develop as a result of respiratory tract infection.
② Healthy adolescents usually do not encounter any serious event in response to respiratory infections.
③ Although the respiratory system undergoes changes during the aging process and there is a decline in respiratory function, complications related to infection are usually not as acute, sudden, or life threatening as with infants.
④ Healthy school-age children usually do not encounter any serious event in response to respiratory infections; however, school-age children generally have respiratory infections more frequently because of exposure to other children.

18 TEST-TAKING TIP ● The word "priority" is the key word in the stem that sets a priority. The phrase "elevation of the clavicles on inspiration" is the clue in the stem.

① The respiratory rate is not the only sign that should be monitored when a patient is receiving oxygen; other changes in vital signs can occur, such as increased depth and character of respirations, increased pulse rate, and elevated blood pressure. Apprehension, decreased level of consciousness, decreased ability to concentrate, behavioral changes, pallor, cyanosis, dizziness, dyspnea, and increased fatigue are also signs that indicate hypoxia. These assessments should be made before, during, and after care is delivered.
② Determining the oxygen flow rate is a dependent function of the nurse and requires a physician's order. In addition, too high a concentration of oxygen will diminish the respiratory drive in some people (individuals with chronic obstructive pulmonary disease) because the respiratory drive is stimulated by a decrease in oxygen in the blood, not an increase in blood carbon dioxide levels.
③ Whether a patient is or is not on bed rest, care will still need to be delivered in a manner that minimizes exertion; pacing care is the priority.
* ④ When the patient uses accessory muscles to increase lung volume during inspiration, the work of breathing increases. This places greater demands on the body and increases the metabolic rate, which in turn increases the need for oxygen; pacing care allows for rest, which reduces the physical demand for oxygen.

19 TEST-TAKING TIP ● The word "most" is the key word in the stem that sets a priority. The words "dramatic increase" are the clue in the stem.

① Although a pregnant woman's metabolic rate is increased, pregnancy does not place as high a demand on the body's need for oxygen as exercise.
② A fever causes an increase in a person's metabolic rate; however, a fever does not place as high a demand on the body's need for oxygen as exercise.
* ③ Most exercise dramatically increases the metabolic rate, which in turn increases the body's demand for oxygen.
④ General anesthesia relaxes the muscles of the body; when muscles are relaxed, the metabolic rate decreases and the demand for oxygen also decreases.

20 TEST-TAKING TIP ● The word BEST is the key word in the stem that sets a priority. Four different combinations of possible assessments are offered to determine the adequacy of peripheral circulation in a patient's lower extremity. If you are able to identify one assessment that determines adequacy of peripheral circulation, you can narrow the correct answer to two options. If you can identify one assessment that does not contribute to an assessment of adequacy of peripheral circulation, you can eliminate two distractors and narrow the correct answer to two options.

① Although the pedal pulses are assessed to determine circulation to the feet, a lack of, not the presence of, hair on the feet and lower legs may be caused by prolonged hypoxia.

* ② Both of these assessments help to determine adequacy of peripheral circulation. Applying pressure to a toenail causes blanching, and when the pressure is released, the normal color should quickly return (within 1 to 2 seconds), indicating adequate arterial perfusion. Assessing pedal pulses measures the adequacy of circulation to the feet.

③ Although lack of hair on the feet and lower legs may indicate prolonged hypoxia, other factors such as genetic endowment may cause a lack of hair. Blood pressure reflects the pressure exerted by the blood as it pulsates through the arteries. Although people with arteriosclerosis may have increased resistance and therefore hypertension, a blood pressure does not evaluate peripheral circulation in the lower extremities as does inspection and palpation.

④ Although capillary refill assesses adequacy of peripheral circulation, blood pressure does not evaluate peripheral circulation in the lower extremities as does inspection and palpation.

21 TEST-TAKING TIP ● The word "most" is the key word in the stem that sets a priority.

* ① A cough forcefully expels air from the lungs and is an effective self-protective reflex to clear the trachea and bronchi.

② An incentive spirometer is a device used to encourage voluntary deep breathing, not to clear an airway; it is used to prevent or treat atelectasis.

③ A nebulizer treatment does not clear an airway; it adds moisture or medication to inspired air to alter the tracheobronchial mucosa. Once the respiratory passages are dilated or mucolytic agents have reduced the viscosity of secretions, the patient can cough more productively.

④ Abdominal breathing does not clear the air passages. It helps to decrease air trapping and reduce the work of breathing. Abdominal breathing is used postoperatively, during labor, and with pulmonary disease to promote relaxation and pain control.

22 TEST-TAKING TIP ● The words "local pressure" and "specifically" are clues in the stem.

① Edema is fluid in the interstitial compartment and is not specifically an adaptation to pressure as is ischemia.

* ② Ischemia is a lack of blood supply to a body part (tissue ischemia) and is directly related to pressure which can occlude blood vessels.

③ Orthopnea is the ability to breathe only in an upright position, such as sitting or standing, and is not a local adaptation to pressure.

④ Hypovolemia is a reduction in blood volume and is not a local adaptation to pressure.

23 TEST-TAKING TIP ● The word "initial" is the key word in the stem that sets a priority. The use of the word "airway" in the stem and in Option 3 is a clang association.

① Inserting an airway with the tip toward the tongue is contraindicated; this can displace the tongue to the posterior oropharynx, which could occlude the airway. An airway should be inserted with the tip toward the roof of the mouth; when the flange touches the teeth, the airway should be rotated 180 degrees into position over the tongue.

② The nurse should avoid putting a finger into the mouth of a patient, particularly an unconscious patient, because the patient may bite down and injure the nurse; an airway should be used only with an unconscious patient because in a conscious patient it stimulates the gag reflex, promoting regurgitation and aspiration.

* ③ Adult, child, and infant sizes are available; the correct size airway must be used to prevent oropharyngeal trauma and promote an open airway.

④ A water-soluble lubricant, not a petroleum-based lubricant, should be used to lubricate the lips.

24 TEST-TAKING TIP ● The word "most" is the key word in the stem that sets a priority. The word "accurately" is the clue in the stem.

① Although hematocrit is the percentage of red blood cell mass in proportion to whole blood, it is not an accurate test for adequacy of tissue oxygenation; a low hematocrit may indicate possible water intoxication, and an elevated hematocrit may indicate dehydration.

② Although hemoglobin is the red pigment in red blood cells that carries oxygen, it is not an accurate test for adequacy of tissue oxygenation; a low hemoglobin is evidence of iron-deficiency anemia or bleeding.

* ③ Arterial blood gases include the levels of oxygen, carbon dioxide, bicarbonate, and pH. Blood gases determine the adequacy of alveolar gas exchange and the ability of the lungs and kidneys to maintain the acid-base balance of body fluids.

④ Pulmonary function tests measure lung volume and capacity; although these are valuable data, they do not provide specific data about tissue oxygenation.

25 TEST-TAKING TIP ● Options 2 and 3 are equally plausible.

* ① Because of the energy required to "fight" an infection, the basal metabolic rate increases, resulting in an increased respiratory rate.

② The body has a need to exhale carbon dioxide, not retain carbon dioxide.

③ Tachypnea occurs in the presence of elevated levels of carbon dioxide and carbonic acid, not decreased carbon dioxide levels.

④ The patient with an infection is more likely to be in metabolic acidosis; tachypnea that progresses to hyperventilation causes respiratory alkalosis.

26 * ① Well-chewed food is broken down and mixed with saliva, forming a bolus of food; a bolus of food is easier to swallow and causes less risk for aspiration.

② The patient has no difficulty chewing; food does not need to be cut up as long as the patient has the time to chew the food adequately before attempting to swallow.

③ This could flush food into the breathing passages rather than down the esophagus.

④ This could increase the risk for aspiration; people should not talk with food in their mouths; people need to inhale before talking and this action could cause aspiration of food when food is in the mouth.

27 TEST-TAKING TIP ● Option 2 is the unique option. It is the only option that refers to positioning. Options 1, 3, and 4 all relate to pathophysiology. Consider Option 2 carefully. In this item, it can be deleted from consideration.

① Sounds caused by fluid in the alveoli are called crackles or rales and sounds caused by fluid or resistance in the bronchi are called rhonchi or gurgles.

② Positioning is unrelated to adventitious sounds (abnormal breath sounds).

* ③ Wheezes occur as air passes through air passages narrowed by secretions, edema, or tumors; these high-pitched squeaky musical sounds are best heard on expiration and are usually not changed by coughing.

④ This is a pleural friction rub; it is a superficial grating sound heard particularly at the height of inspiration and not relieved by coughing; it is caused by the rubbing together of inflamed pleural surfaces.

28 **TEST-TAKING TIP** ● This question focuses on the characteristics of respirations: rate, depth, and rhythm. If you know that Kussmaul respirations are rapid, Options 2 and 3 can be eliminated. Options 1 and 3 are opposites and Options 2 and 4 are opposites; consider these options in relation to each other.

* ① Kussmaul respirations are rapid, deep, and regular; they are the body's effort to correct metabolic acidosis by blowing off excess carbon dioxide.
② Slow (less than 12 breaths per minute), regular respirations are called bradypnea.
③ Slow respirations are called bradypnea. Biot's respiration and Cheyne-Strokes respiration have shallow breaths as part of their characteristics.
④ This describes Cheyne-Stokes respirations; the breathing cycle begins with shallow breaths that gradually increase to an abnormal depth and rate, then the breaths gradually become slower and more shallow until there is a period of apnea, and then the cycle begins again.

29 **TEST-TAKING TIP** ● Options 1 and 4 are equally plausible. They both involve touching the abdomen during the procedure of diaphragmatic breathing; they can be eliminated from consideration.

① The abdomen rises on inspiration.
② These accessory muscles consciously should not be involved with diaphragmatic breathing. The abdomen should rise and fall rather than the shoulders; the chest will naturally expand and recoil.
* ③ Diaphragmatic breathing involves a pattern of a slow deep inhalation followed by a slow exhalation with a tightening of the abdominal muscles to aid exhalation; the patient should hold the breath for 2 to 3 seconds at the height of inhalation, just before the exhalation.
④ Pressure against the abdomen would interfere with the amount of air that could be drawn into the lungs on inspiration.

30 **TEST-TAKING TIP** ● The words "exchange," "perfuse," and "diffuse" all relate to actions that occur at particular sites within the body. The word "transport" refers to the movement of something from one place to another. The identification of Option 1 as the unique option was difficult because the interrelationship of these words was more obscure than most.

* ① The hemoglobin portion of red blood cells carries oxygen from the alveolar capillaries to distant tissue sites.
② Exchange occurs in the capillary beds of the alveoli via the process of diffusion; this is unrelated to anemia.
③ Perfusion relates to the extent of inflow and outflow of air between the alveoli and pulmonary capillaries or extent of blood flow to the pulmonary capillary bed; perfusion is not related to red blood cell levels.
④ Diffusion occurs at the alveolar capillary beds and is not related to anemia.

31 ① Rings do not interfere with the reading.
* ② The ingredients in acrylic nails or black, blue, green metallic, or frosted nail polish will interfere with the reading.
③ It is unnecessary to elevate the site being monitored; however, the pulse oximeter may identify motion as arterial pulsations. It may be necessary to immobilize, not to elevate, the monitoring site to achieve accurate readings.
④ The removal of body hair is unnecessary to achieve an accurate reading.

32 TEST-TAKING TIP ● Options 1 and 2 are equally plausible. Options 1 and 3 are opposites.

① Brisk, low-volume breaths tend to snap the ball to the top and should be avoided. Once the ball reaches the top, it should remain at the top for as long as possible to maintain increased airway pressure at the height of inhalation (maximum sustained inhalation). The patient should not exhale rapidly.

② Although the patient should seal his or her lips around the tube, the inhalation should be done slowly, not rapidly.

* ③ A slow, deep inhalation that is sustained at the height of inspiration ensures adequate ventilation of the alveoli.

④ Although the ball should rise slowly, the ball will drop abruptly when the patient exhales. The focus should be on inhalation, not exhalation.

33 ① A productive cough may or may not produce pain, depending on the patient's underlying condition.

* ② A productive cough is accompanied by expectorated secretions.

③ When a patient raises respiratory secretions and expectorates them, breathing usually improves.

④ When a cough is productive it does not indicate that it is also progressive.

34 TEST-TAKING TIP ● Options 1 and 4 are opposites. Consider these options carefully. One of them is the correct answer.

* ① Intermittent suction is exerted on withdrawal of the suction catheter; this prevents trauma to any one section of the respiratory mucosa because of prolonged suction pressure.

② For wall suctioning to be effective when suctioning an adult, it should be maintained at 110 to 150 mm Hg.

③ The opposite is the acceptable technique. The nasotracheal area is considered sterile and is suctioned before the oropharyngeal area, which is considered clean; this minimizes contamination of the sterile area.

④ Suction is applied on removal, not insertion, of the catheter. Intermittent suctioning is less traumatic to the mucosa than is continuous suctioning.

35 ① Osmosis is the passage of a solvent, not a gas, through a semipermeable membrane from an area of lesser solute concentration to an area of greater solute concentration.

② Invasion refers to metastasis of a tumor by direct extension.

* ③ Diffusion is the movement of gases from an area of greater pressure or concentration to an area of lesser pressure or concentration.

④ Decompression is the lowering of pressure within a space by removing fluid or gas; for example, a nasogastric tube to suction removes gastric contents decompressing the stomach.

286 Administration of Medications

This section includes questions related to the principles associated with the administration of medications via the oral, parenteral (intravenous and intramuscular, intradermal and subcutaneous injections), topical, ear, eye, vaginal, and rectal routes. The questions focus on allergies, untoward effects, toxic effect, developmental considerations, the Z-track method, peak and trough levels of medications, and pain assessment before administering medication for pain.

Questions

1 Before administering a medication that is teratogenic, the nurse should ask the patient:
① "Have you ever had an anaphylactic reaction?"
② "Were you ever addicted to drugs?"
③ "Do you have any allergies?"
④ "Are you pregnant?"
TEST-TAKING TIP ● Identify the equally plausible options. Identify the unique option.

2 Which statement would indicate that the patient needed further teaching regarding care of the eyes and eye medications?
① "Excess medication on the eyelid can be wiped away."
② "I should gaze downward while instilling the eye drops."
③ "I should place one drop of the medication inside my lower eyelid."
④ "The risk of transmitting infection from one eye to the other is high."
TEST-TAKING TIP ● Identify the key word in the stem that indicates a negative polarity.

3 The nurse changes the needle after drawing up the required dosage of a caustic drug. This is done primarily because the needle is:
① Too long for the required route
② Coated with the medication
③ No longer sterile
④ Not sharp
TEST-TAKING TIP ● Identify the key word in the stem that sets a priority. Identify the unique option.

4 When administering a 2-mL intramuscular injection to an adult patient who is in severe pain and lying in the supine position, the site that would be the safest and most therapeutic would be the:
① Deltoid
② Dorsogluteal
③ Ventrogluteal
④ Vastus lateralis
TEST-TAKING TIP ● Identify the key word in the stem that sets a priority. Identify the equally plausible options

5 When using an insulin syringe with a $1/2$-inch needle to administer insulin, the nurse should insert the needle at an angle of:
① 30 degrees
② 45 degrees

③ 90 degrees
④ 180 degrees

TEST-TAKING TIP ● Identify the clue in the stem. Identify the options that are opposites.

6 When administering oral medication to children, the MOST important factor to consider is their:
① Age
② Weight
③ Level of anxiety
④ Developmental level

TEST-TAKING TIP ● Identify the key word in the stem that sets a priority. Identify the clue in the stem.

7 When instilling ear drops into the ear of an adult, the nurse should:
① Gently press a cotton ball into the ear canal
② Pull the pinna of the ear upward and backward
③ Pull the pinna of the ear downward and backward
④ Hold the dropper approximately 2 inches above the canal

TEST-TAKING TIP ● Identify the clue in the stem. Identify the options that are opposites.

8 The nurse would recognize that further teaching was needed about the administration of eye drops when the patient says, "I should:
① Wipe my eye moving from the outer corner toward my nose."
② Hold the eyedropper about $^1/_2$ inch above my eye."
③ Close my eyes after putting the drops in my eye."
④ Put the fluid in a pocket in the lower lid."

TEST-TAKING TIP ● Identify the key word in the stem that indicates negative polarity.

9 A patient is receiving an intravenous piggyback medication every 4 hours. Because the medication has a narrow therapeutic window, the physician orders a peak blood level. The nurse should plan to obtain a blood specimen:
① Three hours after administering a dose
② Halfway between two scheduled doses
③ One hour after administering a dose
④ AT 10 PM in the evening

TEST-TAKING TIP ● Identify the options that are opposites.

10 What should the nurse do when blood appears at the hub of the needle while aspirating an intramuscular injection?
① Remove the syringe and attach a new needle.
② Discard the syringe and prepare a new injection.
③ Interrupt the procedure and notify the physician.
④ Withdraw the needle slightly and inject the solution.

TEST-TAKING TIP ● Identify the options that are opposites.

11 Besides inhibiting microbial growth, an antibiotic may also depress the bone marrow. This response is classified as:
① An overdose
② A side effect
③ An habituation
④ An idiosyncratic effect

TEST-TAKING TIP ● Identify the unique option.

12 Because of the physiological changes associated with aging, when administering drugs to elderly people, the nurse should specifically assess for signs of:
① Toxicity
② Side effects
③ Allergic reactions
④ Drug-food interactions

TEST-TAKING TIP ● Identify the clue in the stem.

13 Which route of administration is used only for its local therapeutic effect?
① Rectum
② Skin
③ Nose
④ Eye

TEST-TAKING TIP ● Identify the clues in the stem.

14 What should the nurse do first when injecting an intravenous medication via an already existing intravenous line?
① Select the port closest to the needle entry site.
② Pinch the tubing above the port being used.
③ Determine patency of the intravenous line.
④ Clean the injection port with an antiseptic.

TEST-TAKING TIP ● Identify the key word in the stem that sets a priority.

15 What should the nurse do when filling a syringe from a multidose vial?
① Keep the needle above the level of the liquid and maintain sterile technique
② Keep the needle below the level of the liquid and change the needle after withdrawing the solution
③ Keep the needle below the level of the liquid and record the date and time on the vial when opened
④ Keep the needle above the level of the liquid and inject air at $1^1/_2$ times the volume of the ordered dose

TEST-TAKING TIP ● Identify the duplicate facts among the options.

16 The nurse can best evaluate that compliance with a drug regimen occurs when:
① A cumulative effect results
② The patient's symptoms subside
③ Physiological dependence results
④ The patient takes the drug as prescribed

TEST-TAKING TIP ● Identify the key word in the stem that sets a priority.

17 When administering an intradermal injection, the nurse should recognize that the patient is at the highest risk for exhibiting an:
① Overdose
② Allergic response
③ Idiosyncratic reaction
④ Interaction with other drugs

TEST-TAKING TIP ● Identify the key word in the stem that sets a priority. Identify the clue in the stem.

18 How can the nurse best protect a patient from aspiration when administering an oral medication?
① Offer extra water
② Crush the medication

③ Position the patient in a sitting position

④ Inspect the patient's mouth after he or she swallows

TEST-TAKING TIP ● Identify the key word in the stem that sets a priority.

19 What position should the nurse instruct the patient to assume when planning to instill a vaginal cream?
① Dorsal recumbent position
② Right lateral position
③ Left lateral position
④ Supine position

TEST-TAKING TIP ● Identify the options that are opposites.

20 The nurse would know that a mother correctly administered nose drops to her child when she:
① Told her child to sniff the medication into the lungs
② Allowed her child to sit upright after its administration
③ Put the remaining fluid in the dropper back into the bottle
④ Held the dropper $1/2$ inch above the nares during instillation

TEST-TAKING TIP ● Identify the clue in the stem.

21 The nurse recognizes that the most dangerous method of administering medication is via:
① Intravenous push
② Piggyback infusion
③ Subcutaneous injection
④ Intramuscular injection

TEST-TAKING TIP ● Identify the key word in the stem that sets a priority. Identify the equally plausible options.

22 Which action is unique when administering medication via the Z-track injection method?
① The skin is pulled laterally before needle insertion.
② Injection sites are rotated along a "Z" on the abdomen.
③ An air lock is established behind the bolus of medication.
④ A "Z" is formed when dividing the buttocks into quadrants.

TEST-TAKING TIP ● Identify the clues in the stem.

23 Which route is considered to be the most accurate and safe when administering medications?
① By mouth
② Topically
③ Intravenous
④ By injection

TEST-TAKING TIP ● Identify the key word in the stem that sets a priority.

24 The physician orders peak and trough levels to monitor an antibiotic. To measure trough levels, the nurse should plan for a blood specimen to be drawn:
① At 8 in the morning
② Halfway between scheduled doses
③ A half hour before a scheduled dose
④ A half hour after drug administration

TEST-TAKING TIP ● Identify the clue in the stem. Identify the options that are opposites.

25 After abdominal surgery a patient asks for medication for pain. Before administering the medication for pain, the nurse should first:
① Obtain the vital signs
② Assess the pain further
③ Review the original order
④ Check when the last dose was given

TEST-TAKING TIP ● Identify the key word in the stem that sets a priority. Identify the clue in the stem.

26 Via what area would the nurse administer a medication in the form of a troche?
① Rectal route
② Buccal cavity
③ Vaginal vault
④ Auditory canal

27 The nurse recognizes that the patient understands the teaching about how to self-administer a rectal suppository when the patient:
① Bears down during insertion of the suppository
② Requests sterile gloves to perform the procedure
③ Allows the suppository to warm to room temperature
④ Inserts the suppository immediately after its removal from the refrigerator.

TEST-TAKING TIP ● Identify the options that are opposites.

28 What is most important for the nurse to do when administering a topical medicated cream to a patient's skin?
① Use medical aseptic technique when applying the medication.
② Wash the area before administering the medication.
③ Pat the medication onto the surface of the skin.
④ Apply a moderate layer of the medication.

TEST-TAKING TIP ● Identify the word in the stem that sets a priority.

29 A transdermal patch for delivery of an analgesic is most effective because it:
① Has an immediate systemic effect
② Affects only the area covered by the patch
③ Releases controlled amounts of medication over time
④ Produces fewer side effects than other routes of administration

TEST-TAKING TIPS ● Identify the word in the stem that sets a priority. Identify the options that are opposites. Identify the specific determiner.

30 Which behavior would indicate an inappropriate technique to use with a metered-dose inhaler (MDI)?
① Shaking the drug before pressing down on the inhaler
② Pressing down on the inhaler while inhaling quickly
③ Holding the breath at the height of inhalation
④ Tilting the head back slightly

TEST-TAKING TIP ● Identify the word in the stem that indicates negative polarity.

31 Which site would most rapidly absorb medication by subcutaneous injection?
① Abdomen
② Buttock
③ Thigh
④ Arm

TEST-TAKING TIP ● Identify the word in the stem that sets a priority.

32 What is the site of choice for administering an IM injection to an infant?
   ① Deltoid
   ② Dorsogluteal
   ③ Ventrogluteal
   ④ Rectus femoris
   TEST-TAKING TIP ● Identify the words in the stem that set a priority.

33 What is the least desirable site for an IM injection in an obese adult?
   ① Vastus lateralis
   ② Rectus femoris
   ③ Dorsogluteal
   ④ Deltoid
   TEST-TAKING TIP ● Identify the word in the stem that indicates negative polarity.

34 Which route of delivery for medication should be questioned if the patient is an older adult who is cachectic?
   ① Intradermal route
   ② Intravenous route
   ③ Subcutaneous route
   ④ Intramuscular route
   TEST-TAKING TIP ● Identify the unique option.

35 Medication administered by the sublingual route is contraindicated when the patient:
   ① Is able to swallow
   ② Is a mouth breather
   ③ Has a lowered level of consciousness
   ④ Has a nasogastric tube to continuous suction
   TEST-TAKING TIP ● Identify the word in the stem that indicates negative polarity.

Rationales

1 **TEST-TAKING TIP** ● Options 1 and 3 are equally plausible. Option 4 is unique. Options 1, 2, and 3 discuss situations that relate to "prior" drug use.

① An anaphylactic reaction is a severe, systemic hypersensitivity to a drug, food, or chemical; in some people this reaction can be fatal.

② Drug addition refers to an uncontrollable craving for a chemical substance because of a physical or psychological dependence.

③ Allergies are unpredictable hypersensitive reactions to allergens such as drugs; it can be a mild to severe reaction and can cause a rash, pruritus, rhinitis, wheezing, hives, and even an anaphylactic reaction.

* ④ "Teratogenic," when used in the context of medication, refers to a drug that can cause adverse effects in a fetus or an embryo.

2 **TEST-TAKING TIP** ● The word "further" is the key word in the stem that indicates a negative polarity. The correct answer is the option that would "not" be an acceptable action when administering eye drops.

① Excess medication is unneeded and can be wiped away; also, it promotes comfort.

* ② The reverse is true; gazing upward moves the cornea upward and away from the conjunctival sac where the medication is to be instilled.

③ Inside the lower eyelid is called the "conjunctival sac" and is the correct location to instill eye drops.

④ Eye infections can be easily transmitted from one eye to the other; however, it must be stressed that if aseptic principles are followed, cross-infection can be minimized.

3 **TEST-TAKING TIP** ● The word "primarily" is the key word in the stem that sets a priority. Option 2 is unique. Options 1, 3, and 4 are all negative statements. In Option 1, "too long" indicates that the needle is "not" the correct length.

① Any size needle can be used to draw up a caustic medication.

* ② Changing to a new needle prevents tracking the medication through the subcutaneous tissue and skin.

③ If all of the principles of sterile technique are followed when preparing an injection, the needle is still considered sterile.

④ Most needles are made of stainless steel with a beveled tip that makes them sharp; they do not need to be replaced due to dullness after drawing up medication because they remain sharp.

4 **TEST-TAKING TIP** ● The word "most" is the key word in the stem that sets a priority. Options 2 and 3 are equally plausible because they both require repositioning the patient.

① The deltoid is not well developed in many adults and children. The radial and ulnar nerves and brachial artery lie in the upper arm along the humerus. The deltoid should not be used for intramuscular injections unless other sites are unavailable.

② To access the dorsogluteal, the patient would have to be repositioned, which could increase pain. Historically the dorsogluteal was the preferred site for an intramuscular injection; however, there is a higher risk of hitting the sciatic nerve, blood vessels, or greater trochanter. Hitting the sciatic nerve can cause partial or permanent paralysis of the leg.

③ To access the ventrogluteal, the patient would have to be repositioned, which could increase pain. The ventrogluteal would be the preferred site after the vastus lateralis; it is safe to use in cachectic patients, infants, and children.

* ④ The vastus lateralis is the preferred site for this patient because it has no major nerves and blood vessels, has rapid drug absorption, and the patient does not have to be repositioned while in pain.

5 **TEST-TAKING TIP** ● The words "½-inch needle" are the clue in the stem. Options 1 and 4 are opposites among the options offered.

① Thirty degrees is too shallow an angle for a subcutaneous injection.

② A 45-degree angle is too shallow for the administration of a subcutaneous injection with a needle that is only ½-inch long. A 45-degree angle would be appropriate if the needle were ⅝ of an inch to 1 inch long.

* ③ A 90-degree angle is appropriate for a subcutaneous injection with a ½-inch needle; it injects the insulin into the loose connective tissue under the dermis.

④ To use a 180-degree angle for any injection would be impossible. Various injection methods are from 15 degrees to 90 degrees, not 180 degrees.

6 **TEST-TAKING TIP** ● The word MOST is the key word in the stem that sets a priority. The word "children" is the clue in the stem.

① Age is not reliable for calculating a pediatric dose of medication; the weight of a child at any age can vary greatly.

* ② Children's body sizes are different, necessitating calculation of drug dosage by weight, rather than by age or developmental level. Weight is an objective, specific, and accurate way to calculate appropriate medication dosages for children.

③ This variable does not influence calculation of dosage of medication for a child.

④ Same as #3.

7 **TEST-TAKING TIP** ● The word "adult" is the clue in the stem. Options 2 and 3 are opposites.

① A cotton ball may be placed in the outermost part of the ear; it should not be pressed into the canal.

* ② Pulling the pinna of the ear upward and backward straightens the ear canal of an adult. This action facilitates the distribution of medications throughout the external ear canal.

③ Pulling the pinna of the ear downward and backward straightens the ear canal of a young child, not an adult.

④ The force exerted by a drop falling from this height could injure the eardrum; the dropper should be held ½ inch (1 cm) above the ear canal, and the drop should fall against the wall of the canal and then flow toward the eardrum.

8 **TEST-TAKING TIP** ● The word "further" is the key word in the stem that indicates negative polarity.

* ① The eye should be wiped moving from the inner to the outer canthus; this promotes comfort, prevents trauma, and moves excess medication away from the nasolacrimal duct, minimizing systemic absorption and infection.

② It is desirable to hold the dropper ½ to ¾ inch above the conjunctival sac. Holding it higher could injure the eye because of the force exerted by the drop; holding it lower increases the risk of contaminating the dropper or injuring the eye.

③ Closing the eyes after administering eye drops is acceptable because it distributes the medication across the eye.

④ Putting the fluid in a pocket in the lower lid (conjunctival sac) is appropriate because it permits an even distribution of the medication.

9   TEST-TAKING TIP ● Options 1 and 3 are opposites, 1 hour before or after the dose.
①   One hour before the next scheduled dose would provide an inaccurate result when testing for a peak blood level.
②   A blood level specimen taken halfway between two scheduled doses would not provide an accurate result when testing for a peak blood level.
* ③   Most medications administered every 4 hours have a peak concentration about 1 hour following administration.
④   A blood level specimen taken at 10 PM would provide inaccurate results for a peak blood level unless the drug was administered at 9 PM; there is no information to indicate that the drug was administered at 9 PM

10   TEST-TAKING TIP ● Options 2 and 4 are opposites.
①   This is unsafe; the fluid in the syringe would be contaminated.
* ②   The equipment should be discarded because the fluid and needle are contaminated and a new sterile syringe should be prepared.
③   It is unnecessary to notify the physician; a small vessel was pierced and the procedure should be interrupted and completed with all new equipment.
④   Same as #1.

11   TEST-TAKING TIP ● Option 2 begins with the word "a" rather than "an." Options 1, 3, and 4 all begin with the word "an."
①   An overdose occurs when a person receives a dosage larger than the usual recommended dose; this is rarely planned and is usually an accident.
* ②   A side effect is a secondary effect; side effects can be harmless or cause injury; if injurious, the drug is discontinued.
③   Habituation is an acquired tolerance from continued exposure to a substance.
④   An idiosyncratic effect is an unexpected effect; it can be an overreaction, an underreaction, or an unusual reaction.

12   TEST-TAKING TIP ● The word "elderly" is the clue in the stem.
* ①   Biotransformation of drugs is less efficient in the elderly than during younger developmental ages; when drugs are not fully metabolized and excreted from the body, toxic levels can accumulate.
②   Harmless or injurious secondary effects are common to people of all ages, not just the elderly.
③   Allergic reactions are common to people of all ages, not just the elderly.
④   Drug-food interactions are common to people of all ages, not just the elderly.

13   TEST-TAKING TIP ● The words "only" and "local" are the clues in the stem.
①   Medication can be administered via this route for either a local or systemic effect; medications can be absorbed through the rich vascular bed in the mucous membranes.
②   Medications can be administered via the skin for either a local or systemic effect.
③   Same as #1.
* ④   Medications are instilled into the eye only for their local effect; part of the procedure for instillation of eye drops is to apply gentle pressure to the nasolacrimal duct for 10 to 15 seconds to prevent absorption of the medication into the systemic circulation.

14   TEST-TAKING TIP ● The word "first" is the key word in the stem that sets a priority.
①   This would be done later in the procedure; determining the viability of the line is the priority.
②   Same as #1.

  * ③ For medication to enter a vein, the intravenous line must be unobstructed; also, for an intravenous medication to be appropriately absorbed, it must be in a vein, not the subcutaneous tissue.

  ④ Same as #1.

15 TEST-TAKING TIP ● Options 1 and 4 contain a duplicate fact and Options 2 and 3 contain a duplicate fact. If you know whether or not a needle should be kept above or below the level of fluid in a vial, you can reduce your final selection to two options.

  ① Although sterile technique should be maintained, the bevel of the needle should be kept below the level of the fluid or the syringe will fill with air.

  ② Although the bevel of the needle should be kept below the level of the fluid, changing the needle would be unnecessary. The needle needs to be changed only when the solution is caustic to tissues.

  * ③ The bevel of the needle must be kept below the level of the fluid to prevent air from entering the syringe. Once opened, medications generally have a recommended period of viability before they should be discarded.

  ④ The bevel of the needle should be kept below the level of the fluid or the syringe will fill with air. The amount of air injected into the vial should equal the amount of solution to be withdrawn; extra air would result in excessive pressure within the closed space of the vial.

16 TEST-TAKING TIP ● The word "best" is the key word in the stem that sets a priority.

  ① If a drug is ineffectively metabolized or slowly excreted, the serum drug concentrations increase with each subsequent dose; this cumulative effect tends to occur in the elderly and people with decreased functioning of the liver, kidneys, or thyroid gland and is unrelated to compliance.

  ② Many factors may cause symptoms to subside; it is inappropriate to come to the conclusion that the symptoms subsided because of the drug.

  ③ Physiological dependence occurs when the patient has a physiological reliance on the drug; failure to take the drug results in withdrawal symptoms.

  * ④ Compliance occurs when the patient follows an ordered course of treatment.

17 TEST-TAKING TIP ● The word "highest" is the key word in the stem that sets a priority. The word "intradermal" is the clue in the stem.

  ① Overdoses are a risk with all types of injections, but the highest risk of overdose is via the intravenous route, not the intradermal route.

  * ② An intradermal injection is given under the skin to test for such things as tuberculosis and allergies; these drugs can cause an anaphylactic reaction if absorbed by the circulation too quickly or if the person has a hypersensitivity to the solution.

  ③ Idiosyncratic reactions are unpredictable effects; they are usually underreactions, overreactions, or reactions that are different from the expected reaction. Idiosyncratic reactions are less likely to occur than allergic reactions with intradermal injections.

  ④ A drug interaction occurs when one drug alters the action of another drug; this is not a possible response to a singular intradermal injection.

18 TEST-TAKING TIP ● The word "best" is the key word in the stem that sets a priority.

  ① Excessive water may promote aspiration.

  ② Although crushing the medication helps some people, it is not the consistency of medication but rather the amount of water taken with the medication that can promote aspiration. Also, multiple crushed particles taken with water can stimulate the gag reflex; crushed medications should be mixed in a soft food such as applesauce to increase safety.

* ③ This position allows the patient to control the flow of fluid to the back of the oropharynx as well as promote the flow of fluid down the esophagus via gravity.

④ This is important after, not when, administering medication.

19 TEST-TAKING TIP ● Options 2 and 3 are opposites

* ① The dorsal recumbent position allows easy access to and exposure of the vaginal orifice. Lying in this position for 10 minutes after the administration of the vaginal cream prevents its drainage from the vaginal canal.

② The right lateral position does not thoroughly expose the vaginal orifice.

③ The left lateral position does not thoroughly expose the vaginal orifice. This position is used for the administration of enemas and rectal suppositories.

④ The supine position does not expose the vaginal orifice.

20 TEST-TAKING TIP ● The word "correctly" in the stem is a clue.

① This action is contraindicated because sniffing will pull the medication to the oropharynx, where it will be swallowed rather than inhaled into the upper respiratory tract. Nose drops should be directed toward the midline of the superior concha of the ethmoid bone as the patient breathes through the mouth.

② This action is contraindicated because sitting up will allow the fluid to drain from the nares rather than be inhaled into the upper respiratory tract. The patient should remain 1 minute with the head and neck hyperextended.

③ Returning the remaining fluid in the dropper to the bottle is a violation of medical asepsis and will contaminate the bottle.

* ④ This position prevents touching the patient, which would contaminate the dropper, and yet is not too high to cause trauma to the tissue by the falling drop.

21 TEST-TAKING TIP ● The word "most" is the key word in the stem that sets a priority. Options 3 and 4 are equally plausible.

* ① An intravenous push (IV push) or bolus administration of medication is the instillation of a medication directly into a vein; this rapid administration of an entire dose of medication places the patient at highest risk for adverse effects.

② Although an intravenous piggyback is a dangerous route, the medication is diluted and it is infused over a time period.

③ A solution instilled into subcutaneous tissue or a muscle is absorbed over a longer period of time than an IV push.

④ Same as #3.

22 TEST-TAKING TIP ● The words "unique" and "Z track" are clues in the stem. Options 2 and 4 are distractors, even though they have a clang association with the "Z" in the stem.

* ① The "Z" in the Z-track method refers to pulling the skin to the side before and during an intramuscular injection. This technique alters the position of skin layers so that once the skin is released and the needle is removed, the injected fluid is kept within the muscle tissues and does not rise in the needle tract, which can irritate subcutaneous tissues.

② An intramuscular site, preferably the dorsogluteal, is used for Z track, not the abdomen, which is used for subcutaneous injections.

③ The air-lock technique also can be done with intramuscular injections. When air is injected behind the medication, the air clears the needle of medication, preventing tracking of the drug through subcutaneous tissue.

④ The "Z" in Z-track injections refers to the displacement of tissue layers during the procedure; when the buttocks (dorsogluteal) are used for intramuscular injections, bony landmarks must be used to identify the correct insertion site.

23 **TEST-TAKING TIP** ● The word "most" is the key word in the stem that sets a priority.
* ① Using the oral route is the safest way to administer medication because it is convenient, it does not require breaking the skin barrier, the medication is absorbed slowly, and it usually does not cause physical or emotional stress.
② Because absorption is affected by a variety of factors, such as the extent of the capillary network and condition of the skin, the topical route is not the most accurate method of administration.
③ The intravenous route carries the highest risk because it breaks the skin barrier and the medication is injected directly into the bloodstream.
④ An injection carries a higher risk than a medication administered via the oral route because the medication is rapidly absorbed and it breaks the skin barrier.

24 **TEST-TAKING TIP** ● The word "trough" is the clue in the stem. Options 3 and 4 are opposites.
① The peak and trough of a blood plasma level depend on the time the last dose was administered.
② This would not be a time period when a drug is at its lowest concentration in the blood.
* ③ "Trough level" refers to when a drug is at its lowest concentration in the blood in response to biotransformation; this usually occurs during the time period just before the next scheduled dose.
④ Many variables affect the time when a drug reaches its peak plasma level within an individual; however, a half hour after the administration of an antibiotic, one could safely plot the antibiotic plasma level on the rising side of the curve of the plasma level profile, not within the trough.

25 **TEST-TAKING TIP** ● The word "first" is the key word in the stem that sets a priority. The word "before" is the clue in the stem.
① This would be done after the pain was assessed further and before administering a narcotic.
* ② Whenever a patient complains of pain, the nurse's initial intervention should be to assess the location, intensity, duration, and characteristics of the pain.
③ This would be done after it was determined that the patient needed pain relief and before administering the medication.
④ Same as #3.

26 ① A suppository is designed for administering medication into the rectum.
* ② A troche (lozenge) is placed in the space between the upper or lower molar teeth and gums (buccal cavity) so that it can dissolve and release medication.
③ A suppository, solution, or cream can be delivered to the vaginal vault by a vaginal applicator.
④ Medication in a suspension can be administered via a dropper into the auditory canal.

27 **TEST-TAKING TIP** ● Options 3 and 4 are opposites.
① Bearing down is contraindicated. When people hold their breath, they tend to perform the Valsalva maneuver. The Valsalva maneuver increases intra-abdominal pressure, which makes it more difficult to insert and retain a suppository; the increased pressure can expel the suppository.
② Inserting a rectal suppository is not a sterile procedure.
③ Allowing a suppository to warm to room temperature would cause it to melt, which interferes with insertion.
* ④ Cold suppositories maintain their shape for ease of insertion; it is safe and easy to insert a suppository that has been refrigerated.

28 TEST-TAKING TIP ● The word "most" in the stem sets a priority.

   ① Surgical asepsis should be used; a sterile glove or sterile tongue depressor prevents the contamination of skin lesions or wounds.

* ② Washing removes skin encrustations, discharges, and microorganisms; this allows the new application of medication to come directly in contact with the area, which promotes absorption.

   ③ A patting motion is contraindicated in sterile technique because it contaminates one area of the lesion or wound by another area; a light stroke with a new sterile applicator should be used for each stroke.

   ④ A thin layer of medication should be applied; more is not better.

29 TEST-TAKING TIP ● The word "most" in the stem sets a priority. Options 1 and 2 are opposites and need to be considered carefully. The word "only" in Option 2 is a specific determiner.

   ① The systemic effect depends on the amount of time it takes for the drug to be absorbed through the skin; this takes longer than parenteral routes.

   ② Transdermal disks or patches deliver medications that produce systemic effects.

* ③ Transdermal disks or patches have semipermeable membranes that allow medication to be absorbed through the skin slowly over a long period of time (usually 24 to 72 hours).

   ④ The medication, not the route of delivery, produces side effects.

30 TEST-TAKING TIP ● The word "inappropriate" in the stem indicates negative polarity. The question is asking what should not be done when using an inhaler.

   ① This is an acceptable practice because it mixes the medication within the solution so that the aerosol drug concentration is even.

* ② When using an MDI, inhalation and exhalation should be slow; this limits bronchial constriction and promotes a more even distribution of the aerosolized medication.

   ③ This is desirable because it allows tiny drops of aerosol spray to reach deeper branches of the airway.

   ④ This is desirable because it maximizes airway exposure to medication from the inhaler.

31 TEST-TAKING TIP ● The word "most" in the stem sets a priority.

* ① Medication injected into the abdomen is more rapidly absorbed than medication injected into the limbs of the body.

   ② Medication injected into the buttock is absorbed at a slower rate than medication injected into the abdomen.

   ③ Medication injected into the thigh is absorbed at the slowest rate.

   ④ Medication injected into the arm is absorbed at a slower rate than medication injected into the abdomen.

32 TEST-TAKING TIP ● The words "site of choice" in the stem set a priority.

   ① The deltoid is contraindicated for IM injections in infants and children. This site has a small amount of muscle mass and little subcutaneous fat, and it lies close to the radial nerve and brachial artery.

   ② The dorsogluteal muscle is contraindicated for an IM injection in children younger than 18 months of age because the muscle mass is inadequate to allow a safe injection. Also, the sciatic nerve and gluteal artery lie close to the site.

   ③ An infant or toddler should not receive an IM injection into the ventrogluteal muscle; the muscle is not well developed until the child begins to walk.

* ④ The rectus formis muscle, which belongs to the quadriceps muscle group, is the site of choice for IM injections in infants and children. It is the largest and most well-developed muscle in infants, is easy to locate, and is away from major blood vessels and nerves.

33 **TEST-TAKING TIP** ● The word "least" in the stem indicates negative polarity.
① This site is appropriate for an intramuscular injection in an obese individual as long as the amount of fluid injected is 5 mL or less.
② Same as #1.
* ③ The dorsogluteal muscle has a thick fat layer and with an intramuscular injection the medication would be deposited into subcutaneous tissue.
④ The deltoid is an appropriate muscle for an intramuscular injection in an obese individual as long as the amount of fluid injected is 2 mL or less.

34 **TEST-TAKING TIP** ● Options 1, 2, and 4 all have the prefix "intra." Option 3 is different.
① An intradermal injection is administered by inserting the needle of a syringe through the epidermis into the dermis where the fluid is injected. This is a safe procedure in an older adult who is cachectic.
② Intravenous medications can be administered safely to cachectic older adults.
* ③ Older adults and cachectic individuals have a decrease in subcutaneous tissue. When a subcutaneous injection is administered to a patient with insufficient subcutaneous tissue, the medication is usually absorbed faster; this could be unsafe.
④ Although muscle mass may be smaller in older adults and cachectic individuals, an intramuscular injection can be administered safely by using a 1-inch rather than a $1^1/_2$-inch needle.

35 **TEST-TAKING TIP** ● The word "contraindicated" in the stem indicates negative polarity.
① This is unrelated to the administration of medication via the sublingual route.
② Same as #1.
* ③ Patients who are confused, disoriented, or have a lowered level of consciousness would not be able to follow directions about keeping the medication under the tongue. The medication could be aspirated, which could be life-threatening, or it could be swallowed and inactivated by gastric acid.
④ Same as #1.

Meeting the Needs of the Perioperative Patient

This section includes questions related to meeting the needs of patients during the perioperative period. The questions focus on physical assessment and on prevention and care related to common complications associated with the perioperative period, such as hemorrhage, wound dehiscence, atelectasis, infection, and thrombophlebitis. The principles of perioperative teaching, meeting patients' emotional needs, sterile technique, and types of dressings and wounds are also tested. In addition, assessment and care of postoperative tubes and wound drainage systems are addressed.

Questions

1 Which intervention is unrelated to the prevention of postoperative thrombophlebitis?
① Massaging the legs
② Ambulating regularly
③ Increasing fluid intake
④ Applying antiembolism stockings

TEST-TAKING TIP ● Identify the word in the stem that indicates negative polarity.

2 When a patient is brought to the postanesthesia unit, the nurse is told that the patient lost 2 units of blood during surgery. Which patient adaptations would be significant in relation to this information?
① Rapid, deep breathing and increased blood pressure
② Rapid, deep breathing and decreased blood pressure
③ Slow, shallow breathing and increased blood pressure
④ Slow, shallow breathing and decreased blood pressure

TEST-TAKING TIP ● Identify the options that are opposites. Identify the duplicate facts among the options.

3 When caring for a postoperative patient who smokes, the nurse should monitor for:
① Airway patency
② Thrombophlebitis
③ Pulmonary emboli
④ Pulmonary hemorrhage

TEST-TAKING TIP ● Identify the clues in the stem.

4 While transferring a preoperative patient to a stretcher to be taken to the operating room, the patient states, "I do not want to be seen without my dentures in my mouth." The nurse should:
① Allow the patient to keep the dentures in the mouth
② Explore the patient's feelings regarding not wearing dentures
③ Explain that it is an important rule that preoperative patients must follow
④ Remove them before anesthesia and replace them as soon as the patient awakens

TEST-TAKING TIP ● Identify the option that denies the patient's feelings, concerns, and needs.

5 Sterile technique is maintained when the nurse:
① Always holds a wet 4 × 4 upward until ready for use
② Changes the gloves if they are positioned below the waist

③ Wipes the wound in a circular motion from the outside inward
④ Cleans the edges of the wound before the center of the wound

TEST-TAKING TIP ● Identify the specific determiner in an option. Identify equally plausible options.

6 What can the nurse do to best help a patient deal with postoperative psychological stress?
① Teach the use of imagery.
② Encourage ventilation of feelings.
③ Promote intellectual adaptive responses.
④ Obtain an order for an antianxiety medication.

TEST-TAKING TIP ● Identify the key word in the stem that sets a priority.

7 A patient adaptation that may first indicate internal abdominal bleeding postoperatively would be:
① Pain in the area of bleeding and an increased urinary output
② Cool, clammy skin and a decreased heart rate
③ Restlessness and an increased heart rate
④ Apathy and a decreased urinary output

TEST-TAKING TIP ● Identify the key word in the stem that sets a priority. Identify the duplicate facts among the options.

8 Which intervention would *best* prevent atelectasis following surgery?
① Oxygen via nasal cannula
② Diaphragmatic breathing
③ Progressive activity
④ Postural drainage

TEST-TAKING TIP ● Identify the key word in the stem that sets a priority. Identify the clue in the stem.

9 When does an infection of a surgical wound usually demonstrate clinical signs?
① Between the 3rd and 5th days following surgery
② Between the 1st and 2nd days following surgery
③ After 7 to 10 days following surgery
④ Within 24 hours following surgery

TEST-TAKING TIP ● Identify the options that are opposites.

10 Leg exercises following surgery are encouraged primarily to:
① Promote venous return
② Limit joint contractures
③ Prevent muscle atrophy
④ Increase muscle strength

TEST-TAKING TIP ● Identify the key word in the stem that sets a priority. Identify the equally plausible options.

11 Nursing care that is unique to a portable wound drainage system such as a Hemovac, which is different from tubes such as a T tube or an indwelling urinary catheter, is the need to:
① Maintain patency of the drainage tube
② Assess characteristics of the drainage
③ Ensure negative pressure
④ Measure output

TEST-TAKING TIP ● Identify the clue in the stem.

12 The nurse recognizes that a patient scheduled for bowel surgery has an enema before surgery primarily to reduce:
① Postoperative peristalsis
② Postoperative constipation
③ Incontinence during surgery
④ Contamination of the operative field

TEST-TAKING TIP ● Identify the key word in the stem that sets a priority. Identify the options that are opposites.

13 When collecting the health history before surgery, the nurse discovers that the patient has been smoking a pack of cigarettes daily. What should the nurse do?
① Inform the surgeon about the patient's smoking
② Ask the patient to stop smoking until after surgery
③ Remove the patient's cigarettes at midnight prior to surgery
④ Advise the patient to join a Smoke Enders Club after discharge

TEST-TAKING TIP ● Identify the options that deny the patient's feelings, concerns, and needs. Identify the unique option.

14 When assessing a postoperative patient for hemorrhage, which adaptations are associated with the compensatory stage of shock?
① Tachycardia and bradypnea
② Tachycardia and tachypnea
③ Bradycardia and bradypnea
④ Bradycardia and tachypnea

TEST-TAKING TIP ● Identify the clue in the stem. Identify the duplicate facts among the options. Identify the options that are opposites.

15 What is the primary purpose of a pressure dressing?
① Prevent pain
② Limit infection
③ Decrease drainage
④ Promote hemostasis

TEST-TAKING TIP ● Identify the key word in the stem that sets a priority. Identify the unique option.

16 When planning preoperative teaching for a patient having an appendectomy, what should be the initial action by the nurse?
① Identify the resources available to the patient.
② Explore the patient's prior surgical experiences.
③ Reassure the patient that an appendectomy is minor surgery.
④ Design a teaching plan appropriate for a patient with an appendectomy.

TEST-TAKING TIP ● Identify the key word in the stem that sets a priority. Identify the option that denies the patient's feelings, concerns, and needs.

17 A major difference in the postoperative regimen for a patient having abdominal surgery versus a patient having breast surgery is that the patient with abdominal surgery needs to:
① Ambulate as soon as possible
② Remain NPO until passing flatus
③ Void within 8 hours after surgery
④ Cough and deep breathe every 2 hours

TEST-TAKING TIP ● Identify the clue in the stem.

18 When planning a preoperative teaching class, the nurse understands that most patients avoid taking postoperative analgesics primarily because they are afraid of:

① Losing control
② Receiving an injection
③ Becoming dependent on them
④ Experiencing negative side effects

TEST-TAKING TIP ● Identify the key word in the stem that sets a priority.

19 After concerns about pain, the question most commonly asked by preoperative patients is, "When will I be able to

① Have visitors?"
② Go home?"
③ Shower?"
④ Eat?"

TEST-TAKING TIP ● Identify the key word in the stem that sets a priority.

20 When caring for a patient after thoracic surgery, the assessment that would be MOST specific to this type of surgery would be monitoring the:

① Blood pressure
② Urinary output
③ Intensity of pain
④ Rate and depth of respirations

TEST-TAKING TIP ● Identify the key word in the stem that sets a priority. Identify the clue in the stem. Identify the unique option.

21 When caring for patients with a variety of wounds, which type of wound would heal by primary intention?

① Surgical incision
② Laceration
③ Deep burn
④ Abrasion

TEST-TAKING TIP ● Identify the clue in the stem.

22 The MOST effective way to prevent dislodging the placement of a nasogastric tube is by:

① Pinning it to the pillow
② Attaching it to the gown
③ Taping it to the patient's nose
④ Instructing the patient not to touch it

TEST-TAKING TIP ● Identify the key word in the stem that sets a priority. Identify the equally plausible options.

23 Postoperatively a patient complains of pain in the calf. What would be the most appropriate intervention by the nurse?

① Alert the physician.
② Implement warm soaks.
③ Administer cool compresses.
④ Apply anti-embolism stockings.

TEST-TAKING TIP ● Identify the key word in the stem that sets a priority. Identify the options that are opposites. Identify the unique option.

24 What should the nurse do when assessing for dehiscence following surgery?
① Assess for hypertension.
② Monitor for hypotension.
③ Observe the wound edges.
④ Palpate around the wound.

TEST-TAKING TIP ● Identify opposites in options.

25 The nurse would know that further preoperative teaching was needed when the patient says, "I should:
① Expect to be in the postanesthesia unit after surgery."
② Apply pressure against the incision when coughing."
③ Ask for medication when I begin to have pain."
④ Lie still while I am on bed rest."

TEST-TAKING TIP. ● Identify the words in the stem that indicate a negative polarity.

26 What would be the most therapeutic statement when assessing a patient's knowledge of surgery?
① "Have you ever had surgery before?"
② "What are your concerns about surgery?"
③ "Surgery can be a frightening experience."
④ "Tell me about your experiences with surgery."

TEST-TAKING TIP ● Identify the key word in the stem that sets a priority.

27 What should the nurse do when assessing for correct placement of a nasogastric tube?
① Auscultate the lungs.
② Aspirate stomach contents.
③ Instill 30 cc of normal saline.
④ Place the end of the tube in water.

TEST-TAKING TIP ● Identify the options that are opposites.

28 Which adaptation is indicative of internal hemorrhage?
① Decreased respiratory rate
② Fall in blood pressure
③ Warm, clammy skin
④ Bradycardia

29 What is the technical name for bloody drainage from a wound?
① Sanguineous
② Hemoptysis
③ Purulent
④ Serous

30 Which patient is at the highest risk when undergoing major surgery?
① Neonate
② Adolescent
③ School-age child
④ Menopausal woman

TEST-TAKING TIP ● Identify the options that are opposites.

31 What should the nurse do to help prevent postoperative wound dehiscence?
① Keep the wound clean and dry.
② Change the dressing every 8 hours.

③ Regularly medicate the patient for pain.
④ Provide incisional support during activity.

TEST-TAKING TIP ● Identify the equally plausible options.

32 Which assessment is <u>most</u> significant when assessing a postoperative patient with a history of heart disease?
① Pain at the site of the incision
② Alterations in fluid balance
③ An irregular pulse rhythm
④ Dependent edema

TEST-TAKING TIP ● Identify the word in the stem that sets a priority. Identify the equally plausible options.

33 Which adaptation indicates postoperative laryngeal spasm after extubation?
① Rales
② Gurgles
③ Crackles
④ Wheezing

TEST-TAKING TIP ● Identify the equally plausible options.

34 What is the most important postoperative assessment of a patient after spinal anesthesia?
① Peripheral circulation
② Level of consciousness
③ Sensation in the legs and toes
④ Orientation to time and place

TEST-TAKING TIP ● Identify the equally plausible options.

35 Which factor places an elderly person more at risk for surgery than a younger person?
① Increased glomerular filtration rate
② Decreased rigidity of arterial walls
③ Higher basal metabolic rate
④ Reduced cardiac reserve

Rationales

1 **TEST-TAKING TIP** ● The word "unrelated" in the stem indicates negative polarity. It is asking which option is not related to preventing thrombophlebitis.
* ① Massaging the legs could traumatize the vessels, contributing to the formation of thrombi.
② Ambulating increases circulation in the lower extremities, which helps prevent thrombus formation.
③ Increasing fluid intake promotes hemodilution, which limits the production of thrombus formation.
④ Antiembolism stockings promote venous return, which prevents the formation of thrombi.

2 **TEST-TAKING TIP** ● The question is testing your knowledge about the type of breathing and the type of blood pressure associated with hypovolemia secondary to blood loss. If you know just one of these facts related to hypovolemia, you can reduce your final selection to between two options. Options 1 and 4 are opposites and Options 2 and 3 are opposites. Although there are two sets of opposites in this item, it is easier and more productive to focus instead on the duplicate facts to help you eliminate distractors. The use of test-taking techniques should not become so complex that it makes the question more difficult to answer.
① Although rapid, deep breathing is associated with hypovolemia, the blood pressure will be decreased, not increased.
* ② With a decrease in circulating red blood cells, the respiratory rate will increase in rate and depth to meet oxygen needs. With a reduction in blood volume, there will be a decrease in blood pressure.
③ With hypovolemia the breathing will be rapid and deep, not slow and shallow, and the blood pressure will decrease, not increase.
④ Although the blood pressure will decrease with hypovolemia, the respirations will be rapid and deep, not slow and shallow.

3 **TEST-TAKING TIP** ● The words "postoperative" and "smokes" are clues in the stem.
* ① Smoking increases mucus production and destroys the protective action of cilia; a smoker is at risk for ineffective airway clearance.
② A patient on bed rest is at risk for thrombophlebitis and a pulmonary embolus, which would result in an ineffective gas exchange.
③ The patient with pelvic surgery or venous peripheral vascular disease is at risk for pulmonary emboli, which would result in an ineffective gas exchange.
④ This is an unlikely occurrence; this can occur with the erosion associated with lung cancer.

4 **TEST-TAKING TIP** ● Option 3 denies the patient's feelings, concerns, and needs.
① It is unsafe to allow dentures to be in the mouth during surgery because dentures could be aspirated while the patient is unconscious.
② Although exploring the patient's feelings might be done, it does not address safety needs.
③ This response denies the patient's feelings and cuts off communication; care can be individualized while still meeting safety needs.
* ④ Removing the dentures immediately before surgery and returning them as soon as possible after surgery meets the patient's self-esteem needs while providing for physical safety.

5 **TEST-TAKING TIP** ● Option 1 contains the word "always," which is a specific determiner. Options 3 and 4 are equally plausible.

  ① Fluid from the wet 4 × 4 can run down the upraised hand. When the hand is repositioned with the fingers downward, the fluid that runs back down the hand may be contaminated, which in turn will contaminate the 4 × 4.

  * ② When sterile gloves are accidentally positioned below the waist, they are considered out of the line of sight and must be changed because they may have become inadvertently contaminated.

  ③ This action can move contaminated material from a more contaminated section to a less contaminated section of a wound. The center of a wound is considered less contaminated than the edges of the wound or the surrounding skin; therefore, the nurse should wipe a wound moving from the center outward using one gauze pad per stroke.

  ④ Same as #3.

6 **TEST-TAKING TIP** ● The word "best" in the stem sets a priority.

  ① Teaching imagery may reduce anxiety temporarily, but it does not address the underlying concerns.

  * ② This provides open-minded communication and allows the patient to explore concerns.

  ③ Intellectual adaptive responses do not take place in the affective domain. The affective domain deals with psychological needs.

  ④ Medication may be unnecessary if the patient's psychological needs are addressed effectively.

7 **TEST-TAKING TIP** ● The word "first" is the key word in the stem that sets a priority. Duplicate facts include a decreased or an increased heart rate and a decreased or an increased urinary output. If you know that any of these facts are true, you can reduce your final choice to two options.

  ① Pain is a later sign because enough blood will have had to collect to cause distention of tissues and organ displacement. With hemorrhage, the reduction in circulating blood volume results in a decrease, not an increase, in the urinary output.

  ② Eventually the skin becomes cool and clammy in response to sympathetic nervous system stimulation and vasoconstriction. The heart rate will increase, not decrease.

  * ③ Restlessness and an increased heart rate are sympathetic nervous system–stimulated responses that occur early in episodes of hemorrhage.

  ④ The patient will be apprehensive and restless, not apathetic. Eventually the urinary output will decrease as a result of vasoconstriction and the decrease in circulating blood volume.

8 **TEST-TAKING TIP** ● The word *best* is the key word in the stem that sets a priority. The words "prevent atelectasis" are the clue in the stem.

  ① Exogenous oxygen increases the partial pressure of oxygen, it does not prevent atelectasis.

  * ② Diaphragmatic breathing expands the alveoli, which prevents atelectasis; it also precipitates coughing, which prevents the accumulation and stagnation of secretions.

  ③ Activity will promote cardiopulmonary and circulatory functioning in general; it does not specifically prevent atelectasis to the same extent that diaphragmatic breathing will.

  ④ Postural drainage promotes the flow of mucus out of segments of the lung; it is not done routinely following surgery to prevent atelectasis.

9 **TEST-TAKING TIP** ● Options 3 and 4 are opposites among the options presented.

* ① Inadequate aseptic technique can precipitate an infection, which manifests itself in approximately 3 to 5 days; erythema, pain, edema, chills, fever, and purulent drainage indicate infection.

② This is too short a time for an infectious process to develop from a surgical incision; a contaminated, traumatic wound could precipitate an infection this early.

③ An infectious process would manifest itself before 7 to 10 days; wound dehiscence or evisceration may occur 5 to 10 days after surgery before collagen formation occurs.

④ Same as #2.

10 **TEST-TAKING TIP** ● The word "primarily" is the key word in the stem that sets a priority. Options 3 and 4 are equally plausible.

* ① Circulatory stasis occurs after surgery because postoperative patients are not as active as before surgery; leg exercises promote venous return and prevent the formation of thrombi and thrombophlebitis.

② Range-of-motion exercises, not leg exercises, are performed to prevent joint contractures.

③ Although this is a benefit of leg exercises, it is not the primary reason for performing leg exercises postoperatively.

④ Same as #3.

11 **TEST-TAKING TIP** ● The word "unique" is the clue in the stem.

① All tubes must be patent for drainage to occur.

② All drainage must be assessed for quantity, color, consistency, and odor.

* ③ Portable wound drainage systems work by continuous low pressure as long as the suction bladder is less than half full; T tubes and indwelling urinary catheters work by gravity.

④ The volume of fluid over specific time periods must be measured for all drainage.

12 **TEST-TAKING TIP** ● The word "primarily" is the key word in the stem that sets a priority. Options 1 and 2 are opposites.

① The natural defense mechanisms of the body and the trauma to the intestines will prevent postoperative peristalsis; usually within 3 days peristalsis will return spontaneously.

② Postoperative constipation is prevented by activity and adequate fluid intake.

③ Although an enema will prevent incontinence during surgery, it is not the purpose of a thorough bowel prep for intestinal surgery.

* ④ If feces are present in the bowel when the intestine is incised, the excrement will spill into the abdominal cavity, causing contamination and increasing the risk of peritonitis.

13 **TEST-TAKING TIP** ● Options 2 and 3 deny the patient's feelings, concerns, and needs. Option 1 is unique because it involves communicating information to the surgeon. Options 2, 3, and 4 involve communicating with the patient.

* ① The physician should be made aware of this fact because it may influence the type of anesthesia used and the perioperative medical regimen.

② If the patient is willing to stop smoking, it should be discontinued before and after surgery to prevent respiratory complications. The nurse should recognize that the patient may need to continue to smoke because it may be a coping mechanism.

③ The nurse does not have a right to take a patient's belongings; the patient should be told where and when smoking is permitted or if the facility is "smoke free."

④ Discussing a Smoke Enders Club would be inappropriate at this time because the patient is concerned with the present situation; this might eventually be done after surgery.

14 **TEST-TAKING TIP** ● The words "compensatory stage" modify the word "shock" and are a clue in the stem. This question is testing two concepts associated with shock, heart rate, and respiratory rate. If you know one fact related to shock, two options can be deleted from consideration. Options 1 and 4 are opposites and Options 2 and 3 are opposites. Consider these options carefully.
  ① Tachycardia is associated with shock, but the patient would have tachypnea, not bradypnea.
 * ② With shock, the sympathetic nervous system (SNS) is activated because of changes in blood volume and blood pressure. The SNS stimulates the cardiovascular system, causing tachycardia, and the respiratory system, causing tachypnea.
  ③ The opposite is true.
  ④ Tachypnea is associated with shock and tachycardia, not bradycardia, is also associated with shock.

15 **TEST-TAKING TIP** ● The word "primary" is the key word in the stem that sets a priority. Option 4 is unique because it comes from a positive perspective, expressed by the word "promote." Options 1, 2, and 3 come from a negative perspective, expressed by the words "prevent," "limit," and "decrease."
  ① Although a pressure dressing may help prevent the accumulation of interstitial fluid, thereby limiting pain, it will not prevent pain; also, this is not the primary purpose of a pressure dressing.
  ② Surgical asepsis, not a pressure dressing, limits infection.
  ③ Dressings absorb drainage, they do not decrease drainage.
 * ④ Pressure causes the constriction of peripheral blood vessels, which prevents bleeding; it also eliminates dead space in underlying tissue so that healing can progress.

16 **TEST-TAKING TIP** ● The word "initial" is the key word in the stem that sets a priority. Option 3 denies the patient's feelings, concerns, and needs.
  ① Although it will be done eventually, determining the patient's resources is not the initial intervention.
 * ② Obtaining relevant data about the patient's past experience identifies influencing factors and learning needs; teaching should be based on the patient's frame of reference.
  ③ Minimizing the seriousness of the surgery denies the patient's feelings and cuts off communication.
  ④ Designing a teaching plan can be done only after data are collected and analyzed.

17 **TEST-TAKING TIP** ● The words "major difference" are the clue in the stem.
  ① Both patients must be active to prevent respiratory and circulatory complications.
 * ② Manipulation of the abdominal organs during surgery produces a temporary paralytic ileus. The patient must take nothing by mouth until intestinal peristalsis returns; only the patient with abdominal surgery had the abdominal organs manipulated during surgery.
  ③ Both patients had anesthesia; therefore, for both patients the nurse must implement measures that prevent postoperative complications such as urinary retention.
  ④ Both patients had anesthesia; therefore, for both patients the nurse must implement measures that prevent postoperative respiratory complications such as atelectasis and pneumonia.

18 TEST-TAKING TIP ● The word "primarily" is the key word in the stem that sets a priority. Do not be distracted by the word "most" because it does not really relate to the question being asked, the "primary" reason why people "do not" take analgesics.

① Although this is a concern of some patients, a fear of dependency is the primary reason why patients avoid or decline medications for pain.

② Same as #1.

* ③ Postsurgical patients avoid or limit the intake of pain medication for fear of becoming physically or psychologically dependent; however, the drug dosage and ordered time intervals are insufficient to cause dependence over a short period of time following surgery.

④ Same as #1.

19 TEST-TAKING TIP ● The word "most" in the stem sets a priority.

① Although this may be important to some patients, pain relief and eating are the most basic, common concerns of the majority of patients.

② Same as #1.

③ Same as #1.

* ④ Eating is a basic human need identified by Maslow and is considered very important by postoperative patients.

20 TEST-TAKING TIP ● The word MOST is the key word in the stem that sets a priority. The word "thoracic" is the clue in the stem. Option 4 is unique because it is the only option with two assessments.

① Monitoring the blood pressure is important following any surgery and not specific to thoracic surgery.

② Although monitoring fluid intake and urinary output is important following all types of surgery, this patient's cardiopulmonary status is the priority.

③ Monitoring the characteristics of pain is required following all types of surgery and is not specific to thoracic surgery.

* ④ Thoracic surgery involves entering the thoracic cavity; respiratory function becomes a major priority.

21 TEST-TAKING TIP ● The words "primary intention" are the clue in the stem.

* ① Primary intention is the normal healing process that consists of the stages of defensive, reconstructive, and maturative healing; it involves a clean wound that has edges that are closely approximated.

② A laceration results from trauma; the wound probably contains microorganisms, and the tissue is torn with irregular wound edges. A laceration generally heals by secondary intention.

③ A burn has wound edges that are not approximated, and the wound is usually wide and open. A burn usually heals by secondary intention.

④ An abrasion is an open wound resulting from friction, and the wound edges are not approximated. An abrasion generally heals by secondary intention.

22 TEST-TAKING TIP ● The word MOST in the stem sets a priority. Options 1 and 2 are equally plausible.

① Pinning the tubing to the patient's gown or bed linen is unsafe; tension on the tube would increase with patient movement, which could result in displacement of the tube.

② Same as #1.

    * ③ Taping a nasogastric tube to the patient's nose anchors the tube and helps prevent the tube from becoming dislodged.

    ④ Although this should be done, it is not the most effective way to prevent dislodgment of the tube because patients tend to touch foreign objects that irritate the body.

23 TEST-TAKING TIP ● The word "most" in the stem sets a priority. Options 2 and 3 are opposites. Option 1 is unique because communicating information to other health team members is an independent function of the nurse. Options 2, 3, and 4 are all dependent functions of the nurse.

    * ① Of the options offered, alerting the physician is the most appropriate response. If the pain is due to thrombophlebitis, the patient is at risk for a pulmonary embolus and the physician should be notified immediately. Of course, a detailed assessment should be performed before notifying the physician.

    ② Warm soaks require a physician's order.

    ③ Cool compresses require a physician's order. In addition, this is not an acceptable intervention for thrombophlebitis because cool compresses cause vasoconstriction.

    ④ Anti-embolism stockings are contraindicated during acute thrombophlebitis. The pressure of applying and wearing these stockings could dislodge the clot, resulting in a pulmonary embolus.

24 TEST-TAKING TIP ● Options 1 and 2 are opposites.

    ① Hypertension is unrelated to dehiscence.

    ② Hypotension is related to hemorrhage, not dehiscence.

    * ③ Dehiscence is a separation of the wound edges at the suture line, which is evidenced by increased drainage and the appearance of underlying tissue; this most frequently occurs 5 to 12 days postoperatively. Dehiscence is precipitated by increased intra-abdominal pressure associated with coughing, vomiting, and distention; obesity is a risk factor.

    ④ Palpation assesses for edema and heat; if these signs occur 3 to 6 days postoperatively, infection, not dehiscence, is suspected.

25 TEST-TAKING TIP ● The word "further" indicates negative polarity. The question is really asking which patient statement is "not correct."

    ① Patients are kept in the postanesthesia unit until reactive and stable.

    ② Applying pressure against an incision is an acceptable practice to minimize incisional pain and prevent dehiscence when performing any activity that raises intra-abdominal pressure.

    ③ Pain relief is more effective when analgesics are administered before pain becomes severe; this prevents excessive peaks and troughs in the pain experience.

    * ④ Remaining immobile is unacceptable following surgery because it promotes cardiopulmonary, vascular, and gastrointestinal complications; the patient needs further preoperative teaching.

26 TEST-TAKING TIP ● The word "most" is the key word in the stem that sets a priority.

    ① This statement is a direct question that can be answered with a "yes" or a "no."

    ② Concerns generally focus on feelings rather than knowledge; this statement is a direct question that the patient may be unable or unwilling to answer.

    ③ This statement could precipitate unnecessary anxiety; feelings should be raised by the patient, not the nurse.

    * ④ This statement is an open-ended question that invites the patient to discuss past experiences. The patient's past experiences may be less anxiety producing than the present situation and they provide a database for future teaching.

27 TEST-TAKING TIP ● Options 2 and 3 are opposites. Consider these options carefully. In this question, one of them is the correct answer.

① The tube is in the stomach, not the lungs.

* ② The tube is in the stomach and application of negative pressure to the tube would cause gastric contents to be pulled up the tube and into the syringe.

③ This is unsafe; if the tube is in the wrong place (e.g., esophagus, trachea), it would result in aspiration of the fluid.

④ This is unsafe; if the tube is in the respiratory system rather than the stomach, a deep inhalation could cause an aspiration of fluid.

28 ① The respiratory rate would increase in an effort to bring more oxygen to body cells.

* ② The patient would become hypotensive with the loss of blood because of hypovolemia.

③ The skin would be cool and clammy because of the sympathetic nervous system response.

④ The heart rate would increase, not decrease, in an effort to increase cardiac output and bring more oxygen to body cells.

29 * ① Sanguineous or bloody drainage indicates fresh bleeding or hemorrhage.

② Hemoptysis is coughing up blood from the respiratory tract.

③ Purulent drainage contains pus and indicates the presence of infection.

④ Serous drainage consists of clear, watery plasma.

30 TEST-TAKING TIP ● Options 1 and 4 are opposites. They can both be deleted from consideration or one of them is the correct answer.

* ① The neonate has immature body systems and a lack of physiological reserve and therefore is at greatest risk for the stresses of surgery.

② This age group usually tolerates surgery well.

③ Same as #2.

④ Same as #2.

31 TEST-TAKING TIP ● Options 1 and 2 are equally plausible; they both reflect action that prevents infection

① This would prevent infection, not wound dehiscence.

② Same as #1.

③ Pain medication promotes comfort; it does not limit the occurrence of dehiscence.

* ④ Pressure against the incision supports the integrity of the approximation of the edges of the wound.

32 TEST-TAKING TIP ● The word "most" in the stem sets a priority. Options 2 and 4 are equally plausible; they both relate to problems with fluid balance.

① Pain at the incisional site is common to postoperative patients and not specific to a postoperative patient with a history of heart disease.

② Although this would be an important assessment, it would not be immediately life threatening.

* ③ This could indicate a life-threatening dysrhythmia.

④ Same as #2.

33 TEST-TAKING TIP ● Options 1 and 3 are equally plausible.

① Rales, more correctly known as crackles, are sounds caused by air passing through vessels containing excessive moisture.

② Gurgles, formerly known as rhonchi, are sounds caused by air moving through tenacious mucus or narrowed bronchi.

③ Same as #1.

* ④ Wheezing, which consists of high-pitched whistling sounds, is caused by air moving through a narrowed or partially obstructed airway.

34 **TEST-TAKING TIP** ● Options 2 and 4 are equally plausible. General anesthesia acts on the cerebral centers to produce loss of consciousness. When recovering from general anesthesia, the patient may be disoriented.

① Spinal anesthesia does not alter peripheral circulation.

② General anesthesia, not spinal anesthesia, alters the patient's level of consciousness.

* ③ Spinal anesthesia causes anesthesia and paralysis of the toes, perineum, legs, and abdomen. When motion and sensation of the legs and toes return, the patient is considered to have recovered from the effects of the spinal anesthetic.

④ General anesthesia, not spinal anesthesia, alters orientation to time, place, and person.

35 ① Elderly people have a decreased, not increased, glomerular filtration rate.

② Elderly people have an increased, not decreased, rigidity of arterial walls.

③ Elderly people have a lower, not higher, basal metabolic rate.

* ④ Cardiac output and strength of cardiac contractions decrease and the heart rate takes longer to return to the resting rate as one ages. Sudden physical or emotional stresses may result in cardiac dysrhythmias and heart failure.

Meeting Patients' Microbiological Safety Needs

This section includes questions on concepts and principles related to topics such as medical asepsis, surgical asepsis, types of isolation, and the chain of infection. Particular emphasis is placed on nursing actions that protect the nurse and the patient from microorganisms, including questions on handwashing and disposal of contaminated equipment and linen. The questions also address risk factors for infection, common adaptations to infection, and patient teaching/learning infection control practices.

Questions

1 Which action would break the chain of infection from a portal of exit from a reservoir?
① Washing the hands
② Disposing of soiled linen
③ Disinfecting used equipment
④ Avoiding talking over an open wound
TEST-TAKING TIP ● Identify the words in the stem that provide a clue.

2 When changing the bed linens, the nurse decides to reuse the blanket because it is still clean. The nurse should:
① Reconsider and replace it with a new blanket
② Store it on the floor of the patient's closet
③ Fanfold it to the foot of the patient's bed
④ Place it on the windowsill, out of the way
TEST-TAKING TIP ● Identify the equally plausible options.

3 Which would best increase a patient's defense against microorganisms?
① Intact skin
② Covering a cough
③ Changing bed linen daily
④ Using an antiseptic mouthwash
TEST-TAKING TIP ● Identify the word in the stem that sets a priority. Which option is unique?

4 What can the nurse do to prevent fungal infections in the hospitalized patient?
① Apply moisturizing lotion to the patient's body.
② Dry the folds of the patient's skin well.
③ Provide a daily bath for the patient.
④ Keep the patient's room cool.

5 The nurse recognizes that further teaching about Universal Precautions is necessary when a relative of an HIV-positive patient says, "Universal Precautions apply when I:
① Clean up body fluids that contain blood."
② Provide perineal care."
③ Change soiled linen."
④ Wipe tears away."
TEST-TAKING TIP ● Identify the words in the stem that indicate negative polarity.

6 What should the nurse do to best help the patient deal with the psychological aspects of strict isolation?
① Draw a smiley face on the mask.
② Wear a gown only when direct contact is expected.
③ Explain the reason for, and importance of, isolation.
④ Talk with the patient often from a slightly open door.

TEST-TAKING TIP ● Identify the word in the stem that sets a priority. Identify the option that contains a specific determiner.

7 What should the nurse do first to remove protective clothing when leaving a contact isolation room?
① Untie the gown at the waist.
② Untie the gown at the neck.
③ Remove the gloves.
④ Remove the mask.

8 When planning care for patients who have AIDS, the nurse recognizes that all these patients have the greatest risk for:
① Environmental disorientation
② Nosocomial infections
③ Secondary cancer
④ Pressure ulcers

TEST-TAKING TIP ● Identify the word in the stem that sets a priority. Identify the word in the stem that is a clue.

9 Which patient behavior demonstrates that a patient with pulmonary tuberculosis (TB) understands infection control measures that contain acid-fast bacilli?
① Calling the nurse to empty the urinal
② Wearing gloves when blowing the nose
③ Flushing the toilet twice after a bowel movement
④ Wearing a particulate respiratory mask during transport

TEST-TAKING TIP ● Identify the clue in the stem.

10 Which would place a patient at greatest risk for a respiratory tract infection?
① Urinary catheter
② Long hospital stay
③ Painful chest injury
④ Nasogastric tube for decompression

TEST-TAKING TIP ● Identify the word in the stem that sets a priority.

11 When assessing a patient for an infection, which is the most common adaptation?
① Dehydration
② Headache
③ Anorexia
④ Fever

TEST-TAKING TIP ● Identify the word in the stem that sets a priority. Identify the word in the stem that is a clue.

12 Which question should the nurse ask a patient with an infection when taking a nursing history as opposed to a medical history?
① "Have you done any traveling lately?"
② "How long has the infection been present?"

③ "When did you first notice your symptoms?"

④ "How does the infection affect your daily routine?"

TEST-TAKING TIP ● Identify the equally plausible options.

13 Which laboratory result needs to be reported to the physician for a patient admitted to the hospital with a medical diagnosis of fever of unknown origin?

① 1.020 urine specific gravity

② 20,000 white blood cells

③ 14.5 hemoglobin

④ 42 hematocrit

TEST-TAKING TIP ● Identify the words in the stem that set a priority.

14 Which patient goal is most appropriate for the nursing diagnosis Risk for Infection Related to Chemotherapy? The patient will:

① Be taught how to wash his or her hands before and after using the toilet.

② Explain three ways to limit exposure to microorganisms.

③ Receive a unit of packed red blood cells.

④ Control the spread of infection.

TEST-TAKING TIP ● Identify the word in the stem that sets a priority.

15 Which action associated with handwashing is guided by a principle of medical asepsis?

① Wash with the hands held higher than the elbows.

② Rinse with the hands held lower than the elbows.

③ Turn the water on with a clean paper towel.

④ Adjust the water to a hot temperature.

16 Further teaching about an isolation mask is indicated when a family member visiting a patient on airborne precautions says, "I must:

① Fold the mask within itself to contain microorganisms before I throw it away."

② Pinch the metal band on the mask snugly around the bridge of my nose."

③ Change my mask whenever it gets wet."

④ Put on a new mask every time I visit."

TEST-TAKING TIP ● Identify the unique option.

17 Which action is a violation of aseptic technique when removing soiled gloves?

① Grasping the outer surface of the left glove below the thumb with the gloved right hand

② Containing the removed glove from the left hand within the fingers of the gloved right hand

③ Using the left ungloved thumb and forefinger to grasp the inside and outside of the cuff of the gloved right hand

④ Discarding the right glove that has been inverted containing the left glove into an appropriate waste container

TEST-TAKING TIP ● Identify the word in the stem that indicates negative polarity.

18 When removing the protective gloves that were worn to start an intravenous solution, a female nurse notices that there is a small amount of the patient's blood on her forearm. What should the nurse do first?

① Wash the exposed area with soap and water.

② Wipe the blood off the forearm with an alcohol-soaked 4 × 4.

③ Flush the forearm from the elbow to the fingers with hot water.

④ Apply a new pair of gloves and absorb the blood with a paper towel.

19 Which nursing action interferes with the chain of infection at the level of transmission?
① Covering the nose when sneezing
② Disposing of any item that touches the floor
③ Turning and positioning a patient every 2 hours
④ Placing used syringes in a moisture-resistant, puncture-proof container

20 Where should soiled linen be placed when it is removed from a bed?
① In a soiled linen hamper
② On the overbed table
③ Into the linen chute
④ On a chair

TEST-TAKING TIP ● Identify the phrase that is a clue in the stem. Identify the equally plausible options.

21 Handwashing before and after voiding can be evaluated as effective when the patient is:
① Able to void
② In fluid balance
③ Free from infection
④ Emotionally comfortable

22 Bacteria rapidly multiply in environments that are:
① Hot
② Warm
③ Cool
④ Cold

TEST-TAKING TIP ● Identify the options that are opposites.

23 Linens that are still clean are often reused by the same patient. The article of linen that is least likely to be reused is the:
① Top sheet
② Bedspread
③ Pillowcase
④ Cotton blanket

TEST-TAKING TIP ● Identify the key word in the stem that indicates negative polarity. Identify the unique option.

24 A patient on contact isolation (precautions) needs a blood pressure reading taken every shift. To keep the sphygmomanometer from spreading microorganisms, the most practical intervention by the nurse would be to:
① Place it in a protective bag
② Keep it in the patient's room
③ Store it in the dirty utility room
④ Wipe it with a germicidal solution

TEST-TAKING TIP ● Identify the key word in the stem that sets a priority. Identify the clue in the stem.

25 After a patient vomits, the nurse should:
① Always contain the vomitus in a medical waste container
② Pour the vomitus down the sink in the dirty utility room
③ Discard the vomitus in the toilet and flush
④ Save a specimen of the vomitus for the lab

TEST-TAKING TIP ● Identify the option that contains a specific determiner.

26 The nurse should remove a dirty sheet from an unoccupied bed by:
① Pushing the sheet together
② Rolling the sheet into itself
③ Sliding the sheet to the side of the bed
④ Fanfolding the sheet to the foot of the bed

TEST-TAKING TIP ● Identify the equally plausible options.

27 Which action would break the chain of infection at the portal of entry to a susceptible patient?
① Maintaining sterile technique when administering an injection
② Wearing gloves when handling secretions
③ Donning a mask when splashing is likely
④ Using a gown in contact isolation

TEST-TAKING TIP ● Identify the clue in the stem. Identify the option that is unique.

28 Which would have the greatest impact on limiting the spread of microorganisms?
① Using disposable equipment
② Double-bagging
③ Wearing gloves
④ Handwashing

TEST-TAKING TIP ● Identify the key word in the stem that sets a priority.

29 A patient who chews tobacco continually spits tobacco juice on the floor. What should the nurse do *first*?
① Keep the tobacco at the nurses' station
② Teach the patient to dispose of saliva safely
③ Encourage the patient to use chewing gum instead
④ Inform the patient that tobacco chewing is unhealthy

TEST-TAKING TIP ● Identify the key word in the stem that sets a priority. Identify the patient-centered option. Identify the options that deny the patient's feelings, concerns, and needs

30 Which action is specific to caring for a patient on airborne precautions?
① Keeping the patient's door closed
② Donning a gown when administering medications
③ Wearing disposable gloves when delivering a meal
④ Instructing the patient to wear a mask when receiving care

TEST-TAKING TIP ● Identify the words in the stem that are a clue.

31 Which action is an unacceptable sterile technique when applying sterile gloves?
① Open the outer glove package, grasp the inner package, and lay it on a waist-high, clean surface.
② With the thumb and first two fingers of the nondominant hand, grasp the inside cuff of the glove for the dominant hand
③ With the gloved dominant hand, pick up the nondominant glove from the inside of the cuff and insert the nondominant hand
④ Apply the first glove with the fingers held toward the floor, and the second glove with the fingers held toward the ceiling

TEST-TAKING TIP ● Identify the word in the stem that indicates negative polarity.

32 Which action violates principles of surgical asepsis?
   ① Recapping a syringe once 3 cc of normal saline are withdrawn from a vial
   ② Holding a wet sterile 4 × 4 with sterile forceps while the handle is higher than the tip
   ③ Failing to wipe the rubber port of a newly opened sterile multiple-dose vial with an alcohol swab
   ④ Pouring Betadine on a 4 × 4 that is lying in its opened sterile paper wrapper while on an overbed table

   TEST-TAKING TIP ● Identify the word in the stem that indicates negative polarity.

33 What should the nurse do first when cleaning an emesis basin containing purulent material?
   ① Wash the basin in hot, soapy water.
   ② Rinse the basin with cold running water.
   ③ Clean the basin with an antiseptic agent.
   ④ Spray the basin with a disinfectant and let it work for 3 minutes.

34 When assessing a wound, which exudate would indicate the presence of an infectious process?
   ① Serous exudate
   ② Purulent exudate
   ③ Sanguineous exudate
   ④ Serosanguineous exudate

   TEST-TAKING TIP ● Identify the unique option.

35 Which action interferes with the chain of infection at the stage of transmission?
   ① Changing a soiled dressing
   ② Using Universal Precautions
   ③ Implementing an immunization program
   ④ Maintaining drainage suction equipment

1   **TEST-TAKING TIP** ● The words "portal of exit" provide a clue in the stem.

    ①   This action is an important means of controlling the transmission of microorganisms from one person or object to another; it does not limit the number of microorganisms directly exiting from a reservoir.

    ②   Same as #1.

    ③   Same as #1.

    * ④   This action would limit the number of microorganisms that exit from a respiratory tract. The respiratory tract is one portal of exit from the human reservoir (source of microorganisms); other human portals of exit include the gastrointestinal, urinary, and reproductive tracts and blood and body tissues.

2   **TEST-TAKING TIP** ● Options 2 and 4 are equally plausible because they address storing the blanket, but both actions violate medical asepsis.

    ①   Linen that is still clean can be reused for the same patient.

    ②   Items should never be stored on the floor of any area because they will become contaminated by microorganisms on the floor.

    * ③   Fanfolding a blanket to the foot of the bed is a safe and practical way to store a blanket; a fanfolded blanket can be easily opened over the patient.

    ④   Used linen should never be placed on the windowsill. The blanket would be considered contaminated.

3   **TEST-TAKING TIP** ● The word "best" in the stem sets a priority. Option 1 is unique. Options 2, 3, and 4 begin with the word ending in "ing." Also, they all involve an action.

    * ①   The skin is a barrier to pathogens and, if broken, serves as a portal of entry.

    ②   Covering a cough would protect others from the patient's microorganisms.

    ③   Although this action may reduce the number of microorganisms present, intact skin is the factor that would best protect the patient from microorganisms.

    ④   Same as #3.

4   ①   Moisturizers soften skin; they do not protect the skin from fungal infection.

    * ②   Fungi multiply rapidly in places where moisture content is high, such as in skin folds. Careful drying of skin folds, especially under the breasts and arms, between the toes, and in the perineal area, helps prevent the development of fungal infections.

    ③   Although bathing daily is helpful in preventing infection, careful drying is most essential to minimize a moist environment that supports the growth of fungi.

    ④   A cool room may reduce perspiration; however, careful drying is most helpful in minimizing the moisture in the folds of the skin that supports the growth of fungi.

5   **TEST-TAKING TIP** ● The words "further teaching . . . is necessary" indicate negative polarity.

    ①   Guidelines for Universal Precautions for the Prevention of Transmission of the Human Immunodeficiency Virus, published by the Centers for Disease Control and Prevention, indicate that Universal Precautions apply to blood, body fluids containing visible blood, semen and vaginal secretions, tissues, and cerebral spinal, pleural, synovial, peritoneal, pericardial, and amniotic fluid.

    ②   Universal Precautions should be followed when providing perineal care because the caregiver may come into contact with vaginal secretions, semen, or body fluids containing blood.

   ③ Soiled linen may be contaminated with semen, vaginal secretions, or body fluids containing blood. The caregiver should follow Universal Precautions when changing soiled linen.

* ④ Additional teaching is necessary because, unless blood is present, it is not necessary to use Universal Precautions when coming into contact with tears.

6 TEST-TAKING TIP ● The word "best" in the stem sets a priority. Option 2 has the word "only," which is a specific determiner.

   ① Nurses often draw a smiley face on the mask when caring for a child. When caring for an adult, the nurse should use humor carefully so as not to offend the patient. A patient may not find this action supportive. A patient may interpret a smiley face as an attempt to minimize the gravity of the illness.

   ② Gowns must be worn at all times when entering the room of a patient on strict isolation precautions and not just when the splashing of body fluids is anticipated.

* ③ Explanations support understanding, acceptance, and compliance with isolation precautions. When people understand the reason for a procedure, fear of the unknown and anxiety are usually reduced.

   ④ The door should be closed at all times except when entering or leaving the strict isolation room.

7 * ① The waist is considered contaminated and should be untied with a gloved hand.

   ② Neck ties are considered clean and should be untied after the gloves are removed.

   ③ Gloves are removed after the contaminated waist ties are untied.

   ④ After the gloves are removed, the mask is removed by touching only the ties. This is done to prevent contamination of the nurse's head, hair, and hands.

8 TEST-TAKING TIP ● The word "greatest" in the stem sets a priority. The word "all" in the stem is a clue. The correct answer must address something that is common to all patients with AIDS. Immunosuppression is common to all patients with AIDS.

   ① All patient who have AIDS do not have central nervous system involvement that may cause cognitive impairment.

* ② Patients who have AIDS are immunosuppressed and have a decreased ability to fight infection; this places them at the greatest risk for nosocomial (hospital-acquired) infections.

   ③ Not all patients with AIDS develop cancer.

   ④ Not all patients with AIDS are bed-bound or cachectic, which places them at risk for pressure ulcers.

9 TEST-TAKING TIP ● The word "pulmonary" modifies the word "tuberculosis" and is the clue in the stem. The word "pulmonary" in the stem and the word "respirator" in Option 4 have a covert interrelationship.

   ① Acid-fast bacilli related to pulmonary tuberculosis are not transmitted via urine.

   ② Although the patient would be taught to blow his or her nose and dispose of tissues properly to contain microorganisms, gloves are not necessary.

   ③ Acid-fast bacilli related to pulmonary tuberculosis are not transmitted via fecal material.

* ④ This is a component of airborne precautions necessary to limit the spread of acid-fast bacilli; this action minimizes air contamination and reduces the risk to persons who come into contact with the infected patient when he or she is being transported outside the isolation room.

10 TEST-TAKING TIP ● The word "greatest" in the stem sets a priority.

① A urinary catheter contributes to the risk for a urinary, not respiratory, tract infection.

② The hospital environment contains many pathogens; however, a person would have to be susceptible to contract an infection. Also, a person who could cough, deep-breathe, and clear secretions would be less likely to develop a respiratory tract infection than a patient who was unable to cough and deep-breathe.

* ③ Coughing and deep-breathing are often avoided by people with painful chest injuries in an effort to self-splint and minimize pain; this allows pooling of respiratory secretions and contributes to an environment that supports the growth of microorganisms in the respiratory tract.

④ A nasogastric tube decompressing the stomach removes fluid from the body, which does not increase the risk for a respiratory tract infection. A nasogastric tube used as a feeding tube would place the patient at risk for aspiration pneumonia.

11 TEST-TAKING TIP ● The word "most" in the stem sets a priority. The word "common" modifies the word "adaptation" and is the clue in the stem.

① Although dehydration can occur in response to a fever or an inadequate intake of fluid, it is not as common a response to infection as is a fever.

② This is a nonspecific manifestation of infection and is not as commonly exhibited by a patient with an infection as is a fever.

③ Same as #2.

* ④ Fever is the most common response of the hypothalamus (thermoregulatory center) to pyrogens that are released when phagocytic cells respond to the presence of pathogens.

12 TEST-TAKING TIP ● Options 2 and 3 both ask questions that identify a time frame in relation to symptoms; these options are equally plausible.

① Although the nurse may ask this question, knowing how the infection affects a person's functional health pattern is the nurse's major concern. The nurse's domain is concerned with identifying the patient's nursing diagnoses and formulating a nursing plan of care, not identifying the medical diagnosis and planning the medical treatment regimen.

② Same as #1.

③ Same as #1.

* ④ The nurse is mostly concerned with how the infection affects a person's functional health patterns. Many Nurse Practice Acts recognize that nurses diagnose and treat human responses.

13 TEST-TAKING TIP ● The words "needs to be reported" in the stem set a priority.

① This is within the normal range of urine specific gravity of 1.010 to 1.025 g/mL and is unrelated to infection.

* ② This is higher than the normal range of 4,500 to 11,000/μL and indicates the presence of an infection.

③ This is within the normal range for hemoglobin, which is 12 to 18 g/100 mL of blood.

④ This is within the normal range for hematocrit, which is 40 to 54 percent for males and 37 to 47 percent for females and is unrelated to infection.

14 TEST-TAKING TIP ● The word "most" in the stem sets a priority.

① This is the nurse's goal, not the patient's, because it identifies what the nurse needs to do. A patient goal might say, "The patient will demonstrate how to effectively wash the hands before and after using the toilet."

* ② This goal is acceptable; it is patient centered, measurable, and appropriate for a patient who needs to be protected from microorganisms.

③ This is a medical intervention, not a patient goal; white blood cells or granulocytes, not packed red blood cells, are administered to patients who have low white blood cell counts.

④ Although this goal is patient centered, it is too general, and the outcome is not measurable.

15 ① The hands should be held lower, not higher, than the elbows. The hands are more contaminated than the arms; water should flow from clean to contaminated surfaces.

* ② Rinsing with the hands lower than the elbows is correct technique; the hands are more contaminated than the arms. Water washes away debris and microorganisms and prevents recontamination of the cleaner surfaces.

③ The hands and the faucet are both considered contaminated and, therefore, it is not necessary to use a clean paper towel to turn on the faucet. A clean paper towel should be used to turn the faucet off after the hands are washed and dried.

④ The nurse should adjust the water to a warm, not hot, temperature; warm water removes less protective oils from the skin, which helps avoid chapping.

16 **TEST-TAKING TIP** ● Option 2 is unique because it is the only option that includes a rationale for the action.

* ① This is an unacceptable action. Only the ties should be touched when removing the mask; this prevents contact of the hands with the contaminated mask.

② Pinching the metal band across the bridge of the nose ensures a snug fit, minimizing the entrance or escape of microorganism around the nose.

③ The effectiveness of a mask deteriorates when it becomes moist. The mask should be changed as recommended by the manufacturer.

④ A mask should be discarded after every use. Masks become ineffective when they become moist.

17 **TEST-TAKING TIP** ● The word "violation" in the stem indicates negative polarity. The question is asking which action is not an acceptable practice when removing soiled gloves.

① The outer surfaces of both gloves are contaminated; this action keeps the soiled parts of the gloves from contaminating the skin of the left wrist or hand.

② This action contains the soiled glove within a small area and prevents inadvertent self-contamination.

* ③ This is a violation of aseptic technique. The outer surface of a soiled glove is contaminated and should not be touched by an ungloved hand. While holding the removed left glove in the right hand, the nurse should insert two fingers of the left, ungloved hand inside the cuff of the right glove. The nurse then pulls the right glove off, turning it inside out, thereby containing the left glove inside the inverted right glove.

④ This action disposes of both contaminated gloves safely; the most contaminated surfaces are inside the inverted right glove and they are contained in an appropriate receptacle for removal from the patient's unit.

18* ① Washing includes the action of wetting, rubbing, and rinsing; soap reduces the surface tension of water; friction mechanically disturbs microorganisms; and rinsing flushes microorganisms from the skin.

② The disinfectant isopropyl alcohol can kill bacteria, but cannot kill spores, viruses, or fungi.

③ Hot water does not disinfect and is unnecessary; it could injure the tissue.

④ This action does not adequately remove the contaminated material from the surface of the skin.

19 ① Covering the nose when sneezing interferes with the chain of infection at the portal of exit stage, not at the transmission stage.

* ② This is an action that interferes with the transmission of microorganisms in the chain of infection. Items that touch the floor are contaminated and must be disposed of in a manner that contains the spread of microorganisms.

③ Turning and positioning contributes to maintaining skin integrity. An intact skin interrupts the chain of infection at the portal of entry stage, not the transmission stage, of the chain of infection.

④ Disposing of used syringes properly interferes with the chain of infection at the reservoir or source of the infection. It interrupts the chain of infection at both the portal of entry and portal of exit stages.

20 **TEST-TAKING TIP** ● The phrase "soiled linen" used in the stem and in Option 1 is a clang association. Options 2 and 4 are equally plausible.

* ① This is a safe and acceptable way to contain microorganisms.

② Placing soiled linen on the overbed table will contaminate this surface and is an undesirable practice; the overbed table is considered a clean surface and should not be used to hold soiled linen.

③ Depositing unbagged soiled linen in the linen chute is an undesirable practice because it would contaminate the chute. Soiled linen should be bagged in an effort to contain microorganisms before it is deposited in a linen chute.

④ Placing soiled linen on a chair will contaminate this surface and is an undesirable practice; a chair is considered a clean surface and should not be used to hold soiled linen.

21 ① Handwashing is done to remove microorganisms, not induce voiding.

② Handwashing is related to reducing microorganisms, not fluid balance.

* ③ Handwashing minimizes self-contamination by soiled hands, which can be a source of infection.

④ Handwashing is related to meeting physical needs, not emotional needs.

22 **TEST-TAKING TIP** ● Options 1 and 4 are opposites.

① Hot temperatures are used to destroy bacteria (i.e., sterilization).

* ② Bacteria grow most rapidly in dark, warm, moist environments.

③ Bacteria grow best in temperatures close to "normal" body temperature (98.6°F), not cool or cold environments.

④ Same as #3.

23 **TEST-TAKING TIP** ● The word least is the key word in the stem that indicates negative polarity. Options 1, 2, and 4 are all similar because they are articles of linen that are generally placed over the patient. Option 3 is unique because it is the only article of linen in the options offered that is positioned under the patient.

① This article of linen is often used again if it is still clean.

② Same as #1.

* ③ The pillowcase comes in contact with the hair, exudate from the eyes, mucus from the nose, and saliva from the mouth. A pillowcase is easily soiled and usually needs to be replaced more often than other linens.

④ Same as #1.

24 TEST-TAKING TIP ● The word "most" is the key word in the stem that sets a priority. The word "practical" in the stem is a clue.

① It is unnecessary to bag the sphygmomanometer if it is left in the room. The outer surface of the bag is also contaminated and, if taken out of the room, would contaminate any surface on which it was placed.

* ② Keeping the sphygmomanometer in the patient's room is the most practical action; when isolation is discontinued, all of the equipment can be terminally disinfected.

③ The sphygmomanometer is contaminated and needs to be disinfected *before* it is removed from the patient's room.

④ Cleansing the sphygmomanometer after each use is safe but time consuming; it is more practical to leave frequently used equipment in an isolation room.

25 TEST-TAKING TIP ● The word "always" in Option 1 is a specific determiner.

① Vomitus should be flushed down a toilet, not contained in a medical waste container.

② It is unnecessary to remove vomitus from the room; vomitus should be poured down a toilet rather than a sink.

* ③ Discarding vomitus in the toilet and flushing is the most practical action when disposing of vomitus; it dilutes and contains it and removes the vomitus from the environment.

④ Saving vomitus for a specimen is generally unnecessary. Although a physician may request that vomitus be assessed, it is rarely sent for laboratory analysis.

26 TEST-TAKING TIP ● Options 3 and 4 are equally plausible.

① This would not secure loose ends; debris could fall on the floor.

* ② Rolling the soiled sheet into itself secures loose ends and keeps debris contained within the center of the sheet.

③ Same as #1.

④ Same as #1.

27 TEST-TAKING TIP ● The words "portal of entry" are the clue in the stem. Option 1 is unique. Options 2, 3, and 4 involve the caregiver wearing a product that provides for self-protection.

* ① Procedures that penetrate the body's natural protective barriers (e.g., skin) provide a portal of entry for microorganisms. The administration of parenteral medication uses sterile technique to minimize the risk of infection.

② This action protects the caregiver from contamination, not the patient.

③ Same as #2.

④ Same as #2.

28 TEST-TAKING TIP ● The word "greatest" is the key word in the stem that sets a priority.

① Although disposable equipment helps reduce the spread of microorganisms, it still needs to be safely handled when used. Handwashing is the most effective measure to reduce the spread of microorganisms.

② Double-bagging is used to dispose of infectious waste. Although double-bagging limits the spread of infection, handwashing is the most effective measure to reduce the spread of microorganisms.

③ Gloves protect the nurse; however, even when gloves are used, hands must be washed before and after use to prevent the spread of infection.

* ④ Handwashing is the most effective measure to reduce the spread of infection because it removes microorganisms from the hands, which come in contact with other patients and objects.

29 **TEST-TAKING TIP** ● The word *first* is the key word in the stem that sets a priority. Option 2 is patient centered. Options 1 and 3 deny the patient's feelings, concerns, and needs.

① Storing the tobacco at the nurses' station denies the "right" of the patient to have possession of personal property and does not change the unsafe behavior; an effort must be made to educate the patient about safe disposal of tobacco juice and saliva.

* ② Teaching the patient provides the information the patient needs to meet acceptable expectations regarding the disposal of tobacco juice and saliva; if infection control principles are followed, the patient can chew tobacco.

③ Encouraging the use of chewing gum instead of chewing tobacco denies the right of the patient to engage in activities of personal preference. The patient has a right to chew tobacco as long as acceptable infection control guidelines are followed.

④ Informing the patient that chewing tobacco is unhealthy must be done nonjudgmentally as when all behaviors associated with values are addressed. Although this might be done later, it does not address the immediate infection control problem of spitting on the floor. The patient must be taught infection control principles or he or she may continue to spit tobacco juice on the floor.

30 **TEST-TAKING TIP** ● The words "specific to" and "airborne precautions" are clues in the stem.

* ① Keeping the door closed prevents the spread of microorganisms that can be transmitted via air currents.

② When administering medications to a patient on airborne precautions, the nurse must wear a mask, not a gown.

③ When delivering a meal tray to a patient on airborne precautions, the nurse must wear a mask, not gloves.

④ The nurse, not the patient, wears the mask for self-protection.

31 **TEST-TAKING TIP** ● The word "unacceptable" is the word in the stem that indicates negative polarity.

① This is acceptable technique. A clean, dry surface prevents contamination of the wrapper; objects below the waist are considered contaminated.

② The ungloved hand is permitted to touch the inner surface of a sterile glove; both surfaces are considered contaminated.

* ③ Attempting to put on the second glove by gripping the inner cuff of the second glove increases the risk of touching the gloved hand against the ungloved hand or wrist, resulting in contamination. The gloved hand should slip fingers underneath the outer surface of the folded cuff of the other glove. This sterile-to-sterile contact maintains sterility.

④ This is acceptable technique. It really does not matter which direction the fingers are facing as long as the hands are kept above the waist, are in view, and do not become contaminated.

32 **TEST-TAKING TIP** ● The word "violates" in the stem indicates negative polarity. The question is asking you to identify what behavior is not acceptable when performing a sterile procedure.

① Recapping a sterile syringe that has not had contact with a patient or a nonsterile surface does not violate surgical asepsis; the needle of a syringe and inside the needle cap are both sterile and pose no microbiological risk of contamination. A used syringe or needle must be placed uncapped in an appropriate collection container to prevent needle-stick injury.

② This is correct technique. Fluids flow in the direction of gravity. When the tip is held lower than the handle, fluid will remain at the level of the 4 × 4 and the tip of the forceps; this area is considered sterile. If the nurse raises the tip of the forceps higher than the handle, fluid will flow up the handle onto the hand and the fluid becomes contaminated. When the tip of the forceps is then lowered, the contaminated fluid will flow back down the length of the forceps, contaminating the forceps and the 4 × 4.

③ When the metal protective ring and cap are removed from around the top of a multiple-dose vial, the rubber port surface is sterile until touched by something nonsterile. The rubber stopper does not have to be wiped with alcohol the first time the vial is accessed with a sterile syringe.

* ④ Although the inside of a sterile 4 × 4 wrapper is sterile, when the wrapper gets wet, capillary action will transfer microorganisms from the nonsterile surface of the table to the inside of the wrapper; the 4 × 4 will then become contaminated, which violates sterile technique.

33 ① Articles contaminated with organic material should be rinsed first in cold water. Hot water coagulates the protein of organic material and causes it to stick to a surface. Once rinsed in cold water, articles can be washed in hot soapy water.

* ② This is a correct action. Hot water coagulates the protein of organic material and causes it to stick to a surface. Therefore cold water should be used.

③ Antiseptics are used to limit bacteria on the skin or in wounds, not for cleaning objects.

④ This is unnecessary. Rinsing with cold water, washing with hot soapy water, and then rinsing and drying well are sufficient steps to clean personal articles kept at the bedside.

34 **TEST-TAKING TIP ●** The words in Options 1, 3, and 4 all begin with the letters "s." Option 2 is unique because it begins with a "p." Consider this option carefully.

① Serous exudate is watery in appearance, is composed of mainly serum, and does not indicate an infection.

* ② Purulent exudate contains material such as dead and living bacteria and dead tissue; it indicates the presence of an infection.

③ Sanguineous exudate indicates damage to capillaries that allows escape of red blood cells from plasma.

④ Serosanguineous exudate consists of clear and blood-tinged drainage seen in surgical incisions.

35 ① This reduces the spread of microorganisms and is an action associated with interfering with the chain of infection at the source of microbial growth (the reservoir). This action interferes with the portal of entry and portal of exit stages of the infection cycle.

* ② This prevents the spread of microorganisms and is associated with interfering with the chain of infection at the transmission stage. The transmission stage is when microorganisms move from the reservoir to the host.

③ Immunization supports host defenses and interferes with the chain of infection at the host stage.

④ This reduces the spread of microorganisms and is an action associated with interfering with the chain of infection at the source of microbial growth (the reservoir). It is most concerned with the portal of exit.

328 Meeting the Needs of the Patient in the Community Setting

This section encompasses questions related to caring for an individual, a family, a subgroup, or the population within a community. The questions include topics such as health care delivery settings (e.g., nursing homes, daycare centers, assisted living residences, occupational settings, and private homes), the focus of nursing actions (e.g., prevention of illness, health promotion, maintenance of safe environments, protection and restoration of health), and specific nursing activities (e.g., screening, health education). The questions also focus on levels of health care services (e.g., primary, secondary, and tertiary health care delivery), levels of disease prevention (e.g., primary, secondary, and tertiary levels of prevention), and community-focused examples related to nursing intervention (e.g., developmental stresses, common health problems, crisis intervention, and the needs of individuals in the community based on Maslow's Hierarchy of Needs).

Questions

1 Which statement regarding cultural diversity is most accurate?
① Cultural stereotyping can be helpful when assessing a patient's needs.
② Cultural differences "melt" as people assimilate into society.
③ Preconceptions need to be recognized and replaced with reality.
④ A person's values are rarely a component of culture.
TEST-TAKING TIP ● Identify the word in the stem that sets a priority.

2 Hospice care lies in which category of health care delivery?
① Primary health care
② Tertiary health care
③ Secondary health care
④ Affordable health care

3 Which nursing intervention would take priority when caring for a patient recently discharged from the hospital?
① Exploring the need to modify the environment to prevent falls
② Teaching a family member how to feed a client who has a decreased gag reflex
③ Encouraging the client to ventilate negative feelings about loss of independence
④ Providing opportunities for the client to make choices concerning the plan of care
TEST-TAKING TIP ● Identify the word in the stem that sets a priority.

4 Community-based nursing is mainly associated with which categories of health care delivery?
① Primary and tertiary
② Secondary and primary
③ Tertiary and rehabilitation
④ Rehabilitation and secondary
TEST-TAKING TIP ● Identify the duplicate facts among the options.

5 Community health nursing is mainly associated with:
① Delivering home health care services
② Assisting economically disadvantaged high-risk groups

③ Addressing the nursing needs of a specific individual or group within the community

④ Providing interventions that help people on the health end of the health-illness continuum

TEST-TAKING TIP ● Identify the clue in the stem.

6 Which population could be expected to experience a maturational/developmental crisis?
① Homosexual adolescents
② Recently divorced men
③ Critically ill children
④ Unemployed adults

TEST-TAKING TIP ● Identify the clue in the stem.

7 An essential aspect of community health nursing is its:
① Emphasis mainly on health promotion
② Focus on the needs of individuals
③ Practice within the home setting
④ Interdisciplinary nature

8 Which is an example of a community health practice that would directly remedy an unhealthy situation?
① Providing health care to the homeless
② Providing for fluoridation of water
③ Supporting rehabilitation services
④ Supporting vaccination programs

9 Which group is covered by Medicare?
① People who receive Aid to Families with Dependent Children
② People who need nurse midwife services
③ People with just a low income
④ People 65 years and older

TEST-TAKING TIP ● Identify the option that contains a specific determiner.

10 Which intervention is an example of secondary disease prevention?
① Watching for early signs of child abuse
② Encouraging the use of a baby car seat
③ Suggesting a smoking cessation program
④ Teaching about sexually transmitted diseases

TEST-TAKING TIP ● Identify the clue in the stem. Identify the unique option.

11 A soon-to-be-discharged patient who has respiratory medications states, "Whenever I have difficulty breathing I'll just take extra puffs on my inhaler." What should be the first response by the nurse?
① "If you cannot breathe, you should call 911."
② "How often do you have difficulty breathing?"
③ "If you cannot breathe, you should call your physician."
④ "Let's review why it's dangerous to take medications more frequently than ordered."

TEST-TAKING TIP ● Identify the word in the stem that sets a priority.

12 Which action is an example of primary disease prevention?
① Recalling contaminated food
② Using grab bars in a bathroom
③ Testing soil for hazardous chemicals
④ Assessing a widow for maladaptive grieving

13 What is the key factor that influences the role of the nurse working in the occupational setting?
① The average age of the work force
② The general health of the employees
③ The stresses of the work environment
④ The policies established by management

TEST-TAKING TIP ● Identify the words in the stem that set a priority.

14 Which action by the nurse in the occupational setting reflects the lowest-level need according to Maslow?
① Identifying hazards in the environment
② Assessing the health status of employees
③ Initiating an ordered immunization program
④ Promoting employees' social adaptation to the job

TEST-TAKING TIP ● Identify the key words in the stem.

15 Which action by the nurse in the occupational setting reflects a second-level need according to Maslow?
① Complying with OSHA regulations
② Assessing health potential of employees
③ Moderating a weight-reduction program
④ Predicting the future health needs of employees

TEST-TAKING TIP ● Identify the key words in the stem.

16 Which is the primary goal of the nurse caring for an older adult in the community?
① Encouraging interaction within the family
② Helping with bureaucratic paperwork
③ Supporting rehabilitation needs
④ Maintaining quality of life

TEST-TAKING TIP ● Identify the word in the stem that sets a priority.

17 Which activity is unrelated to primary prevention?
① Educating
② Promoting
③ Immunizing
④ Rehabilitating

TEST-TAKING TIP ● Look for the word in the stem that indicates negative polarity.

18 Community-based nursing is mainly associated with which category of health care delivery?
① Acute
② Critical
③ Primary
④ Secondary

TEST-TAKING TIP ● Identify the word in the stem that sets a priority. Identify the equally plausible options.

19 Which action supports a situational stress?
① Counseling a parent experiencing the empty nest syndrome
② Encouraging an 82-year-old man to visit the senior center

③ Providing sex education classes to adolescents
④ Providing pain relief for a woman with cancer
TEST-TAKING TIP ● Identify the clue in the stem.

20 Which statement is most accurate about health perception and health status?
① Disability is related to the extent to which one is able to carry out the behaviors of the role chosen.
② Anticipation of the future has minimal impact on the understanding of one's health.
③ The ability to tolerate illness and disability is the same for one person as for another.
④ Assuming the sick role is generally maladaptive and harmful to recovery.
TEST-TAKING TIP ● Identify the words in the stem that set a priority.

21 Which statement most accurately reflects the principle of providing for a client's nutritional needs in the home?
① The client should eat whatever is preferred as long as the serum albumin is normal.
② The client should plan to eat meals at the same time as other family members.
③ Community support groups may be employed to ensure adequate nutrition.
④ Supplements should be taken whenever the client is hungry between meals.
TEST-TAKING TIP ● Identify the words in the stem that set a priority.

22 Which nursing activity in the community would address the most basic need according to Maslow's Hierarchy of Needs?
① Arranging for Meals on Wheels
② Exploring the meaning of one's life
③ Teaching the client to remove throw rugs
④ Encouraging the client to visit with friends
TEST-TAKING TIP ● Identify the clues in the stem.

23 To provide for safety when assisting with medication administration in the home, people should be encouraged to keep:
① Over-the-counter drugs in a separate place from prescription drugs
② All medications in a dark, cool environment
③ Leftover medication in a locked closet
④ Medication in a safe, secure place
TEST-TAKING TIP ● Identify the option that contains a specific determiner.

24 Which phrase is most accurately associated with the concept of community coalition?
① Wellness programs
② Growing diversity
③ Shared purpose
④ Home care
TEST-TAKING TIP ● Identify the words in the stem that set a priority. Identify the clue in the stem.

25 Palliative care is most specifically associated with which area of practice?
① Health maintenance
② Rehabilitation
③ Home care
④ Hospice
TEST-TAKING TIP ● Identify the words in the stem that set a priority.

26 What is the main reason the nurse makes an assessment of a patient's community before the patient is discharged from the hospital?
① Enhance the use of community resources
② Help identify the client's role within the community
③ Contribute to an understanding of the patient's relationship within the family
④ Ensure that the focus is on the whole patient and not just on the patient's physical needs

TEST-TAKING TIP ● Identify the words in the stem that set a priority.

27 Which nursing intervention associated with providing pressure ulcer care in the home is often different from providing pressure ulcer care in the acute-care setting?
① Measuring a wound weekly versus daily
② Changing dressings daily versus three times a day
③ Employing aseptic technique versus sterile technique
④ Using a bulb syringe versus a piston syringe when irrigating

28 Which intervention is associated with tertiary disease prevention?
① Screening for head lice in a grammar school
② Providing first aid at the scene of an accident
③ Monitoring blood pressures at a senior center
④ Assessing serum glucose levels during a yearly physical

TEST-TAKING TIP ● Identify the clue in the stem. Identify the unique option.

29 Home care is designed to assist individuals and families in all realms except:
① Restorative care
② Hospice care
③ Respite care
④ Acute care

TEST-TAKING TIP ● Identify the word in the stem that indicates negative polarity.

30 Which population variable is being assessed in a community profile inventory when the nurse asks, "How many people live within a square mile in the community?"
① Size
② Density
③ Mobility
④ Composition

31 Community health practice, unlike acute health care, is:
① Family focused
② Individual focused
③ Population focused
④ Geographically focused

TEST-TAKING TIP ● Identify the clue in the stem.

32 Which statement reflects the concept of prevalence?
① "On Monday morning, the school nurse identified that six children had measles."
② "On the first day of June this year, ten percent of the population of Middletown had heart disease."
③ "During the last 5 years, 1 percent of the population of the United States had tuberculosis."
④ "Last year, of the people at risk for developing breast cancer, 9 percent actually developed the disease."

TEST-TAKING TIP ● Identify the unique option.

33 Which assessment would be most appropriate when conducting a screening program for the leading cause of death associated with adults 60 years of age or older?
① Apical pulse
② Breath sounds
③ Liver palpation
④ Respiratory rate

TEST-TAKING TIP ● Identify the words in the stem that set a priority. Identify the options that are equally plausible.

34 When assessing adolescents in the community, the nurse should be aware of which problem most commonly associated with this age group?
① Mumps
② Measles
③ Child abuse
④ Substance abuse

TEST-TAKING TIP ● Identify the words in the stem that set a priority. Identify the equally plausible options.

35 An older adult, who needs minimal help with activities of daily living and who takes prescription medication twice a day, is to be discharged from the hospital. Which facility would most appropriately meet this individual's needs?
① Group home
② Nursing home
③ Daycare center
④ Assisted-living facility

TEST-TAKING TIP ● Identify the clue in the stem. Identify the words in the stem that set a priority.

Rationales

1 **TEST-TAKING TIP** ● The word "most" in the stem sets a priority.
   ① Stereotyping is often based on generalizations, misinformation, and preconceptions that can be biased and prejudicial and is never helpful when assessing a patient's needs. Each patient must be assessed as an individual.
   ② Although an individual may assimilate into a new society, it does not mean that cultural differences are "melted" out of a person. People still share a common ethnic and religious heritage that has special interests and needs that set them apart from others.
 * ③ The nurse must be able to identify preconceptions about ethnic groups or cultures that are different from his or her own and rely on objective facts that are valid and actual.
   ④ Each culture or ethnic group has norms that identify standards of acceptable behavior or rules of conduct that support the values and beliefs of the group.

2 ① Primary health care is concerned with promoting health, not supporting dying patients.
 * ② This is correct. Tertiary care involves maintaining optimum health once a disease has developed.
   ③ Secondary health care is concerned with early detection of illness, not supporting dying patients.
   ④ Affordable health care is not a level of health care but is rather a value of the American consumer.

3 **TEST-TAKING TIP** ● The word "priority" in the stem requires the nurse to identify what should be done first.
   ① Exploring the need to modify the environment to prevent falls addresses safety, which is a higher level need than physiological needs according to Maslow.
 * ② This is correct; preventing aspiration and meeting a client's physiological need to ingest adequate nutrition take priority over higher-level needs according to Maslow's Hierarchy of Needs.
   ③ Encouraging clients to ventilate negative feelings helps them believe that they are understood and accepted. Feelings of acceptance are related to Maslow's category of love and belonging. Love and belonging are a higher-level needs than physiological needs, which are more basic according to Maslow.
   ④ Providing opportunities for the client to make choices supports self-esteem and the need to feel more empowered over one's situation. According to Maslow, this is a higher-level need than the need to maintain a patent airway and ingest adequate nutrition.

4 **TEST-TAKING TIP** ● Four concepts of health care delivery are being associated with community-based nursing—primary, secondary, tertiary, and rehabilitation. If you know one concept (either primary or tertiary) that is associated with health care delivery, two options can be deleted from consideration. If you know one concept (either secondary or rehabilitation) that is not related to health care delivery, two options can be deleted from consideration.
 * ① Primary care is associated with health promotion, screening, education, and protection. Although tertiary care is associated with specialized diagnostic and therapeutic care generally delivered in the acute-care setting, it also includes specialized services such as rehabilitation and hospice services, which are most often delivered in

community settings. Both primary and tertiary health care delivery categories are associated with care delivered in community settings.

 ② Although primary health care activities generally take place in the community setting, secondary health care activities take place in the acute-care setting and generally not the community setting.

 ③ Although tertiary care is associated with specialized services such as rehabilitation, rehabilitation is not a category of health care delivery. Rehabilitation is a type of specialized service that is provided in acute-care and community settings.

 ④ Rehabilitation is not considered a category of health care but rather a type of service that is provided in acute and community settings. Secondary health care is associated with hospital-based service (e.g., critical, emergency, and acute care, etc.).

5 TEST-TAKING TIP ● The word "community" in Option 3 is directly associated with the words "community health nursing" in the stem. The word "community" in the stem and in Option 4 is a clang association.

 ① The home setting is traditionally associated with the concept of community nursing. However, in the current health care environment, the community includes settings such as schools, work environments, community centers, neighborhood clinics, and even mobile units that bring services directly to people in a neighborhood.

 ② Community-based health activities are designed to help individuals and groups across all economic levels and low- as well as high-risk groups.

 * ③ This is correct. Community health nursing reaches out to people and groups outside of acute-care facilities. Services are provided in neighborhoods, which includes the home.

 ④ Community-based nursing assists individuals and groups from one end of the health-illness continuum to the other, not just the health end of the continuum.

6 TEST-TAKING TIP ● The word "developmental" modifies the word "crisis" and is the clue in the stem.

 * ① Maturational crises are changes that occur during a period of growth that often require the assumption of a new role. Adolescents experience rapid bodily changes, have a need to be accepted and be part of a group, and attempt to become independent. Most importantly, the adolescent is striving to establish sexual identity. This maturational crisis is compounded in adolescents who recognize that they are homosexual. Most schools and parents are unprepared to deal with this situation, which can often have lifelong emotional effects on the individual.

 ② This is a situational, not maturational, crisis. A situational crisis is an external event that is not part of everyday living. It causes a high degree of anxiety and generally requires learning new coping mechanisms.

 ③ Being critically ill is not an expected part of normal growth and development. It is a situational crisis for the child and the parents.

 ④ Same as #2.

**7 **① Community health nursing focuses on illness prevention, health education, providing support services, hospice care, and rehabilitation, not just health promotion.

 ② Community health nursing focuses on the health care needs of groups and families within the community, not just individuals.

 ③ Community nurses practice in many different settings, including clinics, schools, centers of all kinds, mobile units, and places of employment, not just in the home.

 * ④ This is correct; community health nurses must develop collaborative relationships with other health professionals as well as with individuals and groups in the community.

8 * ① This is correct. It is an unhealthy situation for people not to have access to health care.
② Unfluoridated water is not an unhealthy situation because fluoride can be obtained from other sources.
③ Although rehabilitation services would contribute to an increase in the quality of one's life, the lack of rehabilitation services would not be an unhealthy situation.
④ Supporting a vaccination program would contribute to prevention of disease; but it would not correct an already unhealthy situation.

9 **TEST-TAKING TIP** ● The word "just" in Option 3 is a specific determiner.
① Aid to Families with Dependent Children provides assistance to people during the childbearing years, particularly divorced or single women with children.
② Medicare provides assistance to people 65 years of age or older, not people during the childbearing years.
③ In 1965 Medicaid was established under Title 19 of the Social Security Act. Medicaid is a federal public assistance program for people who require financial assistance, such as low-income groups.
* ④ In 1965 the Medicare amendments (Title 18) to the Social Security Act provided a national and state health insurance program for the aged.

10 **TEST-TAKING TIP** ● The word "secondary" modifies the words "disease prevention" and is the clue in the stem. Option 1 is unique. It is the only option that involves the assessment phase of the nursing process.
* ① This is correct. Secondary prevention activities are associated with early detection and encouragement of treatment when interventions may control or eliminate an already present risk factor, illness, or disease.
② This action is a primary-level disease prevention intervention, not a secondary intervention. Primary prevention is associated with health teaching and actions that relate to specific protection and prevention of disease or injuries. Primary prevention activities precede disease or dysfunction; these activities are usually directed toward a healthy population.
③ Same as #2.
④ Same as #2.

11 **TEST-TAKING TIP** ● The word "first" in the stem sets a priority.
① Although the concept in the statement is true, it should not be the nurse's first response to the patient's statement. The patient's lack of knowledge should be addressed first.
② This question might be asked later. The patient's lack of knowledge should be addressed first.
③ The patient's lack of knowledge should be addressed first. Also, this could be unsafe because it would delay the arrival of help. When it gets to the point where a person cannot breathe, 911 should be called.
* ④ When a patient makes a statement that includes inaccurate information, the person is exhibiting an opportunity for learning. The nurse has a responsibility to teach appropriate self-care. The old adage "Strike when the iron is hot" supports this teaching-learning concept.

12 **TEST-TAKING TIP** ● The word "primary" modifies the words "disease prevention" and is the clue in the stem.
① This is associated with tertiary disease prevention, not primary prevention. Tertiary prevention is associated with attempts to reduce the extent and severity of a health

problem or disease in an effort to limit disability and restore, maintain, or maximize function or quality of life.

  * ② This is correct. This action is a primary-level disease prevention intervention. Primary prevention is associated with health teaching and actions that relate to specific protection and prevention of disease or injuries. Primary prevention activities precede disease or dysfunction.

  ③ This action is associated with secondary disease prevention, not primary. Secondary prevention activities are associated with early detection and encouragement of treatment when actions may contribute to controlling or eliminating an already present risk factor, illness, or disease.

  ④ Same as #3.

13 TEST-TAKING TIP ● The words "key factor" set a priority in the stem.

  ① Although health care needs generally increase as people become older or as the health of the work force declines, the key factor depends on the vision and philosophy of the company's administration. The company establishes the scope of health services because it is paying for the services to be provided.

  ② Same as #1.

  ③ Standards for a safe environment, which help to reduce occupational stress, are set by the Occupational Safety and Health Administration (OSHA) within the Department of Labor.

  * ④ In the occupational setting, health care services provided beyond those required by the Occupational Safety and Health Administration (OSHA) depend on the philosophy and vision of the company's administration. In the occupational setting, nurses work within the legal definition of the practice of nursing and provide services that the company is willing to support.

14 TEST-TAKING TIP ● The key words in the stem are "lowest-level need" and "Maslow."

  ① Identifying hazards in the environment is a health promotion activity that supports the safety of employees. The needs for safety and security are second-level needs according to Maslow's Hierarchy of Needs.

  * ② Assessing the health of an employee includes identifying the physical status of the individual, which addresses a first-level (physical/physiological) need according to Maslow's Hierarchy of Needs. First-level needs such as air, food, water, shelter, rest, sleep, and activity are necessary for survival.

  ③ An immunization program is a specific health protection activity that helps to keep a person safe from a specific disease. The needs for safety and security are second-level needs according to Maslow's Hierarchy of Needs.

  ④ Promoting social adaptation addresses people's love and belonging needs. The need to feel loved and the need to attain a place within a group are third-level (love and belonging) needs according to Maslow's Hierarchy of Needs.

15 TEST-TAKING TIP ● The key words in the stem are "second-level need" and "Maslow."

  * ① The Occupational Safety and Health Administration (OSHA), a governmental agency within the Department of Labor, is responsible for ensuring that working environments are safe and healthy. Providing for environmental safety is a second-level (safety and security) need according to Maslow's Hierarchy of Needs.

  ② Realizing abilities and directing capacities to achieve one's maximum potential is the goal of level five (self-actualization) according to Maslow's Hierarchy of Needs.

  ③ When the nurse intervenes to promote health maintenance through activities such as a weight-reduction program, the nurse is addressing a first-level (physiological) need according to Maslow's Hierarchy of Needs.

④ Predicting the future health needs of employees is a level five (self-actualization) need according to Maslow's Hierarchy of Needs. Programs that plan for the future attempt to maximize the health of employees.

16 TEST-TAKING TIP ● The word "primary" in the stem sets a priority.

① This is only one part of caring for an older adult. The primary comprehensive goals of nursing care for an older adult are to maintain and improve the quality of life.

② Same as #1.

③ Same as #1.

* ④ This option is broad in scope and addresses improvement in all aspects of the life of the older adult. Option 4 inherently includes the interventions identified in Options 1, 2, and 3.

17 TEST-TAKING TIP ● The word "unrelated" is asking for the answer that is not related to primary prevention. The stem has a negative polarity.

① Giving information enables people to make the educated choices that help prevent disease; educational activities are used in all levels of prevention.

② Promoting health helps to prevent disease and is included in the level of primary prevention.

③ Immunizations protect against disease and are in the category of primary prevention.

* ④ Activities that help people maintain or restore function after an illness are in the tertiary prevention category, not the primary prevention category.

18 TEST-TAKING TIP ● The word "mainly" in the stem sets a priority. In Options 1 and 2 the words "acute" and "critical" are equally plausible. "Acute" and "critical" are synonyms because they really have the same meaning.

① Acute care is usually provided in hospitals.

② Critical care is provided in the acute-care setting in the form of intensive care units.

* ③ This is correct. Primary care is concerned with health promotion, screening, education, and protection; these activities are usually provided for well people in the community.

④ Secondary health care activities usually take place in acute-care settings or medical-related facilities.

19 TEST-TAKING TIP ● The word "situational" modifies the word "stress" and is the clue in the stem.

① This is an intervention that supports a person experiencing a maturational, not a situational, stresses. Maturational stresses are situations that occur during a period of growth. Maturational growth requires the mastery of tasks in a relatively predictable order and includes the assumption of new roles, according to Erik Erikson. A person who has difficulty mastering a task or adjusting to a new role will experience a maturational crisis.

② Same as #1.

③ Same as #1.

* ④ A situational stress is an external event that is not part of everyday living; it causes a high degree of anxiety and generally requires learning new coping mechanisms. Physical illness is always a situational stress because it is a physical and emotional assault on the "self," requires the sudden assumption of new roles, triggers behaviors that reflect an attempt to cope, and requires the learning of new coping skills to deal with the stress.

20 TEST-TAKING TIP ● The words "most accurate" in the stem set a priority.

* ① Where people place themselves on the health-illness continuum is a highly individual perception based on personal expectations and values. People generally fulfill numerous roles. In the role performance model of health and wellness, people who are disabled or ill, but are able to carry out their role according to personal expectations, tend to view themselves as closer to the high-level wellness end of the health-illness continuum. When role performance becomes impaired, people are more likely to view themselves as disabled.

② How people anticipate the future has a significant impact on their ability to understand their health. The nurse needs to assess what people believe and feel about their future life. The nurse must work within the context of the person's situation to best assist with the development of coping mechanisms.

③ People react in diversified ways to illness and disability. Every person is an individual, and how an individual reacts depends on many factors, such as age, sex, cultural/ethnic background, religious beliefs, economic status, previous experiences, role in the family, and support systems.

④ Assuming the sick role (passivity, social and psychological regression, and submission to treatment regimens) is adaptive and beneficial if not taken to the extreme. Because illness is a modification in the ability to function, there is always a concurrent need to modify behavior in an attempt to rest and recover, which is adaptive. Assuming the sick role becomes maladaptive and harmful when a person is unable to move on physically and emotionally once the crisis is resolved.

21 TEST-TAKING TIP ● The words "most accurately" in the stem set a priority.

① A serum albumin level reflects only adequate protein intake. Although a diet should be designed with a client's food preferences in mind, the diet chosen needs to address all the nutritional components associated with the client's needs.

② Although eating is considered a social activity and clients may be encouraged to eat with family members, this may not meet the nutritional needs of the client. A variety of issues should be considered: a family meal may be too confusing and distracting; the client may be on a restricted diet that may make the client feel uncomfortable when eating with the family; the client may be receiving a tube feeding and prefer not to be with the family at meal time; or the odor of food may be difficult to tolerate.

* ③ Meeting the nutritional needs of a person living at home requires the nurse to consider all phases of achieving adequate nutritional intake, such as the patient and family's knowledge about nutrition and the ability to shop, buy, prepare, cook, and eat food. Community support such as home-delivered meals, senior center lunch programs, meals provided by missions and shelters, school lunch programs, and community food pantries can help people in need.

④ Supplements should be taken only if nutritional needs cannot be met with the prescribed diet. Supplements are rich in calories, vitamins, and/or minerals and, if taken whenever a person is hungry, they may exceed the person's metabolic needs. This could contribute to complications such as excessive weight gain.

22 TEST-TAKING TIP ● The words "basic needs" and "Maslow's Hierarchy of Needs" are the clues in the stem.

* ① Meals on Wheels delivers meals daily to those at home who need assistance with preparing nutritious meals. Adequate nutrition (food) is essential for survival and is a first-level (physiological) need according to Maslow's Hierarchy of Needs.

② This relates to self-actualization, which is the highest level in Maslow's Hierarchy of Needs.

③ Removing throw rugs protects a client from falls. According to Maslow's Hierarchy of Needs, safety and security needs become significant after basic physiological needs are met.

④ Encouraging socialization helps to support the need to belong to a group, which is a third-level need according to Maslow's Hierarchy of Needs. When people feel that they belong and are appreciated for who they are, love and belonging needs are being met.

23 TEST-TAKING TIP ● The word "all" in Option 2 is a specific determiner.

① There is no need to store over-the-counter and prescription drugs separately. All drug bottles and containers should be clearly labeled and stored in a safe place.

② Not all medications need to be kept in a dark, cool environment. Cool environments may alter the action of certain medications and would be contraindicated.

③ *Leftover* medication should be flushed down the toilet and not stored for future use. People sometimes self-medicate with *leftover* medication that is inappropriate for a problem, which is a dangerous practice.

* ④ All medications in the home environment should be stored in a safe and secure place out of the reach of children. Tamper-proof lids and use of a locked cabinet can help prevent accidental poisoning.

24 TEST-TAKING TIP ● The words "most accurately" in the stem set a priority. The word "coalition" in the stem is related to words such as "alliance," "unification," and "share." The definition of the word "coalition" should lead you to Option 3.

① A "wellness program" and a "community coalition" are two different concepts. A wellness program is a type of health promotion program that focuses on the reduction of risks and the development of positive health habits. A community coalition is a group working toward a common goal. A community coalition may be established to develop and fund a wellness program.

② Growing diversity speaks to the increasing differences in culture and ethnicity in the population. People of different cultures maintain cultural values, traditions, and beliefs that contribute to the texture and complexity of a community. Although a group of people from one cultural or ethnic group may share a common purpose, this concept is different from community coalition, which is when diverse groups share a common purpose.

* ③ Synonyms for the word "coalition" include "alliance," "unification," and "combination." A community coalition is the unification of individuals and groups to address issues related to a shared purpose.

④ "Home care" and "community coalition" are two different concepts. Home care is associated with providing services for a patient in the individual's place of residence. Community coalition is the unification of individuals and groups to address issues related to a shared purpose.

25 TEST-TAKING TIP ● The words "most specifically" in the stem set a priority.

① Health maintenance involves efforts that move healthy people toward optimum well-being or higher levels of wellness.

② Rehabilitation attempts to reduce disability, restore function, and develop new compensatory skills.

③ Home care nursing is a specialty within community health care nursing. It refers to all the services provided to people in their homes to maintain, restore, or promote their physical, mental, and emotional health.

* ④ Palliative care involves relieving or reducing uncomfortable symptoms. Hospice care attempts to maintain quality of life, keep people as comfortable as possible, and provide support and instruction to caregivers so that people can die with dignity.

26 TEST-TAKING TIP ● The words "main reason" in the stem set a priority.

* ① Community assessment varies in levels of complexity. The nurse who provides acute care in a hospital setting uses community assessment primarily as it relates to meeting the individual needs of patients in the context of the community. Therefore, the nurse might conduct a focused community assessment to determine available, accessible, and appropriate resources for referral.

② Although this may be a true statement, particularly when the nurse performs a comprehensive community assessment, it is not the main reason why the nurse makes an assessment of a hospitalized patient's community.

③ Same as #2.

④ Same as #2.

27 ① Pressure ulcers should be measured at least weekly whether the patient is in the hospital or in the home. It may be done more frequently depending on the needs of the individual.

② The frequency of changing the dressing on a wound is individualized depending on the patient's needs. The setting is irrelevant.

* ③ Sterile technique is used when a hospitalized person needs a wound dressing change to prevent the occurrence of a nosocomial infection. The risk of infection for a hospitalized person is increased at several stages of the chain of infection; for example, hospitalized people are sick and usually more susceptible to infection and there are many microorganisms in the hospital environment. Medical aseptic technique alone often is used when changing a wound dressing in the home. People are usually further along in recovery and less susceptible to infection, and people have built up a resistance to the "familiar microorganisms" in the home environment.

④ Both bulb and piston syringes can be used in either home or acute-care settings.

28 TEST-TAKING TIP ● The word "tertiary" modifies the words "disease prevention" and is the clue in the stem. Options 1, 3, and 4 all involve the collection of data, which is the assessment phase of the nursing process. Option 2 is unique because it involves an intervention, which is part of the implementation phase of the nursing process.

① This action is associated with secondary disease prevention, not tertiary prevention. Secondary prevention activities are associated with early detection and encouragement of treatment when intervention may contribute to controlling or eliminating an already present risk factor, illness, or disease.

* ② This is correct. Tertiary prevention is associated with attempts to reduce the extent and severity of a health problem or disease in an effort to limit disability and restore, maintain, or maximize function or quality of life.

③ Same as #1.

④ Same as #1.

29 TEST-TAKING TIP ● The word "except" in the stem indicates negative polarity.

① Efforts that seek to reduce disability and restore function are related to rehabilitation. Recovering lost functions or developing new compensating skills commonly is accomplished in the home setting.

② Hospice care offers services that enable dying persons to stay at home with the support needed to die with dignity.

③ Respite care provides services so that caregivers can get relief from the stress of their responsibilities. Respite care can be provided in the home or nursing home setting.

* ④ Acute care is provided by institutions with the highly skilled, intensive, specialized services that are provided by hospitals.

30 ① The size of a community is the total number of people in the community.
* ② Density refers to the number of people who live within a square mile. High- and low-density areas have their own commonalities (e.g., high-density areas are usually more stressful; low-density areas may have a decreased availability of health services).
③ Mobility refers to how frequently people move in and out of the community.
④ The composition of a community includes factors such as the age, gender, marital status, and occupations of people in the community.

31 **TEST-TAKING TIP** ● The word "unlike" is a clue in the stem. It is requiring you to differentiate between community health practice and acute health care.
① The family is included in both acute care and community health care.
② Acute care focuses on the physical and emotional needs of the individual.
* ③ A characteristic of community health is that it focuses on the health status of people in an aggregate, people who, as a group, form a distinct population.
④ Although some populations may be within a geographic area, community health care focuses on groups of people. Groups can be identified by a variety of factors such as common interests (e.g., citizens concerned about air pollution) or similar problems (e.g., homelessness, single-parent families).

32 **TEST-TAKING TIP** ● Options 2, 3, and 4 all include percentages. Option 1 is unique. Consider this option carefully. In this question it is a distractor.
① This represents a simple count of the number of people with a disease.
* ② Prevalence refers to all people with a health condition existing in a given population at a given point in time. It is calculated by the formula:

$$\text{Prevalence Rate} = \frac{\text{Number of Persons With a Characteristic on a Particular Day}}{\text{Total Number in the Population}}$$

③ Calculating the prevalence rate over a period of time is called a period prevalence rate. It is calculated by the formula:

$$\text{Period Prevalence Rate} = \frac{\text{Number of Persons With a Characteristic During a Period of Time}}{\text{Total Number in the Population}}$$

④ This reflects an incidence rate. It is calculated by the formula:

$$\text{Incidence} = \frac{\text{Number of Persons Developing a Disease}}{\text{Total Number at Risk Per Unit of Time}}$$

33 **TEST-TAKING TIP** ● The words "most appropriate" in the stem set a priority. Options 2 and 4 are equally plausible because they both relate to respiratory assessments.
* ① The leading cause of death in the older adult is heart disease. Assessments of rate and rhythm of heartbeats are essential.
② Although chronic obstructive pulmonary disease (COPD) is a major health problem in older adults, it is not the leading cause of death.
③ Chronic liver disease is a common cause of death in adults 45 to 64 years of age.
④ Same as #2.

34 **TEST-TAKING TIP** ● The words "most commonly" in the stem set a priority. Options 1 and 2 are equally plausible. They are both communicable diseases.
① Measles and mumps occur most often in toddlers and young school-age children. With the MMR vaccine, the incidence of these diseases has declined considerably.

② Same as #1.

③ Although child abuse occurs in teenagers, it is most commonly identified in toddlers and young school-age children.

* ④ Substance abuse (e.g., alcohol, cigarette, illegal drugs, inhalants) is a health problem commonly associated with adolescents. Complex physical, emotional, cognitive, and social changes, along with the desire to take risks and the need to develop a self-identity, all influence behavior.

35 TEST-TAKING TIP ● The concept "activities of daily living" is associated with the concept of "assisted living." The words "most appropriately" in the stem set a priority.

① Group homes are for specific populations, such as people who are developmentally disabled, mentally ill, or recovering from alcohol or drug abuse.

② A nursing home provides skilled nursing care, which this patient does not need.

③ This patient needs more care than can be provided in a daycare center. This person would need assistance with toileting, grooming, dressing, eating, and transport, which all occur *before* arrival at the daycare center.

* ④ Assisted-living facilities help with activities of daily living, prepare meals, and dispense medications as needed.

344   Pharmacology

This section encompasses questions related to how drugs physiologically and biochemically affect the body (pharmacodynamics) and how drugs are absorbed, distributed, metabolized, and eliminated from the body (pharmacokinetics). The questions include such topics as the therapeutic and side effects of classifications of drugs, medication toxicity, peak and trough values, factors affecting drug action, common assessments before and after drug administration, use of the nursing process in drug therapy, and the role of the nurse in drug compliance and patient teaching.

Questions

1 A patient has an order for morphine sulfate 10 mg, subcutaneously, q4h for pain after abdominal surgery. The nurse would know that the morphine was effective when the patient:

  ① Does not ask for another injection for pain
  ② Is able to cough with minimal discomfort
  ③ Requests another injection in 3 hours
  ④ Has a decrease in the respiratory rate

  TEST-TAKING TIP ● Identify the options that are opposites.

2 Which is an age-related alteration in the older adult that may affect the absorption of an oral hypoglycemic?

  ① An increase in hydrocholoric acid production
  ② An increase in mesenteric blood flow
  ③ A decrease in abdominal body fat
  ④ An increase in cardiac output

  TEST-TAKING TIP ● Identify the unique option.

3 Which cathartic acts as a stool softener and is most effective in preventing straining during defecation?

  ① Colace
  ② Dulcolax
  ③ Mineral oil
  ④ Milk of magnesia

  TEST-TAKING TIP ● Identify the word in the stem that sets a priority.

4 Which drug would be most effective in the immediate treatment of anaphylaxis?

  ① Prednisone
  ② Solu-Cortef
  ③ Epinephrine
  ④ Solu-Medrol

  TEST-TAKING TIP ● Identify the word in the stem that sets a priority. Identify the word that is a clue in the stem. Identify the options that are equally plausible. Identify the unique option.

5 A patient receiving a cardiac glycoside is digitalized. The nurse recognizes that digitalization means:

  ① Large doses of the drug were administered to reach the therapeutic window quickly.
  ② An excessive amount of the drug was given and unacceptable side effects occurred.

③ Blood levels of the drug have been maintained at acceptable levels over time.
④ The therapeutic window was exceeded and toxicity has occurred.

TEST-TAKING TIP ● Identify the equally plausible options.

6 Which group of drugs would most likely be ordered when a patient has the nursing diagnosis of Sleep Pattern Disturbance?
① Benzodiazepines
② Barbiturates
③ Analgesics
④ Narcotics

TEST-TAKING TIP ● Identify the word in the stem that sets a priority.

7 When administering prednisone, a glucocorticoid, the nurse should monitor the patient's electrolytes for:
① Hypokalemia and hyponatremia
② Hypokalemia and hypernatremia
③ Hyperkalemia and hyponatremia
④ Hyperkalemia and hypernatremia

TEST-TAKING TIP ● Identify the duplicate facts among the options. Identify the options that are opposites.

8 Which group of medications has a high risk for a drug interaction with digoxin (Lanoxin)?
① Glucocorticoids
② Sulfonamides
③ Antibiotics
④ Antacids

TEST-TAKING TIP ● Identify the options that are equally plausible.

9 After administering a cathartic, the nurse will know that the drug is effective when the patient:
① Has a bowel movement
② Describes pain relief
③ Falls asleep
④ Voids urine

10 Which undesirable clinical response would indicate the need to discontinue heparin therapy?
① Prothrombin time two times the control
② Platelet count of 100,000/mm^3
③ Hematuria
④ Gastritis

TEST-TAKING TIP ● Identify the word in the stem that indicates negative polarity.

11 Which classification of drugs can precipitate superinfections?
① Diuretics
② Antibiotics
③ Vasopressors
④ Thrombolytics

12 The physician orders kanamycin (Kantrex) 500 mg IVPB q12h. What time should a blood sample be drawn to determine a trough level for this patient when the drug is administered at 2:00 PM?

① 4:00 AM
② 9:00 AM
③ 1:30 PM
④ 2:30 PM

TEST-TAKING TIP ● Identify the options that are opposites.

13 A patient response that would indicate that an antitussive was effective would be decreased:

① Fever
② Nasal congestion
③ Mucus viscosity
④ Frequency of coughing

14 When performing a health history a patient states, "I take 1 package of Metamucil every day no matter what." The most appropriate nursing diagnosis for this patient would be:

① Chronic pain
② Disuse Syndrome
③ Fluid Volume excess
④ Perceived constipation

TEST-TAKING TIP ● Identify the word in the stem that indicates a priority.

15 The patient is receiving gentamicin, which has a 4 to 10 μg/mL therapeutic range, an optimum peak value of 8 to 10 μg/mL, and a minimum trough level of 0.5 μg/mL. A value that would require the nurse to notify the physician would be a:

① Peak value of 5
② Peak value of 9
③ Trough value of 0.3
④ Trough value of 0.7

TEST-TAKING TIP ● Identify the words in the stem that indicate negative polarity.

16 An adaptation that would indicate that a patient was experiencing a therapeutic response to an antiemetic would be a decrease in:

① Nausea and anxiety
② Vomiting and nausea
③ Coughing and anxiety
④ Vomiting and coughing

TEST-TAKING TIP ● Identify the duplicate facts among the options.

17 Which adaptation would indicate that a patient was experiencing a therapeutic response to an expectorant?

① Reduced fever
② Productive cough
③ Relieved nasal congestion
④ Dilation of respiratory airways

18 The blood serum level of the therapeutic range for gentamicin is 4 to 10 μg/mL (micrograms per milliliter). What is the implication of a peak level of 12 μg/mL?

① The drug dose is safe.
② The drug dose is subtherapeutic.

③ The patient would be at risk for drug accumulation.
④ The patient's next dose should be given over 1 hour and not 30 minutes.

TEST-TAKING TIP ● Identify the unique option.

19 Which physiological change in the older adult contributes to prolonged drug half-life?
① Increased gastric emptying
② Reduced glomerular filtration rate
③ Decreased hydrochloric acid production
④ Diminished gastrointestinal absorptive surface

TEST-TAKING TIP ● Identify the unique option.

20 Extrapyramidal symptoms are the most significant undesirable responses associated with neuroleptic drugs and include which adaptations?
① Respiratory depression and diarrhea
② Akathisia and respiratory depression
③ Spasm of the muscles of the face and akathisia
④ Diarrhea and spasms of the muscles of the face

TEST-TAKING TIP ● Identify the duplicate facts among the options.

21 Which is the main expected outcome of an analgesic?
① Temperature below 100°F.
② Less labored breathing.
③ Nausea has subsided.
④ Pain is tolerable.

TEST-TAKING TIP ● Identify the word in the stem that sets a priority.

22 The patient is receiving gentamicin, which has a 4 to 10 μg/mL therapeutic range, an optimum peak value of 8 to 10 μg/mL, and a minimum trough level of 0.5 μg/mL. When monitoring the patient's response to therapy, which value would be acceptable?
① Peak value of 8 μg/mL
② Peak value of 11 μg/mL
③ Trough value of 0.1 μg/mL
④ Trough value of 0.3 μg/L

23 Which statement by the patient receiving digoxin (Lanoxin) 0.25 mg every day would indicate that further teaching is necessary.
① "I should not take antacids with digoxin."
② "I should call the doctor if I have nausea, vomiting, or weakness."
③ "If I forget to take my digoxin, I should take two pills the next day."
④ "I should not take the digoxin if my apical pulse is below 60 beats per minute."

TEST-TAKING TIP ● Identify the words in the stem that indicate negative polarity.

24 The nurse understands that narcotic analgesics limit pain by:
① Diminishing peripheral pain reception
② Modifying the patient's perception of pain
③ Competing with receptors for sensory input
④ Closing the gating mechanism for impulse transmission

25 Postural hypotension is a common side effect of most of the medications in which classification of drugs?
① Antibiotics
② Antiemetics

③ Antihistamines
④ Antihypertensives

TEST-TAKING TIP ● Identify the clues in the stem.

26 When collecting a health history for a patient who will be receiving IV heparin therapy, which statement by the patient needs further exploration?
① "I stopped taking my daily aspirin tablet about 5 days ago."
② "I always experience heavy menstrual periods."
③ "I eat a lot of green leafy vegetables."
④ "I may be pregnant."

TEST-TAKING TIP ● Identify the words in the stem that indicate a negative polarity.

27 To best promote intestinal peristalsis, a patient should be encouraged to:
① Use a bulk cathartic weekly
② Take castor oil once a month
③ Eat whole-grain foods every day
④ Self-administer a stool softener daily

TEST-TAKING TIP ● Identify the word in the stem that sets a priority. Identify the option that is unique.

28 Which drug is palliative in its therapeutic action?
① Calcium
② Demerol
③ Penicillin
④ Synthroid

29 Which is most important to have readily available on the unit when a patient is receiving heparin IV?
① Potassium chloride
② Protamine sulfate
③ Prothrombin
④ Plasma

TEST-TAKING TIP ● Identify the word in the stem that sets a priority. Identify the clues in the stem.

30 When can the nurse generally expect an initial therapeutic response to most antidepressant medications?
① 2 hours
② 2 days
③ 2 weeks
④ 2 months

TEST-TAKING TIP ● Identify the word in the stem that is a clue.

31 Which statement is most accurate when teaching a patient about the use of sublinguinal nitroglycerin for angina pectoris (chest pain related to transient cardiac ischemia)?
① "Take only 1 dose of nitroglycerin. If pain continues call 911."
② "Take 1 dose every 3 minutes as often as necessary until pain is relieved."
③ "Double the dose of nitroglycerin 5 minutes after the first dose if there is no relief from pain."
④ "You can repeat the dose of nitroglycerin every 5 minutes for 3 doses. If pain is unrelieved, get immediate medical attention."

TEST-TAKING TIP ● Identify the word in the stem that sets a priority. Identify the option that contains a specific determiner.

32 Because many antineoplastic drugs cause myelosuppression, the nurse should monitor patients receiving these drugs for signs of:
① Diarrhea
② Infection
③ Constipation
④ Dysrhythmias
TEST-TAKING TIP ● Identify the options that are opposites.

33 Antipsychotics potentiate the effects of:
① Amphetamines
② Anticoagulants
③ Narcotic analgesics
④ Oral hypoglycemics

34 Which patient response would require a dose of digoxin to be withheld?
① Respiratory rate of 30
② Apical heart rate of 56
③ Irregular pulse rhythm
④ Blood pressure of 110/60

35 When administering vincristine sulfate (Oncovin), an antineoplastic drug, the patient should be assessed for which neurologic system side effects?
① Decreased red and white blood cells
② Alternating constipation and diarrhea
③ Electrolyte imbalances and renal failure
④ Peripheral neuropathies and paralytic ileus
TEST-TAKING TIP ● Identify the word in the stem that provides a clue.

Rationales

1 **TEST-TAKING TIP** ● Options 1 and 3 are opposites. Consider these options carefully. In this question they are both distractors and can be deleted from consideration.
  ① Some people are stoics and/or do not request medication for pain. Patients' pain should be assessed and pain medication offered if necessary.
  * ② The main purpose of pain relief medication is to enable the patient to comfortably engage in necessary activity.
  ③ The patient is experiencing pain before the next scheduled dose; this indicates that the patient is in pain and the intervention was ineffective.
  ④ This is a side effect, not a therapeutic effect; opiates decrease respiration by depressing the respiratory center in the brainstem.

2 **TEST-TAKING TIP** ● Options 1, 2, and 4 all relate to concepts that increase something. Option 3 is unique.
  ① Hydrochloric acid production decreases as the body ages.
  ② Mesenteric blood flow decreases as the body ages.
  * ③ As the body ages, there is a decrease in fat in the extremities and an increase of fat in the abdominal area.
  ④ Cardiac output decreases as the body ages.

3 **TEST-TAKING TIP** ● The word "most" in the stem sets a priority.
  * ① Dioctyl sodium sulfosuccinate (Colace) is a detergent that lowers the surface tension of feces, allowing penetration by water and fat, which soften stool.
  ② Bisacodyl (Dulcolax) is a stimulant cathartic because it irritates the intestinal mucosa, increasing intestinal motility.
  ③ Mineral oil is a lubricant that softens the fecal mass; regular use interferes with the absorption of the fat-soluble vitamins A, D, E, and K.
  ④ Magnesium hydroxide (milk of magnesia) is a saline or osmotic agent that draws water into the fecal mass.

4 **TEST-TAKING TIP** ● The word "most" in the stem sets a priority. The word "immediate" in the stem is a clue. Options 1, 2, and 3 are all plausible because they are all corticosteroids. Option 2 is unique because it is the only option that is not a corticosteroid.
  ① This is a corticosteroid. Corticosteroids, which have an anti-inflammatory action, are generally administered to prevent the late recurrence of symptoms.
  ② Same as #1.
  * ③ Epinephrine (adrenalin) is administered subcutaneously as soon as possible after a person demonstrates adaptations of systemic anaphylaxis or as a preventive measure in a person who is highly allergic and who has been exposed to an allergen. Epinephrine quickly stimulates α and β adrenergic receptors of the autonomic nervous system, causing vasoconstriction and bronchodilation.
  ④ Same as #1.

5 **TEST-TAKING TIP** ● Options 2 and 4 are equally plausible because they both relate to toxicity.
  * ① Large loading doses are administered quickly to promote the desired clinical effects. The therapeutic blood level for digoxin is 0.8 to 2.0 ng/mL. Values that are 2.4 ng/mL or greater indicate toxicity.
  ② Toxicity occurs when the therapeutic range is exceeded and is associated with unacceptable side effects.

③ This relates to maintenance doses of the drug; a maintenance dose is sufficient to replace the amount of drug eliminated from the body between doses.

④ Same as #2.

6 TEST-TAKING TIP ● The word "most" in the stem sets a priority.

* ① Benzodiazepines, such as temazepam (Restoril) and zolpidem (Ambien), are a group of nonbarbiturate sedative-hypnotics. They influence the neurons in the central nervous system that suppress responsiveness to stimuli, thereby decreasing levels of arousal.

② Barbiturates, such as sodium pentobarbital (Nembutal) and secobarbital (Seconal), have many side effects and have been replaced by benzodiazepines as the first drugs of choice to induce sleep.

③ These drugs are primarily administered to reduce pain, not induce sleep.

④ Same as #3.

7 TEST-TAKING TIP ● The question is asking about potassium and sodium imbalances as a result of glucocorticoid therapy. If you know at least one electrolyte imbalance that can occur, two options can be eliminated from consideration. Options 2 and 3 are opposites. Consider these options carefully. In this question, one of them is the correct answer.

① Although hypokalemia may occur, hypernatremia, not hyponatremia, may occur.

* ② Prednisone, a glucocorticoid, has significant water- and sodium-retaining (mineralocorticoid) activities. As sodium is retained, potassium is depleted.

③ The opposite may occur. The patient may experience hypokalemia and hypernatremia.

④ Although hypernatremia may occur, hypokalemia, not hyperkalemia, may occur.

8 TEST-TAKING TIP ● Options 2 and 3 are equally plausible. Sulfa drugs are antibiotics.

* ① Prednisone, a glucocorticoid with mineralocorticoid activity, can percipitate hypokalemia. Hypokalemia increases the myocardium's sensitivity to digitalis. Hypokalemia can precipitate digitalis toxicity, even if digoxin serum levels are in the therapeutic range of 0.4 to 2.0 ng/mL.

② These drugs do not interact with digoxin.

③ Same as #2.

④ Same as #2.

9 * ① Cathartics, also called laxatives, induce defecation.

② Analgesics relieve pain. Also, some cathartics may cause slight abdominal discomfort due to increased intestinal peristalsis.

③ Sedatives and hypnotics promote sleep.

④ Diuretics increase urinary output.

10 TEST-TAKING TIP ● The word "undesirable" in the stem indicates negative polarity.

① A prothrombin time (PT) value is done to assess the effectiveness of warfarin sodium (coumadin) therapy, not heparin therapy. An activated partial thromboplastin time (APTT) is one test done to assess effects of heparin therapy.

② A low platelet count (thrombocytopenia) occurs in 5 to 10 percent of patients receiving heparin therapy. Platelets can fall to 100,000 units from the normal range of 195,000 to 400,000/mm³. This often resolves without intervention even with continued heparin therapy.

* ③ Hematuria (blood in the urine) is a serious side effect of heparin therapy that requires the temporary termination of therapy. If severe bleeding is identified, protamine sulfate is administered as an antidote.

④ Heparin is administered parenterally, not by mouth, and does not cause gastritis.

11 ① Diuretics increase the formation and excretion of urine; they can cause dehydration and electrolyte imbalance, not precipitate superinfection.

* ② Prolonged or inappropriate use of antibiotics can stimulate bacterial growth as normal flora of the gastrointestinal tract and skin are destroyed. Infections that occur while a patient is receiving antimicrobial therapy are called superinfections.

③ Vasopressors constrict the blood vessels; they cause hypertension, not superinfections.

④ Thrombolytics dissolve thrombi or emboli; they also prolong normal coagulation processes, which may increase the risk of bleeding. Thrombolytics do not precipitate superinfections.

12 TEST-TAKING TIP ● Options 3 and 4 are opposites. One is 30 minutes before the drug is administered and the other is 30 minutes after the drug is administered.

① This is too soon. The drug would not be at its lowest concentration in the blood at this time.

② Same as #1.

* ③ The blood level of an antibiotic is at its lowest level just before the next ordered dose.

④ Once the drug is administered, the blood level of the drug rises. A value taken at this time will no longer reflect the lowest serum level, which is the purpose of identifying a trough level.

13 ① Antipyretics reduce a fever; antitussives do not.

② Nasal decongestants reduce nasal congestion; antitussives do not.

③ Mucolytics reduce mucus viscosity; antitussives do not.

* ④ Antitussives reduce the frequency and intensity of a cough. They act on the central or peripheral nervous system or on the local mucosa.

14 TEST-TAKING TIP ● The word "most" in the stem sets a priority.

① An analgesic, not a laxative, would be ordered to manage pain.

② Disuse syndrome relates to prescribed or unavoidable musculoskeletal inactivity. It is not related to disorders of the intestines.

③ A diuretic, not a laxative, would be prescribed for fluid volume excess.

* ④ Perceived constipation is the state in which a person self-prescribes the daily use of a laxative to ensure a daily bowel movement.

15 TEST-TAKING TIP ● "Notify the physician" are the words that reflect negative polarity. The physician should be notified if the blood level results are not acceptable.

① Although this falls below the optimal peak value of 8 to 10 μg/mL, it is within the therapeutic window of 4 to 10 μg/mL, which is acceptable.

② This falls within the optimal peak value range of 8 to 10 μg/mL.

* ③ The physician would need to be notified to increase the dose of gentamicin. A value 0.3 μg/mL is below 0.5 μg/mL, which is the lowest trough value of gentamicin necessary to inhibit bacterial growth.

④ A value of 0.7 μg/mL is higher than 0.5 μg/mL, which is the minimum trough value necessary for a dose to be effective.

16 TEST-TAKING TIP ● This question presents four possible responses (nausea, vomiting, coughing, anxiety) to an antiemetic. If you know just one response, you can delete two options from consideration.

① Although antiemetics reduce nausea, anxiolytics reduce anxiety.

* ② Antiemetics block the emetogenic receptors to prevent or treat nausea or vomiting.

③ Anxiolytics reduce anxiety. Antitussives reduce the frequency and intensity of coughing.

④ Although antiemetics reduce vomiting, antitussives reduce coughing.

17 ① An antipyretic reduces a fever; an expectorant does not.

* ② Expectorants cause a cough to be more productive by decreasing viscosity of mucus and increasing the flow of respiratory tract secretions.

③ A nasal decongestant relieves nasal congestion; an expectorant does not.

④ A bronchodilator dilates airways of the respiratory tract; an expectorant does not.

18 **TEST-TAKING TIP** ● Option 3 is unique. It is the only option that does not include the word "dose."

① The drug dose is not safe. A peak level of 12 μg/mL indicates that the drug dose is too high and needs to be reduced by the physician. The optimum peak value should be between 8 to 10 μg/mL.

② The drug dose is excessive, not subtherapeutic. If the value were subtherapeutic, it would be below 4 μg/mL.

* ③ A value of 12 μg/mL is 2 μg/mL higher than is necessary to be effective and will contribute to drug accumulation and toxicity if it continues for 3 to 5 days.

④ The dose is too high; it needs to be reduced by the physician and not just given at a slower rate.

19 **TEST-TAKING TIP** ● In Options 2, 3, and 4 the words "reduced," "decreased," and "diminished" are related. Option 1 is unique because it is the only option that is related to an increase in something. Consider this option carefully. In this question, the unique option is a distractor.

① In the older adult there is a decrease, not an increase, in gastric emptying.

* ② Reduced glomerular filtration rate will contribute to reduced excretion of a drug, thereby prolonging drug half-life.

③ Drugs that rely on gastric acid for absorption are less effective when there is a reduction in hydrochloric acid production in the elderly.

④ Diminished absorptive surface reduces the absorption of drugs.

20 **TEST-TAKING TIP** ● This question is associating four possible effects of neuroleptics: respiratory depression, diarrhea, akathisia, and spasms of the muscles of the face. If you know just one effect, unrelated or related to neuroleptics, you can delete two options from consideration.

① Respiratory depression is associated with opioid analgesics, not neuroleptics. Constipation, not diarrhea, is a common anticholinergic effect of neuroleptics.

② Although akathisia can occur with neuroleptics, respiratory depression is often seen with opioid analgesics, not neuroleptics.

* ③ This is correct. Spasms of the muscles of the face (tardive dyskinesia) and restlessness/agitation (akathisia) occur in response to dopamine blockage or depletion in the basal ganglia. These undesirable responses will occur within the first few day of therapy and are common to most neuroleptic drugs.

④ Although tardive dyskinesia occurs with neuroleptics, constipation, not diarrhea, is a common anticholinergic effect of neuroleptics.

21 **TEST-TAKING TIP** ● The word "main" in the stem sets a priority.

① Antipyretics are a group of drugs designed to reduce fever. Although some analgesics also may have an antipyretic effect, when given as analgesics, they reduce pain.

② Bronchodilators dilate respiratory airways, facilitating breathing.

③ Antiemetics are designed to minimize nausea and vomiting.

* ④ Analgesics are given mainly to reduce pain and discomfort. There are three types of analgesics: non-narcotic and nonsteroidal anti-inflammatory drugs (NSAIDS), narcotic analgesics or opioids, and adjuvants or coanalgesics.

22 * ① This value is acceptable because it is within the therapeutic range of 4 to 10 µg/mL and optimum peak value of 8 to 10 µg/mL.

② This value is not acceptable because it exceeds the therapeutic range and optimum peak value of 10 µg/mL.

③ This value is not acceptable because it is below the minimum trough level of 0.5 µg/mL.

④ Same as #3.

23 **TEST-TAKING TIP** ● The words "further teaching is necessary" in the stem indicate negative polarity.

① Antacids can interfere with the absorption of digoxin and should not be taken at the same time.

② These are signs of toxicity. The patient will need a test to determine digoxin serum blood levels.

* ③ This action is unsafe and could lead to toxicity. If a dose is missed, the patient should call the physician for instructions.

④ This is true. Digoxin slows the heart rate and strengthens cardiac contractions. If the apical pulse is below 60, the dose should be held.

24 ① Local anesthetics, not narcotics, diminish localized sensation and the perception of pain by inhibiting nerve conduction.

* ② Narcotics act on the higher centers of the brain to modify pain perception.

③ This is the theory related to using distracting sensory input to inhibit pain perception.

④ Narcotics do not close synaptic gates; stimulation of large nerve fibers, via methods such as transcutaneous electrical stimulation, close synaptic gates.

25 **TEST-TAKING TIP** ● The words "postural hypotension" and "common" in the stem are clues.

① Postural hypotension is not a common side effect of these drugs.

② Same as #1.

③ Same as #1.

* ④ Most antihypertensives contribute to postural hypotension because of actions such as peripheral vasodilation, decreased peripheral resistance, decreased heart rate, and decreased cardiac contraction.

26 **TEST-TAKING TIP** ● The words "needs further exploration" in the stem indicate negative polarity.

① Although aspirin can prolong bleeding time when given with heparin, 5 days is a long enough time of being aspirin-free to safely administer heparin.

* ② This could be a contraindication for the use of heparin because of an increased risk of prolonged bleeding during menstruation.

③ This could contribute to the ineffectiveness of warfarin sodium (coumadin), not heparin sodium.

④ Heparin does not cross the placental barrier and has no effects on the fetus or newborn.

27 TEST-TAKING TIP ● The word "best" in the stem sets a priority. Options 1, 2, and 4 all focus on taking a cathartic (laxative) to promote intestinal peristalsis. Option 3 is unique because it promotes a dietary approach to prevent constipation and promote defecation.

   ① The routine intake of cathartics (laxatives) should be avoided to prevent dependence.

   ② Same as #1.

 * ③ Whole grains provide fiber and bulk, which distend the bowel lumen, promoting intestinal peristalsis.

   ④ Same as #1.

28 ① Mineral supplements are considered restorative, not palliative; they return the body to health.

 * ② Demerol is a narcotic that relieves the symptoms of a disease (palliative action), but does not alter the disease process itself.

   ③ Penicillin is an antibiotic that kills pathogenic organisms; a drug that kills an organism is considered to have a curative, not palliative, action.

   ④ Synthroid replaces the thyroxine that is deficient in hypothyroidism. When a drug replaces body fluids or substances, it is substitutive, not palliative, in its therapeutic action.

29 TEST-TAKING TIP ● The word "most" in the stem sets a priority. The words "readily available" and "heparin" in the stem are clues.

   ① Potassium chloride is used for the treatment or prevention of potassium deficiency and is unrelated to heparin therapy.

 * ② Protamine sulfate can chemically combine with heparin, neutralizing its anticoagulant action; it should be kept readily available for the treatment of heparin overdose.

   ③ Prothrombin is a plasma protein coagulation factor synthesized by the liver, not a drug that should be used as an antidote to heparin.

   ④ Plasma is a blood product that may be ordered to treat hypovolemia caused by blood loss; however, if a patient is bleeding in response to heparin therapy, protamine sulfate is generally ordered first. Packed red blood cells would more likely be ordered than plasma.

30 TEST-TAKING TIP ● The word "initial" modifies the words "therapeutic response" in the stem and is a clue. Do not be distracted by the word "most" in the stem. It is not setting a priority.

   ① This is too short a time to achieve a therapeutic response. Plasma drug levels can be used as guides for dosage determination if a patient is still clinically unresponsive after one month.

   ② Same as #1.

 * ③ Generally patients demonstrate an initial response 1 to 3 weeks after the start of antidepressant therapy; it takes this long to establish a therapeutic plasma level.

   ④ A month or two may be necessary to achieve a maximal response to antidepressant therapy.

31 TEST-TAKING TIP ● The word "most" in the stem sets a priority. The word "only" in Option 1 is a specific determiner.

   ① Sublinguinal nitroglycerin has a rapid onset and a relatively short duration of action. Transient cardiac ischemia needs to be relieved through cardiac vasodilation that may require up to three doses of sublinguinal nitroglycerin.

   ② This is unsafe. Unrelieved chest pain after three doses of sublinguinal nitroglycerin within a 15-minute time period may indicate the presence of an acute cardiac event that requires emergency medical intervention.

③ This is unsafe. Doubling the dose may precipitate severe or even life-threatening hypotension.

* ④ Sublingual nitroglycerin has a rapid onset and a relatively short duration of action. Three doses may be necessary to achieve a desired therapeutic response. However, if pain persists beyond 15 minutes, it may indicate the presence of an acute cardiac event that requires emergency medical intervention.

32 TEST-TAKING TIP ● Options 1 and 3 are opposites. Review these options carefully. In this question they are both distractors.

① Although diarrhea does occur frequently as a side effect of antineoplastic drugs, it is not related to myelosuppression.

* ② Most antineoplastic drugs depress bone marrow function. When there is a reduction in the number of white blood cells or leukocytes (leukopenia), the patient is at high risk for infection.

③ Most antineoplastic drugs cause diarrhea, not constipation.

④ Although some antineoplastic drugs can cause cardiotoxicity, it is not related to myelosuppression.

33 ① Antipsychotics decrease the effectiveness of drugs in this classification.

② Same as #1.

* ③ Antipsychotics potentiate the effects of other central nervous system depressants.

④ Same as #1.

34 ① This patient reaction has no bearing on whether digoxin is held.

* ② Digoxin causes a negative chronotropic effect (deceleration of the rate of the heart). This drug must be held if the apical heart rate taken over a full minute falls below 60. Take the patient's apical pulse rate in 1 hour and if it is still below 60, notify the physician.

③ Same as #1.

④ Same as #1.

35 TEST-TAKING TIP ● The word "neurologic" in the stem is a clue. The word "neurologic" in the stem and the word "neuropathies" in Option 4 are closely related. Consider Option 4 carefully. In this question it is the correct answer.

① Red and white blood cells are part of the hematopoietic system.

② Constipation and diarrhea are related to the gastrointestinal system.

③ Electrolyte imbalances and renal failure are related to the renal system.

* ④ A peripheral neuropathy occurs in almost every patient, particularly depression of the Achilles tendon reflex. Decreased enervation of the bowel causes a paralytic ileus, resulting in constipation or opstipation.

Index

. . .